Implementing Health/Fitness Programs

IMPLEMENTING HEALTH/FITNESS PROGRAMS

Robert W. Patton
North Texas State University
Texas College of Osteopathic Medicine

James M. Corry
Mt. Sinai School of Medicine

Larry R. Gettman
Vita Life Enhancement Center

Joleen Schovee Graf
Joleen Schovee Graf and Associates, Inc.

Human Kinetics Books
Champaign, Illinois

Production Editor: Andrea Cava
Interior Design: Andrew H. Ogus
Cover Design: Julie Szamocki
Copy Editor: Lyn Dupré
Print Buyer: Barbara Britton
Technical Illustrators: Joan Carol and Salinda Tyson
Illustrations on pages 198, 201, 203: Pamela Manley
Cover Illustration: DJ Simison

Printed in the United States of America
3 4 5 6 7 8 9 10—90 89
ISBN 0-87322-038-2

Library of Congress Cataloging in Publication Data
Main entry under title:

Implementing health/fitness programs.

  Includes bibliographies and index.
  1. Health promotion.   2. Preventive health
services—Administration.   I. Patton, Robert W.
RA427.8.I47   1986   613'.068   85—10660
ISBN 0-87322-038-2

Human Kinetics Books
A Division of Human Kinetics Publishers, Inc.
Box 5076, Champaign, IL 61825-5076
1-800-DIAL-HKP
1-800-334-3665 (in Illinois)

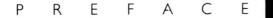

In 1978 the late John Knowles edited a book called *Doing Better and Feeling Worse*, which profiled the health-care industry in the United States. The image presented was that of a rapidly growing, almost uncontrollable nonsystem of health care, the annual costs of which constituted a greater portion of the gross national product than the year before. One reason given for this problem was that consumers utilize the system and pay for health care in seemingly free dollars provided by insurance companies or by federally sponsored programs such as Medicare and Medicaid. The companies that underwrite their employee health care costs also are being strapped by this escalation. General Motors, for example, spent more in one year for employee health care than for the purchase of steel. Because of the high demand on the system, the expected increase in demand, and the inherent high cost of a highly technical acute-care form of medical care, Knowles and others believe that drastic steps must be taken to reduce pressures on the system in order to slow the rising costs. If the rise in costs cannot be stemmed, Knowles and others warn, a crisis of health care will result wherein many people will be unable to afford medical care.

Among the proposals to slow the rise in costs is a plan to reduce utilization of the medical system by helping Americans stay healthier, longer. Health promotion service and education is considered a key ingredient in an overall strategy to help them use the medical system more wisely. This plan of health promotion and education to reduce health-care costs has been adopted recently by both the community and corporate sectors. Commercial health/fitness programs and hospital wellness programs also are being developed. Health/fitness programs are being established at a significant rate in the corporate, community, commercial, and clinical settings. Although preliminary studies regarding cost-containment of health care are positive, much needs to be done to improve and refine the evaluation of such programs.

Concurrent with the concern for corporate health-care cost containment is the concern of the general public for enhanced health and fitness levels. The number of Americans who have recently began a new diet or exercise program is staggering. Entrepreneurs are quick to take advantage of this new consumer market. Community-based programs and commercial fitness centers are presently enjoying record numbers of participants. Indeed, many of the new health/fitness program providers offer corporate memberships for the employee wellness programs too small to warrant their own facilities.

Professional preparation for the practitioners of health/fitness programs is lagging well behind the demand for personnel. Certification programs are being developed by cognate associations, and licensure may be on the horizon. In the meantime, guidelines are needed for implementing health/fitness programs. Specifically, this book is intended to help educators in professional preparation programs and professional practitioners establish effective health/fitness programs to aid their constituencies in becoming healthier.

The book is divided into three parts. Part 1 serves as an introduction to the field of health promotion. It provides a brief profile of the economic crisis in the health field and ways in which health/fitness programs can help ameliorate the crisis. From this rationale, the section discusses the many possibilities of a healthy lifestyle and the typical components of a comprehensive health/fitness program. This profile and rationale will help health/fitness professionals sell programs to their superiors more easily.

Part 2 describes a model of implementation for health/fitness programs that allows health/fitness professionals to evaluate and develop their programs. The implementation model is explained and then the key components of the model are laid out. Health/fitness professionals can adapt each component to fit into their pro-

grams, or they can adapt only those components that seem most useful.

Part 3 focuses on the organizational, administrative, and political issues that the health/fitness professional must consider in establishing an effective, long-lived health/fitness program. This section is based on the principles of administration and the practical experience of the authors in setting up programs. The appendixes include useful information on facility design, buyer's guides, and related associations.

We would like to acknowledge the contributions of all those who made this book possible, but space permits only a brief recognition. Appreciation is extended to Elad Levinson, who authored the stress management chapter, and to the many graduate students who contributed significantly to the development of the program implementation chapters. Finally, to Nancy Taylor, Phil Cecchettini, and Andrea Cava, our sincere appreciation for coping above and beyond the call of duty.

R.W.P.
J.M.C.
L.R.G.
J.S.G.

CONTENTS

■ PART 2: Implementation of Health/Fitness Programs

PART 3: Management of Health/Fitness Programs

PART I
INTRODUCTION TO
HEALTH/FITNESS PROGRAMS

A PROPOSAL FOR
HEALTH/FITNESS PROGRAMS

During the last decade, many U.S. businesses and community agencies have initiated health/fitness programs to grapple with serious sociomedical problems. For example, over 31% of the nation's companies with more than 100 employees now provide exercise programs,[1] and approximately 90% of these programs are scheduled or underwritten by the company.[2] There are over 2000 community YMCA programs providing individual, family, and corporate memberships. Many organizations use the Y programs as their off-worksite program. There is also a recent trend for government agencies to offer health/fitness programs for employees. For example, 20 colleges and universities in Texas now offer faculty/staff wellness programs as a result of an expanded definition of the state's position on employee training and development. In the private commercial sector, there are now over 5000 health clubs providing health/fitness programs. Hospitals are rapidly expanding the concept of health care to include health promotion as well as disease management; facilities to provide employees' and patients' health-promotion activities are being constructed at an accelerated rate each year. The manner of program delivery in each of these settings differs greatly. We will briefly illustrate the diverse nature of these programs to get a better perspective on this booming trend.

Examples of Health/ Fitness Programs

An example of a health/fitness program in the corporate sector is that of the Pepsico Company in Purchase, New York. The program began modestly, with a small percentage of employees attending and a limited number of health/fitness activities. It grew into a comprehensive program that now enrolls a majority of the employees. The program components include physiologic stress testing, exercise prescription, supervised workouts, aerobic activities, health counseling, and health education. Evaluations of employees have demonstrated improved fitness levels. Other indicators of success include employees' self-reported feelings of improved well-being, energy level, and morale. Cost–benefit studies, although still incomplete, indicate the program saves Pepsico approximately $3 for every $1 spent.

In Salem, Oregon, the Department of Education has sponsored health/fitness education fairs for its own employees, and it has also tried to facilitate implementation of health/fitness programs throughout the school districts of the state. Len Tritsch, health education specialist for the Oregon Department of Education (ODE), reports that the staffers of the ODE in Salem have responded positively to the program, with many staffers continuing to exercise and practice health-enhancing behaviors. At the school-district level, a two-step strategy was used. First, the teachers and administrators of the schools were helped to become more fit and healthy through an annual summer program called the *Seaside Conference*. They then were taught to launch extensive health-education and fitness programs for the students in their home school districts.

Evaluations of this statewide effort revealed surprisingly good results. Local school administrators reported better morale, increased energy, and improved group cohesiveness among their employees. The school children also noticed a positive difference in their teachers, and consequently the emotional atmospheres of the schools seem brighter and happier. Lastly, the school children reported they felt better from their own health/fitness programs.[3]

Health/fitness programs do not have to be at the worksite or be comprehensive. This situation is typical of small companies, which employ the majority of workers in the United States. For many small companies, if not most, a comprehensive program would be impractical because of space requirements for changing, workout, instructional, and assessment areas. Relatively small companies therefore may hire outside consultants to provide specific services, or may pay for memberships at already established organizations such as the Aerobics Center, the Houstonian Club, the YMCAs, or Vista International's Executive Health/Fitness Program.

Some small companies encourage employee health without offering a formal program of assessment, prescription, and supervision. For example, the Nike shoe company permits individual retailers to set flexible hours for store employees so they can exercise during the day.

The Nike philosophy of health and wellness is passed on to workers not through formal programming but through example.

The Mendocino School District in California encourages employee wellness by means of economic incentives and access to its fitness facilities. It provides health insurance for employees that has a high deductible (over $500), which permits savings for the district in insurance premiums. The district then grants to each employee $500 to handle medical bills not met by the insurance plan. The wellness incentive lies in the fact that employees may keep any portion of the $500 grant not used during a 1-year period. Thus, employees are encouraged to be conservative in their use of medical services by staying fit, healthy, and safe. The school district also encourages wellness by allowing employees to use school facilities to exercise during the day.

These organizations vary tremendously in how they approach the problem of the health status of their constituents. The ODE may have as the ultimate goal for its efforts improving education and well-being of school children. Pepsico may have as a primary goal lowering health-care costs, improving worker productivity, and decreasing morbidity and mortality rates among its employees. Whatever the motivation and details of the individual program, however, the decision makers in these organizations and in thousands of other businesses and communities throughout the United States have grappled with the common problems of rising medical costs and poor morbidity and mortality figures, and have chosen to institute some kind of program to promote health and wellness.

In this chapter we will examine some of the possible motivations that have prompted health/fitness programs to be adopted throughout the United States. We designed this chapter as a *proposal* for your consideration. We chose this format because we hope readers will adapt the first chapter for their own use in their own organization. The rest of this book offers an implementation plan that should prove useful in beginning or improving a health/fitness program.

■ T A B L E I . I ■

Percentage of Deaths in the United States by Cause

Cause	1900	1975	1980
Cardiovascular	21	52.5	48.5
Cancer	5	19.3	20.9
Accidents	6	5.4	10.7
Pneumonia and influenza	19	2.9	2.7
Diabetes	7	1.9	1.7
Other	42	18.0	15.5

Source: Final Monthly Statistics 1980, Washington, DC: Monthly Vital Statistics Report, National Center for Health Statistics, 1980.

■ Background

The Nature of Morbidity Today

Morbidity and mortality statistics in the United States have changed dramatically during the 20th century. Rising from about 47 years in 1900, the average life expectancy in 1984 is about 74 years and is expected to go higher.[4] The primary causes of death also have changed: the great majority of Americans today die from chronic degenerative disease rather than infectious disease (Table 1.1).

Today, people generally suffer and die from lifestyle-related chronic degenerative diseases such as cardiovascular disease, cerebrovascular problems, and cancer, all of which are expensive to treat. These diseases account for nearly 70% of all deaths. The top "maimers," "killers," and "wealth drainers" are statistically correlated with certain lifestyles and exposure to health-risk factors: there is a statistical indication that prudent persons should avoid certain health risks and behaviors to lessen their odds of being hurt or dying from specific problems.

In one study in which lifestyle and risk factors were linked to morbidity and mortality, 7000 people's lifestyles and vital statistics were examined over a 10-year span.[5] The investigators found that certain key behaviors (eating three meals per day, not snacking, eating breakfast every day, engaging in moderate exercise two or three times per week, sleeping 8 hours each night, not smoking, drinking little or no alcohol, and maintaining moderate weight)

were linked to life expectancy: a 45-year-old male with only three of these behaviors had a remaining life expectancy of 21.6 years, whereas an age-matched cohort with six or seven of them had a remaining life expectancy of more than 33.1 years.

Another longitudinal study of middle-aged and older men linked exercise to increased longevity.[6] Researchers have followed the medical histories and living habits of 16,936 Harvard Alumni since 1960. They found that exercise seemed to be linked to fewer deaths from all causes, but was most substantially correlated with lower risk of cardiovascular disease, especially in alumni who used 2000 or more calories per week in walking, climbing, and sports play.

The Costs of Disease

There are apparent as well as hidden costs associated with disease. For example, *heart attacks* are variously estimated to result in between 32 and 132 million lost working days per year,[7,8,9] which the National Chamber Foundation estimates results in actual costs to industry of approximately 150% of daily wages.[10] The editors of *Business Week* magazine estimate that the wages of employees felled by heart disease total $8.6 billion annually and that over $700 million is spent annually recruiting for executives to replace heart attack victims.[8]

Pacific Mutual Life estimates the illness cost of *poor nutrition* to be $30 million annually.[10] Pearson estimates that *backaches* annually result

T A B L E 1 . 2
Costs to American Economy for Cigarette-Induced Major Illnesses, 1964–1983

Health-care costs for cigarette-induced cancer	$ 56,200,000,000.00
Productivity lost due to cigarette-induced cancer	186,300,000,000.00
Subtotal—cancer	242,500,000,000.00
Health-care costs for cigarette-induced cardiovascular disease	108,300,000,000.00
Productivity lost due to cigarette-induced cardiovascular disease	265,600,000,000.00
Subtotal—cardiovascular disease	373,900,000,000.00
Health-care costs for cigarette-induced chronic lung disease	120,000,000,000.00
Productivity lost due to cigarette-induced chronic lung disease	195,400,000,000.00
Subtotal—chronic lung disease	315,400,000,000.00
Total cost	$931,800,000,000.00

Source: National Interagency Council on Smoking and Health. Cigarette-induced medical costs exceed $930 billion. *Smoking and Health Reporter* 1:1, 1984. © 1984 National Interagency Council on Smoking and Health. Reprinted by permission of the National Interagency Council on Smoking and Health.

in $225 million in workers' compensation.[9] *Alcoholism* is estimated to cost industry between $15.6 billion and $25 billion annually.[8,10] These figures result from lost worktime, health and welfare services, and accidents. The rate of absenteeism of alcoholic workers is 250% that of nonalcoholics, and the accident rate for alcoholic workers is 3.6 times that of nonalcoholics. North American Rockwell estimates their annual cost per alcoholic employee at $50,000,[10] and the United California Bank of Los Angeles spends $1 million annually for their 10,000 alcoholic employees.[10]

Drug abuse is estimated to cost about $26 billion per year in lost productivity.[11] The National Interagency Council on Smoking and Health estimates the average one-pack-per-day *smoker* costs his or her employer more than $600 per year. The American Council on Science and Health estimates that since the release of the surgeon general's report on smoking in 1964, more than $930 billion in medical costs directly attributed to smoking tobacco have been incurred (Table 1.2).[12]

Although there is no good estimate of the total tax dollars lost to government when people are disabled, common sense indicates that the figure is several billion dollars annually. Add to this the financial burden communities take on to underwrite social-service needs related to illness (anything from altering buses and curbs for disabled people to providing income subsidies, mental-health services, and other services for ill people) and you can see that the hidden costs of illness to society and industry are high indeed.

Americans are estimated to spend $10 billion annually on legal *drugs* and $4 billion more on illegal drugs.[13] People in the United States spent over $2 billion on quackery in 1976, largely on *alternative treatment modalities*, which often do not cure an ailment, delay the onset of proper treatment, and can necessitate a more difficult and expensive treatment regimen when the patient finally undertakes standard therapy. Quackery has enjoyed a substantial renewal in the United States lately, and the right of quacks to offer so-called *alternative medicine* has even fallen under the protection of the law in various states.[14] Americans spend about $5 to $10 billion per year on *devices*, such as slenderizing machines, headache machines, and negative-ion generators, that offer no proven therapeutic benefit.[14] Most people are unable to afford *dental insurance* and *dental care*: one study found that 52% of all Americans had not been to a dentist in the preceding year, and 20% of people 5 years of age or older had not been to a dentist in 5 years.[14] Americans are finding it increasingly difficult to afford any *medical insurance*; this is especially true of people who earn under $15,000 per year, and the elderly. People waste untold amounts of money through *inappropriate use of medical services*, such as using a hospital emergency room for primary care.

Absenteeism and Reduced Productivity

In addition to these obvious health costs, absenteeism and reduced productivity are less obvious but still substantial costs of poor health. For example, one author estimated the costs to industry in the United States due to lost productivity to be $25 billion in 1977.[7] Another estimated that backaches alone result in a $1 billion loss in productivity per year.[9]

One interesting study analyzed the costs of poor health for an individual company in medical costs and absenteeism. Gettman, in testimony before the House Ways and Means Select Revenue Measures Subcommittee, said:[2]

> Fitness programs are related to lower medical costs, lower absenteeism rates and increased productivity. In 1982, Mesa Petroleum employees who did not participate in the fitness program averaged $434 per person in medical costs, paid by Mesa. However, employees who participated in the fitness program averaged only $173 per person (see Figure 1.1). This difference in medical costs between nonparticipating and participating employees amounts to a projected reduction in medical expenses of nearly $200,000 per year.

Although these findings may reflect bias in the sense that participating employees were self-selected, the finding of lower costs among participants argues that employees should be vigorously encouraged to participate in health/fitness programs.

A review of the literature revealed a dearth of truly experimental research designs used to evaluate industrial-based health-promotion programs (Table 1.3). However, the author pointed out that health/fitness professionals should not despair of finding positive relationships between health/fitness programs and good health. He offers the criteria used in the 1964 surgeon general's report as one possible method to solidify the link between formal health/fitness programs and good health (Table 1.4, p. 10).[15]

> Absenteeism rates also were lower for participating employees in 1982. Mesa's nonparticipating employees averaged 44 hours of sick time, whereas the participating employees averaged only 27 hours of sick time.
>
> Tenneco, Inc., Houston, Texas, found a highly significant relationship between exercise participation and job performance among 3231 employees. Employees with high ratings of job performance also had high exercise participation indicating that productivity is related to fitness.

This profile of the indirect costs and industrial losses related to disease does not reflect the costs of health *care*, which, according to a five-part *New York Times* series, continue to rise so high as to constitute a threat to the health status we enjoy.[16] We will examine this proposition in more detail.

The Threat Posed by Rising Health-Care Costs

As has that of all other salable items, the cost of health care has risen steadily since the 1930s. What is troublesome, however, is that health-care costs have become a greater portion of the gross national product (GNP) every year for the last 52 years. Today health-care costs are nearly 11% of the GNP and are still rising, although there was an encouraging drop in the rate of increase of the medical-care price index for the

Figure 1.1 Medical cost versus activity level of Mesa Petroleum employees in 1982.

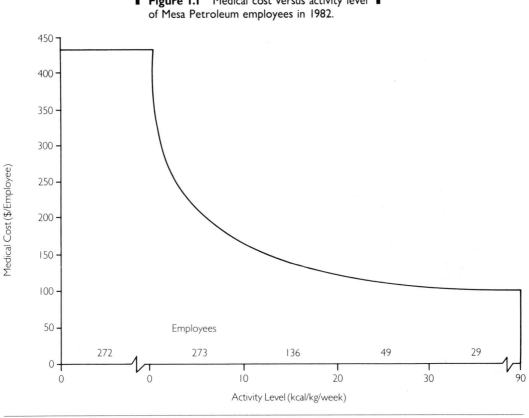

first 5 months of 1984 (Figure 1.2, p. 11).[16]

Economists are concerned because of the economic dislocations inherent in rising health costs. Specifically, they point to the nonproductive nature of health services, paid for by insurance dollars or public money, as being key factors contributing to inflation and thus forcing up medical prices and all other prices. Because insurance premiums usually are paid by an employer, and these costs are passed on to consumers, the current form of insurance (low deductibles but rising premium costs) results in an inflationary pressure, as does excessive inappropriate use of medical services. The most telling descriptor of the cost to industry of health care is that *50% of the total health bill for the nation, which totaled over $380 billion in 1984 and* *constituted 11% of the nation's GNP, was paid for by industry.*[17] Perhaps a more graphic illustration of this is that the Chrysler Corporation estimates that health benefits for its employees add $600 to the cost of each car.[18] Because businesses try not to run in the red, these costs either are directly passed on to consumers or are written off on the corporate tax return, another way of passing them on to consumers. The total effect is ultimately to create an economic climate wherein people find it impossible to purchase consumer products. This economic dislocation is possibly the most troublesome of all, because U.S. companies find it difficult to compete with foreign ones and may face bankruptcy when their sales drop. Thus, widely available insurance that is used freely forces prices higher,

■ T A B L E 1.3 ■
Examples of Industrial Health Promotion Program Outlines

Setting	Program	Outcome	Design Classification
Consulting firm (38)	3-month program in which employees selected health behavior changes	"Affordable" with apparent employee satisfaction and attainment of self-selected goals	Preexperimental
Davidson Louisiana	Voluntary exercise program for employees with individualized prescription with credit toward expense-free vacation for attainment of fitness goals	Apparently successful and ongoing	Preexperimental
Campbell Soup	Smoking cessation	$500 expenditure per successful "quitter"	Preexperimental
Metropolitan Life	Smoking cessation	Less than $200 expenditure per successful "quitter"	Preexperimental
Massachusetts Mutual Life	Hypertension control	In 3 years, fewer hospitalization days required for hypertensives compared with normotensives	Quasi-experimental
New York Telephone	Alcohol rehabilitation, smoking cessation, fitness, cholesterol reduction, stress management, cancer screening, and "healthy back" programs	Estimated $2.7 million saved in 1 year	Preexperimental
Metropolitan Life	Multifaceted center with employee health information, appraisal, screening, fitness activities, and blood pressure monitoring	N/A	N/A
IBM	"A Plan for Life" comprehensive health-education program	Very high employee satisfaction	Preexperimental
AT&T	Educational program on breast-cancer detection, diagnosis, treatment, and rehabilitation	Knowledge of breast cancer improved and retained even after 5 months. Monthly practice of breast self-examination increased	True experimental

Kaiser-Permanente	Employee health-promotion program instituted with blood-pressure screening and education, nutritional awareness, and freedom-from-smoking campaign	Only descriptive and anecdotal assessments of blood pressure screening and nutritional awareness programs were available	Preexperimental
Xerox Corporation	Xerox Health Management Program (XHMP): helping employees become more responsible for their own health	"... not sure whether XHMP had any influence on self-confidence, attitude, job motivation, aspirations, or ambition ... believe ... positive influence upon interpersonal relations"	Preexperimental
American Hospital Association; Anheuser-Busch; Blue Cross and Blue Shield of Indiana; Ford Motor Company; Internorth; Kimberly-Clark; Trans World Airlines, United Healthcare; Wyerhaeuser (not previously reviewed)			With the exception of Ford, Johnson & Johnson, and Kimberly-Clark (all apparently quasi-experimental) company programs used preexperimental designs.
Industrial workers who smoked	Twice yearly health advice and health education; multifactorial prevention	Smokers decreased by 6.5% over a 2-year period compared with controls	True experimental
Land O'Lakes	Computer program to generate awareness and interest in diet and exercise	No evaluation	Preexperimental
Speedcall	Cash incentive for employees to stop smoking	Increase in business volume from $900,000 to $1,200,000 in 1 year without increasing the number of employees; also fewer employee illnesses and shorter periods of absenteeism	Preexperimental

Source: Chen. M. Proving the effects of health promotion in industry: An academician's perspective. *Health Education Quarterly* 10:235, 1983. References omitted. Reprinted by permission of John Wiley & Sons, Inc.

■ T A B L E 1 . 4 ■

Ideal Evidences for Demonstrating the Effectiveness of Health Promotion Programs in Industry

Surgeon General's Causality Criteria	Types of Evidence Used by Surgeon General	Types of Evidence Needed to Demonstrate Causality for Health-Promotion Programs
Consistency of association	29 retrospective studies (examinations of past records comparing cancer patients with controls); 7 prospective studies (studies of smokers versus nonsmokers followed through time to determine those who died from lung cancer versus other causes).	Retrospective studies may not be feasible because of incomplete record keeping in early health-promotion programs. However, a variety of prospective studies might be conducted with participants compared with nonparticipants (e.g., true experimental and quasi-experimental designs to ascertain the degree of consistency between health-promotion programs and their outcomes).
Strength of association	Calculated ratio of the number of observed lung cancer cases in smokers compared to the expected number of lung cancer cases (based on nonsmokers' rate of lung cancer).	From the variety of prospective studies, calculate the ratio of observed cases of participants deriving a prescribed health-promotion–program benefit with the expected number who would have derived the same prescribed benefit (based on nonparticipants' experience).
Specificity of association	Could the relative risk ratios of cigarette smokers acquiring lung cancer (averaging 900%–1000%) compared to nonsmokers be explained by any other factor? No other factor has yet been demonstrated.	Could the relative risk ratios of benefits acquired by health promotion program participants compared to nonparticipants be explained by any other factor?
Temporal relationship of association	Individuals were exposed to cigarette smoking (became cigarette smokers) before they acquired lung cancer.	Individuals must have participated in industrial health-promotion programs prior to having achieved the purported benefits.
Coherence of association	Agreement with known facts about cigarette smoking and lung cancer, such as the rise in lung cancer cases associated with increase in per capita cigarette consumption and a dose–response relationship (e.g., more cigarettes smoked, more likelihood of lung cancer).	The outcomes of the industrial health-promotion programs must be logically related to such factors as the increase in health awareness by employees, improved employees' health, and reduced employer-financed hospitalization claims.

Source: Chen, M. Proving the effects of health promotion in industry: An academician's perspective. *Health Education Quarterly* 10:235, 1983. Reprinted by permission of John Wiley & Sons, Inc.

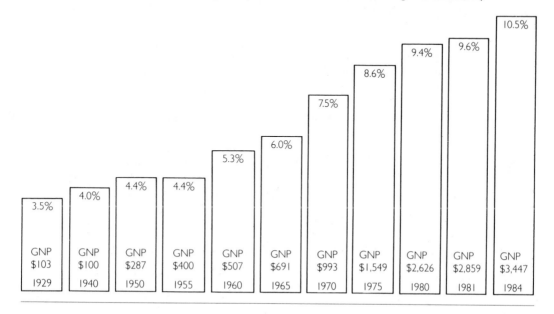

Figure 1.2 Chart shows how, as gross national product (GNP) increases, the portion spent on health care rises. Figures in boxes show GNP for each year, rounded in billions of dollars. 1984 figure is for fiscal year ended September 30; all others are for calendar years. (Data from Health Care Financing Administration.)

which results in higher premiums and more inflation, ad infinitum.

The situation is a neat but vicious circle, and medical planners fear that consumers (both employers and employees) no longer will be able to afford medical insurance or medical care. This has already occurred among certain groups (many families earning under $15,000 annually, the elderly with modest incomes, employees of small companies, and many self-employed people) and may escalate.[19] The real threat to our health has been noticed by government leaders, who have responded by establishing commissions to study the problem. Several reasons why the costs have risen so high and so fast have been cited, and recommendations to control these costs have been made.

Reasons for Rising Medical Costs

The most widely reported reasons for rising medical costs include: unhealthy lifestyle or specific behaviors related to health; the acute-care model of medical care applied to chronic degenerative disease; widely available insurance; inappropriate use of the medical system; the physician acting as agent for the patient; and the increased number of elderly who require medical services.

Unhealthy Lifestyle Many Americans eat too much, smoke too much, drink alcohol too much, neglect to wear seatbelts, avoid exercise, and in general neglect personal health maintenance. The 1980 edition of *Health: United States* listed approximate levels of health-destroying behaviors engaged in by various groups of Americans (for example, smoking by age, sex, and ethnic group; use of medical facilities; and adherence to therapeutic regimens).[20] The publication warned of the absolute necessity to do more in disease prevention and health promotion or face the prospect of continually rising medical costs.

Acute-Care Model The acute-care model of health care, which harnesses tremendous resources and hurls them at various illnesses, has been extraordinarily successful in fighting communicable diseases, trauma, poisoning, and similar acute problems. This model may not be the correct one, however, given the prevailing nature of disease today. The fact that so many people suffer from preventable chronic degenerative diseases, which are catastrophic in treatment time and expense, suggests that preventive medicine should be allotted resources equal to those spent on acute-care medicine.

Widely Available Insurance Widely available insurance results in a greater use of medical services. Most Americans are now covered by either private insurance or public insurance (Medicare and Medicaid; Figure 1.3) and few people must go without medical care when they are sick—although this may not be true in the future.

Inappropriate Use of Medical Services Inappropriate use of medical services, which seem to be free because of extensive insurance coverage, forces up the cost of medical care. Examples of inappropriate use of medical care include: use of hospital emergency rooms for primary care for ordinary sickness; failure to seek preventive services, such as prenatal care, innoculations, and periodic physical and dental checkups; and doctor hopping.

Physician as Agent of the Patient The physician acts as the agent for the ill patient. As such, the physician orders whatever tests and therapies he or she deems necessary, no matter how costly they may be. Also, because services are billed on a fee-for-service basis, there is no incentive to hold back treatment services.

Increase in the Elderly Population The graying of America taxes the medical system because the elderly generally have more episodes of disease than do younger populations, and their ailments usually are more catastrophic.

The Problem

The overriding problem is how best to improve the health of Americans and thus increase longevity, decrease illness, reduce absenteeism, increase productivity, and lower medical-care costs while maintaining the generally high quality of available medical care. How can the general level of health enjoyed by Americans be raised so as to reduce demand on medical services and health insurance? How can programs that educate about health and provide fitness experiences be implemented to increase productivity, decrease absenteeism, lower medical costs, and still be economically feasible? What is the experience of companies and communities that have implemented health/fitness programs regarding effectiveness and cost savings?

Cost Controls and Health/Fitness Programming

Health experts offer two apparently divergent approaches to solving the problem: health and cost controls and health/fitness programming.

Cost Controls

Three recent innovations in health-care cost control and health-care delivery hold hope of reducing the rise in health-care costs without compromising the quality of health care in this country: prospective payment via diagnostic-related groups (DRGs), preferred provider organizations (PPOs), and health maintenance organizations (HMOs).[17]

Prospective Payment and DRGs Prospective payment is a policy, recently instituted in many states, that establishes predetermined payments for illnesses suffered by Medicaid and Medicare patients. Rather than reimbursing on a fee-for-service basis, which covers all reasonable health services provided to a patient, prospective payment sets a maximum dollar amount for care of a patient with a given diagnosis. *Diagnostic-related groups (DRGs)* is the term given to the

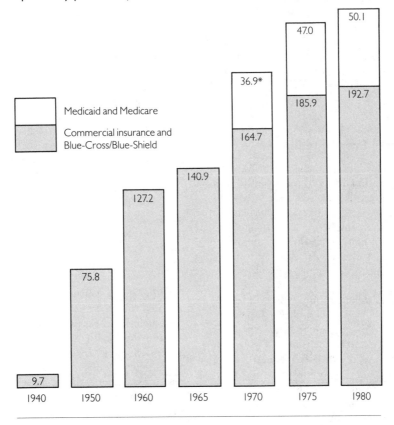

■ **Figure 1.3** Number of people in the United States covered by private health ■ insurance, Medicaid, and Medicare, in millions. Medicaid programs for the poor began in 1965 and Medicare for the elderly in 1966. Many people covered by government programs also have private insurance coverage. (Based on data from Health Insurance Association of America, in *The New York Times*, March 31, 1982. Copyright © 1982 by The New York Times Company. Reprinted by permission.)

reimbursable expenses for over 400 recognized diagnoses. Under this plan, when a diagnosis is made on a particular patient, the hospital or other care-giving institution is reimbursed not on an unlimited basis but rather only up to a maximum amount. Thus there is an economic incentive to control costs and reduce unnecessary procedures to prevent financial losses. Early experience with this form of reimbursement shows hospitals releasing patients earlier to reduce costs. Also, physicians are being counseled to provide cost-effective quality care.

PPOs PPOs, although not precisely defined, generally are agreements between group purchasers (usually corporations) and individual practitioners, institutions, or combinations thereof. The practitioner or institution agrees to discounts of their fees and utilization review in return for the group purchaser's agreement to advertise the provider's services and to encourage employees to use the listed practitioner, often through economic incentives such as lower copayments, lower deductibles, and higher levels of benefits. It should be emphasized that the agreements are between the sponsoring group purchaser and individual practitioners or institutions, thereby avoiding the risk of antitrust liability.

HMOs   HMOs are group practices that accept annual prepayment from individuals for health services. Employees of HMOs usually accept a salary rather than fees based on services, so the HMO can better predict its labor costs. Also, through preventive medicine HMOs can decrease the onset of catastrophic diseases in their clients, thereby avoiding having to provide costly care.

Health/Fitness Programming

Health/fitness programming is a newly popularized but traditional way to increase the well-being of participants through planned health education and fitness experiences. Participants also are helped to higher levels of health by individualized needs assessment, customized programming, and the provision of support services such as counseling and regular exercise classes.

In the remainder of this chapter and in the rest of this book, we will describe health/fitness programming implementation, provision, and evaluation, rather than focusing on strict cost-containment practices. It is our belief that significant cost savings, as well as increased vigor, productivity, and longevity of participants, result from health/fitness programming. We will begin our discussion by defining the relevant terms.

Health Promotion   Health promotion is a combination of health education and related organizational, economic, or political interventions designed to facilitate behavioral or environmental changes conducive to health.[21]

Health/Fitness Programs   Health/fitness programs are combinations of health education, health counseling, health assessment, and fitness-promoting experiences designed to facilitate

behavioral changes conducive to health. Health/fitness programs do not necessarily include economic and political interventions.

Health/Fitness Specialist   A professional man or woman with training in exercise physiology, health education, or related fields who administers or delivers health/fitness programs is a health/fitness specialist.

Health/Fitness Education   Health education, according to Green, is any combination of learning opportunities designed to facilitate voluntary adaptions of behavior conducive to health.[21] Green's definition is meant to be broad; he would include as learning opportunities cognitive, affective, and behavioral experiences as well as mass communication campaigns, appeals to people's underlying motives, and so on. The emphasis on design implies that there has been a diagnosis of learner deficits, values, and other factors related to health and that therefore the strategies selected have an excellent chance of helping a learner change his or her behavior to enhance health.

Health/Fitness Services   Those medical and nonmedical services that complement and reinforce health/fitness programs and are designed to raise the health status of individuals to the highest level within their genetic limits are called health/fitness services. Examples include health assessments and counseling, supervised fitness or workout sessions, dietary counseling, and behavioral modification programs in weight control and substance abuse.

Objectives of Health/Fitness Programs

The Corporate Sector

Given that a corporation has a captive audience of workers, an opportunity to deliver extra support services beyond simple education, and an ability to influence the decisions of employees (to

■ T A B L E I . 5 ■
Objectives of Health/Fitness Programs in the Corporate Sector

Primary Objectives (Net Cash Value)	Secondary Objectives (Nonfinancial Benefits)
Reduced illness	Improved morale of workers
Reduced absenteeism	Improved company image
Reduced accidents	Reduced inflation
Reduced health insurance premiums	Reduced turnover of disgruntled employees
Increased productivity, energy, and creativity of workers on a daily basis	Greater ability of employees to cope with new or otherwise stressful situations
Greater continuity of performance; reduced training of new employees to replace ill or deceased employees	Greater ability of employees to manage personal life with consequent reduction in stress at work
Increased competitiveness of corporation	Increased employer recruitment potential
More profit to stockholders	Improved employee interactions

some degree) by appeals for teamwork and corporate image, it is no surprise that adherence rates in some well-run corporate health/fitness programs are high. Also, many data about employees, to which a community-based organization would have no access, are available to corporations; this permits more precise needs assessment, goal setting, and evaluation than in most community programs. Expected outcomes are easier to state and evaluate for a corporate program. Some of the expected primary and secondary objectives of corporate programs are listed in Table 1.5.

Community-Based Programs

There are many organizations and agencies that serve clients in community-based, as opposed to corporate, settings. Examples of these community-based programs include: *voluntary health agencies* (American Heart Association, American Cancer Society, YMCA, YWCA, YMHA, YWHA, American Red Cross, American Lung Association, March of Dimes, and others); *schools* (health and physical education programs, health services, and health environment); *churches* (Seventh Day Adventist nutrition-education and smoking-cessation programs; various church-

sponsored fitness programs, recreational programs, and parenting classes); *private social service agencies* (Henry Street Settlement House in New York City; various drop-in centers); *medical agencies* (patient education, visiting nurses, drug rehabilitation programs, health maintenance organizations, outpatient clinics, nursing homes); *insurance companies* (health promotion offices); and *centers for the elderly.*

In all of these settings, various versions of health/fitness programming have been tried because the objectives for the programs vary depending on the mission of the organization. Also, the success of the program may be nebulous because the organization may have other, unspoken goals that impinge on the health/fitness endeavor. For example, the smoking-cessation program of the Seventh Day Adventist Church may achieve only a modest success rate in getting people to stop smoking, yet the church continues to offer the program. Why? The answer lies in the spiritual goals of the organization, namely to spread the view of the church about good health and the body as a temple of the Holy Spirit. Some of the expected primary and secondary objectives of health/fitness programs in community agencies are listed in Table 1.6.

■ T A B L E 1 . 6 ■
Expected Outcomes of Community Health/Fitness Programs

Type of Agency and Programs	Primary Objectives	Secondary Objectives
Voluntary health organizations (health promotion)	Improve health status of clients; defeat disease	Increase volunteers; increase private donations; increase political influence
Schools (health promotion)	Improve health status of students; fulfill legal requirements; facilitate full development of students	Improve psychological atmosphere of school to make it more conducive to learning; increase attendance; improve funding based on school attendance
Churches	Improve spiritual life	Improve ability to cope; increase membership and church attendance; improve psychological atmosphere of congregation; increase political power; help church members fulfill their religious obligations
Private social service agencies	Improve health status of clients	Increase private donations; increase volunteers; increase attendance at center

Commercial Health/Fitness Enterprises

Commercial or for-profit health/fitness enterprises have existed for many years in the United States, but it was not until the 1980s that these commercial enterprises began an explosive growth period. This coincided with the wellness movement, which has flourished in the United States and has become a lucrative market for investors and entrepreneurs. *Business Week* magazine has estimated health/fitness enterprises will become a $1 billion industry by 1991.[22] An obvious primary objective for commercial health/fitness centers is profit. Secondary objectives are customer satisfaction and manageable growth, which in turn dictate the establishment of safe, effective exercise environments and classes. Table 1.7 lists typical objectives for commercial health/fitness centers.

Government Health/Fitness Programs

Health promotion initiatives from government agencies take many forms ranging from issuing regulations to supporting research or funding demonstration projects. Encouraging health/fitness endeavors falls within this range and has occurred via the issuance of regulations (for example, when a state board of education mandates physical education courses for school-age children), via funded research programs (for example, a series of studies on health promotion has been funded by the Health Education Bureau), and via funded demonstration projects. Whichever form the government chooses to promote health/fitness programs, it has certain objectives, which are listed in Table 1.8.

Hospital Health/Fitness Centers

Recently, many hospitals have identified the need to provide more health education and fitness experiences as part of their delivery systems. Because there are many types of hospitals with diverse objectives, and because there are varying reimbursement plans in the different states, the types of health-education and fitness experiences vary greatly.[23] For example, hospitals can be private or public, for-profit or nonprofit, designed to serve the general community

■ T A B L E I . 7 ■
Objectives for Commercial Health/Fitness Centers

Primary	Secondary
Obtain reasonable profit on capital invested	Encourage manageable, sustained growth of the client base, staff, and number of outlets
	Increase customer satisfaction
	Provide a safe, supervised exercise environment to reduce legal risks and meet health standards of regulatory agency
	Assure customer satisfaction by providing effective and entertaining health/fitness experiences

or special populations. Also, although the federal government is rapidly forcing the DRG reimbursement formula on the states, some states are exempt from this policy because they already have cost-containment control boards. Lastly, many hospitals are financially at risk and thus have no incentive to reduce their patient populations. Hospitals thrive financially with full occupancy rates; any health education offerings probably will be designed to increase compliance with treatment regimens but not necessarily to improve wellness and fitness levels. Table 1.9 lists some primary and secondary objectives for hospital health/fitness programs.

Meeting Health/Fitness Objectives ■

Organizations can meet their particular health/fitness objectives—be they improved productivity and morale, improved spirituality, or decreased medical costs—by following a careful implementation plan such as the one we will describe in Chapter 4. By defining its needs and assessing its resources, an organization can plan intelligently a custom-suited, cost-effective program, rather than blithely contracting with a vendor to provide services or simply adopting another organization's plan. Health/fitness programs can flop royally if the participants are not consulted beforehand and their needs,

■ T A B L E I . 8 ■
Objectives for Government Health/Fitness Programs

Primary	Secondary
Promote the health of citizens to secure the future of the United States	Reduce excess medical costs
	Reduce inflation
Meet constitutional obligations	Promote voter satisfaction
	Establish demonstration programs that spread throughout the nation
	Support research on safe, effective methods to improve the health/fitness levels of citizens
	Develop regulations that tend to promote health/fitness of citizens

■ T A B L E   I . 9 ■
Objectives for Hospital Health/Fitness Centers

Primary	Secondary
Improve compliance of patients with treatment regimens (nonprofit and for-profit, private and public community hospitals)	Create a marketing vehicle to develop good will with the community
	Recruit clients for the hospital (inpatient and outpatient)
Gain reasonable profit for services rendered to community and corporate worlds (community and private for-profit hospitals)	Provide an entertainment device for ambulatory-care patients
	Improve the general health of the community as part of hospital's overall role
Render services to the community on a cost-recovery basis (community hospitals)	
Meet accreditation standards of the Joint Commission (all hospitals)	
Provide employee health/fitness programming to reduce hospital costs and increase productivity (all hospitals)	

cultural differences, and preferences duly recorded.

Assuming you follow a careful implementation plan, it might then be useful to compare your organization's method of achieving objectives to that of other organizations. Profiles of various organization's health/fitness programs can be found in Chapter 9.

■ Possible Outcomes of Health/Fitness Programs

Benefits

The benefits of a long-standing employee health/fitness program are demonstrated by the results obtained by NASA, which began its program in 1968 in Washington, DC. After initial examinations, 259 men aged 35 to 55 years exercised three times per week. After 1 year, they underwent a second medical examination and were quizzed on their experience. The findings were: 50% reported better job performance and better attitudes toward work; 12% who took part occasionally reported similar effects; most regu-

lar exercisers reported feeling better; 89% reported improved stamina; 40% reported sleeping better; 60% lost weight; 50% reported paying more attention to their diet; and there was a highly consistent and positive relationship between perceived benefits of the program and the results of medical tests.[24]

Another health/fitness program for the New York State Education Department was studied for 5 years; the findings demonstrated that the program reduced risk factors in the participants, eased health problems, and cut down employee absenteeism by 55%.[24]

According to *Building a Healthier Company*, produced by Blue Cross/Blue Shield, the President's Council on Physical Fitness and Sports, and the American Association of Fitness Directors in Business and Industry, "studies of health/fitness programs in Russia have documented the economic benefits of exercise programs . . . because people who exercise produce more, visit the doctor less frequently and are far less prone to industrial accidents."[24]

The Safeco Insurance Company program called *Self Help* has resulted in the following effects for 650 employees who were surveyed:

53% were the same weight, 35% lost weight, and 13% gained unwanted weight; 63% said they paid more attention to caloric intake and fat intake and made eating decisions accordingly; 7% of smokers quit, 63% were exercising, and 67% reported "changes" or "real changes" in their lifestyle.[25] Kimberly-Clark's extensive health-promotion program, which includes health-risk identification and reduction, physical fitness, health education, and counseling, has had excellent results in identifying employees who have dangerous risk factors and referring them to their employee-assistance program. Their findings, reported over the last 5 years, include: a 65% rehabilitation rate for their alcohol and drug-abuse program; a significant reduction in weight for employees enrolled in the obesity-control program; and a reduction in blood pressure and triglyceride levels for employees in their health-promotion program.[25]

Employee-assistance programs (often a part of comprehensive health/fitness programs) often report success. Kimberly-Clark's employee-assistance program showed a 70% reduction in accidents for the year after participation as compared to the year before.[10] Bethlehem Steel reported a 60% rehabilitation rate in its alcoholism program.[10] Dow Chemical reported a 70% success rate for participants of a smoking-cessation program 1 full year after attendance.[10] Various risk-reduction programs (for example, North Karelia, Finland preventive medicine program; Western Electric Company's 20-year study; the Multiple Risk Factor Intervention Trial or MR FIT) have demonstrated success in reducing or eliminating risk factors accompanied by lowered incidence of stroke and reduced rates of acute myocardial infarction.[10] Campbell Soup reported a 25% success rate in their smoking-cessation program.[26] New York Telephone reported an 85% success rate in its alcoholic-rehabilitation program, a form of secondary prevention. Kennecott Copper's *Insight* mental health counseling program helped reduce absenteeism by 52% and hospital, surgical, and medical service by 55%. Johnson & Johnson's *Love of Life* program was evaluated over a 2-year

period and early reports revealed that participants were absent from work less frequently, were more satisfied with their jobs, and were better able to handle job strain than non-participants.[27] General Motors' employee assistance program enrolled 44,000 employees and, after 1 year of the program, they reported a 40% reduction in lost time and a 60% reduction in grievances; the alcoholism program reported a 49% reduction in lost worktime and a 20% reduction in disability costs. Control Data's *Staywell* program has shown that health-care costs are lower for participants than for other employees.[27] New York Telephone calculated its annual savings from nine health-promotion programs (smoking cessation, cholesterol reduction, hypertension control, fitness training, stress management, alcohol-abuse control, colorectal-cancer screening, breast-cancer screening, and healthy-back program) at $5,540,000. Their costs for the programs ran at $2,840,000 for a net gain of $2,700,000 annually. A study done in Canada compared two similar white-collar employee groups and found a net medical and hospital cost savings of $84 per individual per year in the company as a result of a fitness and lifestyle program.[28] Former heart-attack victims who were taught to reduce their stressful Type A behavior had a statistically significant lower rate of recurrent heart attacks than did similar victims who were given only standard cardiological advice (9% versus 19%).[29] Table 1.10 lists some cost savings for selected programs.

Costs

Initiating health/fitness programs featuring education interventions, fitness programming, counseling, health-hazard appraisal, referral, and elaborate exercise facilities can be expensive. The Kimberly-Clark program—which has a $2.5 million exercise facility, several medical and fitness specialists, an employee-assistance program, a risk-reduction program, and expensive diagnostic and exercise equipment—is a costly undertaking. The director of this *Health*

■ T A B L E I . 1 0 ■
Cost Savings Reported for Some Employee-Assistance Programs

Company	Number Employees	Number Using Program	Rehabilitation Rate (%)	Annual Cost Savings[a]
University of Missouri	7,000	1,002	80	$ 67,996[b]
Scovill Manufacturing	6,500	180	78	186,550
Illinois Bell Telephone (family)	38,490	1,154	80	254,448[c]
U.S. Postal Service	83,000	100	75	2,221,362
Kennecott Copper (with dependents)	7,000 28,000	1,200/yr.	0	448,400[d]
New York Transit	43,000	?	75	2,000,000
E.I. du Pont (with spouses)	16,000	176/yr.	70	419,200[e]
New York Telephone	80,000	300/yr.	85	1,565,000

Source: Berry, C. A. *An approach to good health for employees and reduced health care costs for industry.* Washington, DC: Health Insurance Association of America, 1981, p. 21. Used by permission.

a Number rehabilitated × average salary.
b Plus a 40% decrease in use of health benefits.
c 31,806 disability days were saved; off-duty accidents decreased 42.4% and on-duty accidents decreased 61.4%. There also were savings in health insurance utilization and job inefficiency.
d The total included absenteeism, sickness, and accident disability and health insurance use. Absenteeism decreased 53%, weekly indemnity costs (sick accident) 75%, and medical costs 55%. Rehabilitation rate not calculated as varies with type of case and definition. Plan to compare number discharged with number seen. Conservative calculation found a $5.78 return on $1.00 invested in program.
e Only alcohol program.

Management Program estimates a payback period of approximately 9.5 years on the fitness center and equipment; 3 years for the employee-assistance program; 6.5 years for the risk-reduction program; and 10 years to show significant dollar savings. They have a staff-to-participant ratio of 1:62 and annual costs per employee of $435.[30]

Contrast this with organizations that offer minimal services such as free hypertension screening and perhaps offer to pay for a course on stress management at the local YMCA. Total costs might well run under $50 per employee, but have a questionable payback feature because the program is not comprehensive and therefore *may* not have any lasting effect on behavior.

Costs vary tremendously among programs. This variation may reflect many things, such as location of the company or organization, climate, existing materials and facilities, community resources, and the number of people to be served. The common denominator to be used in comparing these programs, however, should not be the cost, but rather the cost-effectiveness.

Cost–Benefit Analysis and Cost-Effectiveness Studies ■

Cost–benefit (C–B) analysis is an attempt to quantify the worth of a program in dollar amounts. Usually stated as a ratio of cost to benefit, a positive C–B ratio would be: $1 to $1 plus *x*. However, several points must be noted. First, a perplexing problem in this form of evaluation is the lack of standardized criteria for data to be entered in the model. For example, how many dollars is a human worth? An uneducated human? One possessing an advanced degree? Should the value be in terms of that person's income-producing ability minus his or her income, projected *x* amount of years into the future? How would a nonsalaried but important volunteer in an organization be valued? How can indirect and nontangible effects of a program such as an obvious boost in morale be quantified? And is it even fair to attribute any measured effects to a program knowing the complicated nature of humans and the many uncontrolled variables in their lives?

Individual companies will accept as positive and useful widely varied C–B ratios. For example, one company organized into profit centers may seek immediate and substantial paybacks of any money invested into a health/fitness enterprise. In another company, health/fitness programming may be supported for the good of the employees even if it does not generate a positive C–B ratio.

The field simply has not matured sufficiently for companies to be fully confident of any one model. However, a useful C–B model devised by Phillips and Hughes is discussed in Chapter 4. Of course, only those benefits that are readily measurable can be entered in a C–B model.

Although fitness may prolong life, this benefit may not be easily demonstrable. An assay of medical costs, days lost from work, and production levels, although less exciting, may be more verifiable. Claims of benefit therefore should be limited to these or similar quantifiable variables.

Cost-effectiveness (C-E) studies determine how effectively and efficiently a program meets its goals, and whether altering the methodology of the program would result in less cost (more efficiency). Again, the goals stated for the program should be measurable and the costs tied to the program. C-E studies determine to what degree the goals are met, how much it costs to meet these goals, and whether another method that is less costly could be employed to meet those goals. Thus, a C-E analysis may ask how much it will cost to increase knowledge about cancer risk by 50% in 75% of all employees. A C–B study might then answer the question: What is the benefit of increasing knowledge of cancer risk by 50% in 75% of employees and is this benefit a positive one when cost is considered?

Summary ∎

Health/fitness programs that help participants adopt health-enhancing behaviors have tremendous potential. They can (1) increase an individual's health while preventing disease; (2) improve the psychological atmosphere of organizations; (3) contribute to the primary and secondary goals of organizations, especially decreased absenteeism and raised productivity; (4) reduce medical costs; and (5) reduce an important source of inflationary pressure on the economy, namely, rising medical costs. When combined with more global health promotion endeavors (planned economic, political, and organizational changes that also tend to protect and promote health), health/fitness programming improves the overall status of various organizations and people within the organizations.

References ∎

1. National Heart, Lung and Blood Institute (NHLBI). *Annual report to the nation.* Washington, DC: NHLBI, 1984.

2. Gettman, L. *Testimony on HR 3525 "Permanent Tax Treatment on Fringe Benefits Act of 1983."* Ways and Means Select Revenues Subcommittee, August 1, 1983. *Employee Benefits Plan Review,* November 1983.

3. Davis, L. Evaluation of the seaside conference. *Health Education* May–June 1984, pp. 12–15.

4. Center for Disease Control. Behavioral risk factor surveillance. *Morbidity and Mortality Weekly Reporter: Surveillance Surveys* 33:2–10, 1984.

5. Belloc, N. B., and Breslow, L. The relation of physical health status and health practices. *Preventive Medicine* 1:409, 1972.

6. Paffenbarger, R., et al. A natural history of athleticism and cardiovascular health. *Journal of the American Medical Association* 252:491, 1984.

7. Edwards, M. A. Introduction in *Fitness and industry: Proceedings of a symposium.* Pittsburgh, PA: Health Education Center

of the Health and Welfare Planning Association, 1978, p. 5.

8. Goldberg, P. *Executive health.* New York: McGraw-Hill, 1978, p. xi.

9. Pearson, C. The emerging role of the occupational physician in preventive medicine, health promotion and health education. *Journal of Occupational Medicine* 22:104–106, 1980.

10. National Chamber Foundation. *A national health care strategy: How business can promote good health for employees and their families.* Excelsior, MN: Interstudy, 1978.

11. Feighan, E. F. When a drug king rules abroad. *The New York Times*, August 10, 1984, p. A25.

12. National Interagency Council on Smoking and Health. Cigarette induced medical costs exceed $930 billion. *Smoking and Health Reporter* 1:1, 1984.

13. Corry, J., and Cimbolic, P. *Drugs: Facts, decisions, alternatives.* Belmont, CA: Wadsworth, 1985.

14. Corry, J. *Consumer health: Facts, skills and decisions.* Belmont, CA: Wadsworth, 1983.

15. Chen, M. Proving the effects of health promotion in industry: An academician's perspective. *Health Education Quarterly* 10:235, 1983.

16. Growth in insurance coverage. *The New York Times*, March 31, 1982, p. A1.

17. Stewart, G. Doctors are entering a brave new world of competition: The medical cost crunch—and a healthy supply of MDs—make times tougher. *Business Week*, July 16, 1984, 56–61.

18. Koenig, R. HMOs shed socialized image gaining acceptance on Wall Street? *The Wall Street Journal*, August 10, 1984, p. 27.

19. Associated Press. Health care in the 1990's: Only rich to get top care. *The Advocate*, August 16, 1984, p. A7.

20. U.S. Department of Health and Human Services (DHHS), Public Health Service, Office of Health Research, Statistics and Technology. *Health United States 1980.* Hyattsville, MD: DHHS, 1980.

21. Green, L., et al. *Health education planning: A diagnostic approach.* Palo Alto, CA: Mayfield, 1980.

22. Employee fitness shapes up as a business. *Business Week*, July 6, 1981, p. 34BD.

23. Bader, B. S., et al. *Planning hospital health promotion services for business and industry.* Chicago, IL: American Hospital Association, 1982.

24. Blue Cross Association; Blue Shield Association; President's Council on Physical Fitness and Sports; and the American Association of Fitness Directors in Business and Industry: *Building a healthier company.* Chicago, IL.

25. Berry, C. A. *An approach to good health for employees and reduced health care costs for industry.* Washington, DC: Health Insurance Association of America, 1981.

26. Wear, R. F. *Health promotion programs in Campbell Soup Co.* Presented at "Health Education and Promotion for the Eighties," Atlanta, GA, March 16–18, 1980.

27. Lee, C. Companies sponsor diet programs to help workers shed pounds, raise productivity. *The Wall Street Journal*, August 9, 1984, p. 31.

28. *Employee fitness "the how to."* Ontario, Canada: Ministry of Culture and Recreation, Sports and Fitness Branch, 1979, p. 4.

29. Friedman, N., et al. Alterations of type A behavior and reduction in cardiac recurrences in post myocardial infarction patients. *American Heart Journal* 108:237, 1984.

30. Berry, C. A. *An approach to good health for employees and reduced health care costs for industry.* Washington, DC: Health Insurance Association of America, 1981, p. 27.

CHAPTER 2

WELLNESS

Although the boom in health/fitness programs in the United States is gratifying to those who work in the field, a potentially troublesome issue is the potential proliferation of unethical and ineffective programs. In this chapter, we will briefly explore ethical issues related to health/fitness programming, a philosophical position that we believe is ethical and effective, an approach to health/fitness programming called *wellness* that embodies this philosophical position, and some specific practices used in wellness programs.

■ Ethical Issues

Sackett has offered four criteria to determine when it is ethical to increase compliance of patients via behavioral, organizational, and educational techniques:[1] (1) the diagnosis must be correct; (2) the therapy must do more good than harm; (3) there must be mutual responsibility of patient and physician for prescribing and taking any medication; and (4) the patient must be an informed, willing partner in execution of any maneuver designed to alter compliance behavior. Although health/fitness professionals may prefer a different word than *compliance* and are involved with participants, not patients, they are just as concerned with having participants in their programs comply with, adhere to, or remain in the health/fitness program long enough to receive benefits and have a chance

of reaching health goals. Therefore, because health/fitness professionals are concerned with compliance, and because the health/fitness intervention undoubtedly will change the participant's life, we submit that health/fitness professionals must be concerned with the ethical criteria offered by Sackett.

For example, the first criterion implies two things: assessment is customized or individualized, rather than all participants getting the same program, and assessment is scientific—that is, some statistical analysis of the assessment mechanism has demonstrated the reliability and validity of the technique.

The second criterion is certainly relevant to the health/fitness professional. For example, administering a "canned" exercise program, such as following a video cassette of a vigorous aerobic dance workout, may potentially do more harm than good for unscreened individuals with preexisting medical problems, or even for healthy individuals who are just beginning to exercise. False, faddish, or unscientific information about nutrition may cause financial and health harm to participants; should this faddish information be presented in an antiscientific manner, participants may become swayed by other unscientific, quackish approaches to health.

The third criterion perhaps does not pertain to health/fitness professionals. However, we can consider a transliteration: there must be mutual responsibility of the participant and health/fitness professional for setting fitness and health goals and a health-enhancement plan, as well as for adhering to the plan. Paternalism in medicine or in health promotion often is self-defeating as well as unethical, because the patient–participant is kept dependent; he or she is not able to be self-responsible.

The fourth criterion implies that the participant in a health/fitness program must be fully informed, must not be cajoled or coerced into entering the program, and must genuinely volunteer to be part of the program. For example, if a health/fitness professional were to use behavior modification techniques to foster adherence but did not inform the participant of this approach, this would be unethical. However, if there was a detailed discussion of this approach prior to the start of the program, and the participant agreed that this would be a good way to aid his or her adherence until exercise (or some other behavior) became a self-reinforcing habit, this would be ethical.

Allegrante offers two other ethical considerations: the dilemma of conflicting loyalties and the dilemma of victim blaming.[2] Allegrante warns that health/fitness professionals must be wary of violating the trust of participants in a program because of conflicting loyalty to their employers. For example, should health/fitness professionals keep detailed and personal notes of health counseling sessions knowing that they may later be called for by the employer?

Victim blaming is the potential shifting of blame for ill health entirely to the participant as a byproduct of a health-promotion effort that emphasizes self-responsibility. What are the limits of one's ability to affect one's health? What role does the workplace play in poor health? Should the health/fitness professional offer educational experiences that will enable participants not only to improve their personal lifestyles but also to fight environmental insults and threats coming from the workplace? How accountable should participants be for their health status, knowing there are many uncontrolled hazards to health in the environment?

A philosophy that may arise from these ethical considerations is an approach to health/fitness programming called *wellness*.

A Philosophy of Health/Fitness

The earmarks of a philosophy of health/fitness that is ethical as per the criteria discussed and that is also cost-effective are (1) participants are seen as worthy and capable, with great human potential that can be expanded through cooperation or partnership; (2) the health/fitness program is available to potential participants on a voluntary rather than a coercive basis; (3) the health/fitness program involves the participants in decision making about their health-promotion plans; (4) the techniques used in the health/fitness program are scientifically correct, safe, and appropriate for the individual as determined by needs assessment; (5) compliance or adherence techniques are fully explained to the participant, who agrees to engage voluntarily in these activities; (6) health/fitness professionals are properly trained; and (7) the use of health/fitness records is explained to the participants—any potentially adverse use of records, such as to justify employment termination, is revealed before participation in the program.

These hallmarks of an ethical health/fitness program are exemplified in a wellness approach to health promotion.

Wellness Defined

The term *high-level wellness* is synonymous with the more familiar terms *robust health, excellent health*, and even simply *health*. However, *wellness* is a term coined by Dunn in a deliberate attempt to fashion a new way of thinking about a person's health status; Dunn wished to differentiate the realm of disease—dominated by the medical system—from that of health promotion and human excellence—dominated by social scientists, educators, coaches, and others generally outside the world of medicine or therapy.[3] The term *health* leads many people immediately to think of disease, illness, and doctors. Dunn decided to employ *wellness* or *high-level wellness* to describe the state of some humans who are operating at or near their potential because of the lifestyle they have adopted.

Rather than disease treatment or even prevention being the primary goal of a wellness program, Dunn saw wellness as the style of living that permits or facilitates human excellence, high energy levels, and optimal functioning. Disease prevention can and does result from wellness programs, but this is a secondary function. Dunn's definition of wellness is an integrated *method* of functioning. By fostering high-level wellness, Dunn believes, we can help people to experience "upward direction, greater potential of functioning, an ever-expanding tomorrow and an integration of mind, body and spirit.[3] Dunn's view of wellness and health is dynamic, not static. Dunn sees health as a way of living that helps us continuously to uncover our potential. This concept is similar to that of humanistic psychologist Maslow's *self-actualizing personality*, the person who continuously grows and strives toward new knowledge and as a result experiences happiness and ever-expanding potentials.[4]

Hochbaum, a noted health educator, also believes that achieving the health state or even an optimal health state per se is wasted effort. He believes we need to view health as a balanced lifestyle, a *process* that allows us to enjoy life and to reach the potential of which we are capable.

These dynamic views of health or wellness, with an emphasis on self-responsibility and health as a method of living, are useful to the health/fitness professionals who are defining the proper goal(s) for their programs. Although it is true that some people may view disease prevention and cost savings as the only worthy goal of a health/fitness program, this may be a shortsighted approach. Think of the corporation, for example, that adopts the disease intervention/prevention approach exclusively. We believe they miss an opportunity to foster personal growth and lifelong discovery and

creativity in their employees. By adopting a wellness approach, the corporation can develop a cadre of employees who continuously renew themselves, are highly energetic, live close to the potential for which they were hired, and whose lifestyle serves as an innoculation against many debilitating conditions such as mental depression, alcoholism, obesity, self-doubt and despair, myocardial infarctions, and ulcers.

Self-Responsible and Goal-Oriented Nature of Wellness

Don Ardell notes that "a wellness system intends to maximize good health, moving a person to higher levels of health from any point of initial contact. In contrast, the illness system seeks only to minimize the impact of disease— arresting its progress, minimizing its complications, sustaining a person when the disease process is irreversible."[5] The difference he visualizes is shown in Figure 2.1. Notice that in an illness system all efforts (indicated by the arrows) are directed toward the disease; the goal is to defeat the disease. By focusing exclusively on illness, medical therapists have accomplished enormous breakthroughs in curing disease. They have not, however, traditionally been concerned with human excellence or facilitating optimal health. Note also that traditional disease-prevention programs often do not include *enabling* exercises, which help participants to be more self-responsible and capable of growth. Instead, they focus on steps to avoid disease, often telling people what *not to do*, rather than what *to do*.

Health/fitness professionals, on the other hand, look beyond the mere absence of disease symptoms. They emphasize *self-responsibility*. Whereas in an illness system the therapist may perform all the tasks and hope that the participant will not ruin these efforts (will comply), a wellness system assumes the participant is responsible for his or her own improvement plan. The health/fitness professional is available as a resource for the participant and provides assessment, health information, safe fitness experience,

■ **Figure 2.1**   Goals of wellness and illness systems differ. (From Ardell, D. High- ■
level wellness strategies. *Health Education,* July–August 1977, pp. 2–4. Reprinted
by permission of the Association for the Advancement of Health Education, an
association of the American Alliance for Health, Physical Education, Recreation, and
Dance.)

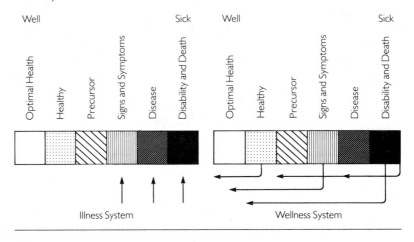

An Illustration of Wellness

counseling, motivation or encouragement, monitoring of a behavior-modification contract and so on. Wellness-oriented health/fitness programs have a philosophical basis similar to that of humanistic psychology and humanistic education, which recognize self-responsibility as being integral to genuine self-growth. All three systems have derived noncoercive techniques that help the participants in personal growth and equip them to work on fulfilling their potential.

An Illustration of Wellness

Recently, a 43-year-old planner for a major electronics firm earned a promotion to corporate director after a whirlwind 5-month campaign that resulted in the directors adopting the planner's proposal for a new corporate division. The campaign began with the planner's insight into future computer needs in new buildings, progressed through literature searches, intensive needs assessment, and documentation, and was followed by development of a business plan. The 5 months were punctuated by transcontinental flights, 19-hour business days, and

long, grinding meetings during which the planner sold company executives his new idea and his plan for implementing it with no financial outlay by the company.

The executives noticed that, in conversations with this planner, one overriding quality probably helped his campaign more than anything else: boundless energy and enthusiasm. Obviously, the idea was a winner, but the tremendous work done to document the feasibility of the concept, carry it throughout the corporate structure to win support, and finally develop a financing and implementation plan testified to the stamina of this man. Further conversation elicited complementary qualities that assured success: a happy lifestyle that emphasized creativity, personal growth, confidence, and a positive outlook on life, the characteristics mentioned in *In search of excellence: Lessons from America's best run companies.*[6] Besides self-confidence and a clear set of values, regular exercise permitted the planner to have a superior level of energy that not only seemed to contribute to his daily survival but also prompted him to explore his potential and to renew himself regularly. Because he was pleased with his life, he took steps to safeguard his health and safety by following a comprehensive health-maintenance plan.

In our opinion, this man's lifestyle is high-level wellness, which Dunn defined as "*an integrated method of functioning* which is oriented toward maximizing the potential of which the individual is capable within the environment where he or she is functioning."[3] This definition emphasizes self-responsibility and a lifestyle or method of functioning that is holistic.

Today, corporate America realizes that employees are a prized commodity to be protected, encouraged, and helped to grow. In some well-run companies, wellness programs have been phased into the corporate culture to protect the health of employees while facilitating their growth.

Comprehensive Nature of Wellness

The goals of wellness programming are to improve all parts of human health to the point where a person can live life to the fullest. This means program participants have ample energy for work, play, and continuous self-improvement, are relatively free from minor illnesses, and are well protected (within genetic limitations) from serious acute and chronic degenerative diseases. Their mental and physical health status complement and reinforce each other.[7] They are energetic, can meet life's demands, and have reserve energy for play and self-discovery. They are healthier; they also feel renewed, energetic, and ready for life's challenges. This may occur as a function of *physiological* events, such as greater oxygen uptake, increased muscular tone, homeostatic balance of neurotransmitters, reduced muscular and nervous tension,[8,9,10,11,12] or it may result from *mental* events, such as clearer values systems, greater ability to cope with stress by thinking through situations, ability to alter consciousness to improve mental health through biofeedback or meditation, or ability to manage time and stay in the present moment.[13] It may result from *social* events, such as ability to resolve conflict constructively, to communicate better and with greater trust, or to reach out to loved ones.[14]

Spiritual events also may evoke this new level of wellness, such as ability to shift consciousness to experience rapture and awe; ability to find peace, meaning, and a way of life in religion; or ability to find inspiration.[4,15]

Whatever the initial source of the good feelings, the participant feels better, and often converts to a new, healthier lifestyle. In other words, an improvement in the level of one dimension may positively affect all the other dimensions. As far as the health/fitness professional is concerned, programs that employ techniques to facilitate positive interactions among the physical, mental, social, and spiritual sides of participants will tend to increase wellness. A program director will increase the probability of behavioral change and improved wellness if the participant is challenged: (1) in all the various learning domains, and (2) in a sequential and planned fashion. Also, if wellness-enhancing behaviors and skills are covered in the mental, social, physical, and spiritual domain, chances are improved that positive synergistic interactions will occur to move participants into higher levels of wellness. If Maslow was correct in his assertions that self-growth and self-actualization take on a momentum of their own, then health/fitness professionals who tangibly improve the wellness status of participants while equipping them to undertake eventually their own lifelong self-improvement projects will have done their job. One simple technique to convey the self-responsibility and continuous growth concepts to participants is the use of *wellness inventories* and *health-hazard appraisal instruments*. Participants use these inventories to self-assess the many aspects that constitute health, and typically target one or two factors they wish to add to their lives, or identify those behaviors they already perform. This is an ethical approach to health promotion because the participant makes the changes. The role of the health/fitness professional is to help the participant choose realistic and needed changes, and to reinforce these changes or adaptions (with the full knowledge and permission of the participant) through education, motivational appeals, counseling, and behavioral-management plans (contingency management).

A Look at Sample Wellness Inventories

High-Level Wellness Behavior Inventory

The High-Level Wellness Inventory was developed at North Texas State University. It has a reading level of age 16 years and has been judged to be valid by a panel of experts who were asked if the behaviors in the inventory were indeed health enhancing for participants with no underlying pathology. It was also found to be reliable by a test-retest procedure.

Notice that the inventory asks about only *behavior*—it does not assess a person's current or future level of health, how many years of life they project given their health statistics, and so on. It has a scale for the participant to target an increase in health-enhancing behaviors. It also has a contingency-management plan (or behavior-modification contract) to help the participant successfully adopt the new behavior(s).

The underlying tenet for this instrument is that it is easier to add a positive behavior than it is to stop a negative, health-destroying behavior. This idea originated with Festinger, who formulated the concept of *cognitive dissonance*.[16] Becker and coworkers also tested this idea using their *Health Belief Model* and showed that behaviors can be added more easily than they can be expunged.[17] Eventually, new behaviors squeeze out old behaviors simply because there is a finite amount of time in the day.

The contingency-management instrument should help to add healthy behaviors to a participant's lifestyle. More important, once the participant begins to feel the extra energy, greater confidence, and clearer thinking that reflect high-level wellness, this becomes a critical reinforcer to his or her decision to adopt a healthier lifestyle. Eventually, when the original target behaviors become habits, the participant may add one or two more behaviors. This can continue ad infinitum.

Research on compliance indicates that combinations of educational, motivational, communicative, behavioral, and organizational strategies are significantly more effective than is one

approach used alone.[18] Therefore, the use of wellness inventories probably is necessary but not sufficient to ensure complete compliance to recommended health behaviors.

Assessing Health-Related Behaviors Figure 2.2 is an inventory of behaviors that tend to enhance a person's health. The underlying assumptions in this inventory are that the person has no serious preexisting illnesses and that the behaviors are undertaken in a reasonable, noncompulsive manner. If, for example, a positive behavior of regular exercise becomes an obsessive behavior of exercise for several hours each day, and if this exercise prevents the individual from coping with other aspects of life, then the behavior is not health producing. Balance is the key to a good wellness plan. Obsessive, faddish, unbalanced lifestyle alterations cause more problems than they solve.

The behaviors listed in Figure 2.2 are *ideal* behaviors; that is, the healthiest level of involvement for each behavior (whenever that behavior is performed) is 100% of the time (or always). For example, when exercising it is best to warm up and limber up before actually getting into the workout (question 2). The behavior inventory covers many areas of life—physical, social, spiritual, and mental. With it you can assess your present behaviors as well as ones you would choose for the future. The behaviors are suggested by health-promoting agencies such as the American Heart Association, the California Department of Public Health, the World Health Organization, the American Cancer Society, and the Office of Health Information, Health Promotion and Sports Medicine. To determine the rating for each question, consider whether you participate 100% (all the time). If not, estimate how much of your time is spent in that behavior and select the rating closest to your practice. If you wish to improve the level of a particular behavior, mark the appropriate box in the second column.

Using a Behavior-Modification Contract After you have identified some target behaviors to add

Figure 2.2 Sample page from high-level wellness behavior inventory. (From Corry, J. M. *Consumer health: Facts, skills and decisions.* Belmont, CA: Wadsworth, 1983, pp. 360–367.)

High-Level Wellness
Behavior Inventory

Rate yourself in each of the following behaviors. Figure the percentage or amount of time spent when you perform the behavior.

Use these ratings:
Answer both for now and future:

My Present Status
Now

100% Always	99%–81% Most of the time	80%–61% Frequently	60%–41% Occasionally	40%–21% Sometimes	20%–1% Rarely	0% Never	Can't answer: Need more information
7	6	5	4	3	2	1	0

I should change to this rating:

Enhancement Plan
Future

100% Always	99%–81% Most of the time	80%–61% Frequently	60%–41% Occasionally	40%–21% Sometimes	20%–1% Rarely	0% Never
7	6	5	4	3	2	1

I. Physical Health Behaviors

A. Exercise

A.1 Vigorous workouts for 25 minutes at least four times weekly (.75 × (maximum heart rate − resting heart rate) + resting heart rate).

A.2 Warm up with flexibility exercises before workout? Limber up?

A.3 Supplement workouts with stretching and strength exercises?

A.4 Regularly check fitness status to prevent staleness due to overwork?

A.5 Let your mind drift and really enjoy exercising to the point that you consider it "playing"?

B. Nutrition

B.1 Enjoy your meals in a pleasant setting, relaxed, at regular times?

to your lifestyle, it is useful to create a system that will help you comply with your intentions. Behavior modification is a systemized technique to aid you in voluntarily changing your behavior. A contract form is shown in Figure 2.3. For the system to work, it must be realistic in the goals set and the rewards used. It must also be simple to follow. First, you should delineate clearly and specifically each behavior you wish to add or increase, including how many times per day or week you wish to do it. Second, plan to reward yourself for immediate success as well as long-range improvement (Figures 2.4 and 2.5). In fact, you may give yourself a small reward im-mediately after the behavior, and then, when the behavior becomes a habit, give yourself a big reward. For example, for 15 minutes of exercise in 1 day, you might allow yourself 30 minutes of television watching; if you exercise 4 or more days in 1 week, you might go to a movie. If you develop a regular exercise habit, you might re-ward yourself with a handsome new running outfit. The rewards should be fair and appropri-ate. Do not over- or underreward.

If punishment is used to shape your be-havior, this too should be fair and specific. If you use a point system (behaviors earn certain points, points buy certain rewards), you need to

▌ **Figure 2.3** Self-contract planning form. (From Corry, J. M. *Consumer* ▌ *health: Facts, skills and decisions.* Belmont, CA: Wadsworth, 1983, pp. 368–370.)

1. Name _____

2. Monitors to help you _____
   _____

3. Health behaviors you wish to add or increase (in-cluding specific units of time per day or week; some behaviors may require practice, such as practicing good listening 20 minutes per day)
   a. _____
   b. _____
   c. _____
   d. _____
   e. _____

4. What is your long-range expectation for doing these behaviors, aside from any rewards you build into this contract?
   _____
   _____
   _____

5. What activities make up your typical day?
   _____
   _____
   _____

6. What activities do you typically do on a weekend?
   _____

_____
_____

7. How can you add behaviors to your weekday and weekend activities?
   _____
   _____

8. List 20 things you love to do (or consult the checklist at the end of the form):
   a. _____   k. _____
   b. _____   l. _____
   c. _____   m. _____
   d. _____   n. _____
   e. _____   o. _____
   f. _____   p. _____
   g. _____   q. _____
   h. _____   r. _____
   i. _____   s. _____
   j. _____   t. _____

9. What kinds of things do you hate to do?
   a. _____   f. _____
   b. _____   g. _____
   c. _____   h. _____
   d. _____   i. _____
   e. _____   j. _____

(continued)

10. Your Plan:

Behaviors	Consequences (Reward and Punishment)	Date Begun?	Date Finished?
a. _____	_____	_____	_____
	_____	_____	_____
	_____	_____	_____
	_____	_____	_____
b. _____	_____	_____	_____
	_____	_____	_____
	_____	_____	_____
	_____	_____	_____
c. _____	_____	_____	_____
	_____	_____	_____
	_____	_____	_____
	_____	_____	_____
d. _____	_____	_____	_____
	_____	_____	_____
	_____	_____	_____
	_____	_____	_____
e. _____	_____	_____	_____
	_____	_____	_____
	_____	_____	_____
	_____	_____	_____

11. Fun Things

_____ shopping
_____ party
_____ go to movies
_____ swimming
_____ go to beach
_____ surfing
_____ camping
_____ date
_____ attend sport events
_____ play musical instrument
_____ ride bikes
_____ ride motorcycles
_____ drive a car
_____ go horseback riding

_____ go to a play
_____ visit a museum
_____ go target shooting
_____ fishing
_____ gardening
_____ climb
_____ skate
_____ dance
_____ disco
_____ hunt
_____ backpack
_____ photography
_____ making toy models
_____ play with animals
_____ cook
_____ make love

_____ watch TV
_____ listen to radio
_____ read novels
_____ eat
_____ write poems
_____ sing
_____ attend church
_____ do volunteer work
_____ go boating
_____ go scuba diving
_____ go wind surfing
_____ sailing
_____ skiing
_____ water skiing
_____ walking
_____ suntanning

_____ carpentry
_____ hang gliding
_____ fly airplane
_____ write short stories
_____ skateboarding
_____ running
_____ picnicking
_____ softball
_____ Frisbee
add your own:
_____ _____
_____ _____
_____ _____
_____ _____
_____ _____

Figure 2.4 Contract management chart (A). (From Corry, J. M. *Consumer health: Facts, skills and decisions*. Belmont, CA: Wadsworth, 1983, pp. 372–373.)

(Daily Rewards, Weekly Totals)

Points Earned / Behaviors	Units of Reward or Points to Be Earned for Doing a Behavior	Units of Reward or Points to Be Lost*	Total Points Earned M T W Th F S Sn	Units and Points Used / Reward	Reward Costs in Points or Units*	Monday's Spending	T W Th F S Sn	Total Spent	Total Remaining (to be used) for major reward at end of program (transfer to)
1.				1.					
2.				2.					
3.				3.					
4.				4.					
5.				5.					

Total Earnings: _____

Total Spending: _____

*Units can be units of time (e.g., 30 minutes of TV) or units of convenient measure (e.g., ounces of soda, dimes).

Punishment for Deficit Spending = Punishment in Units of Time or Point Values (e.g., 20 deficit points = 1 hour of repetitious dish washing).

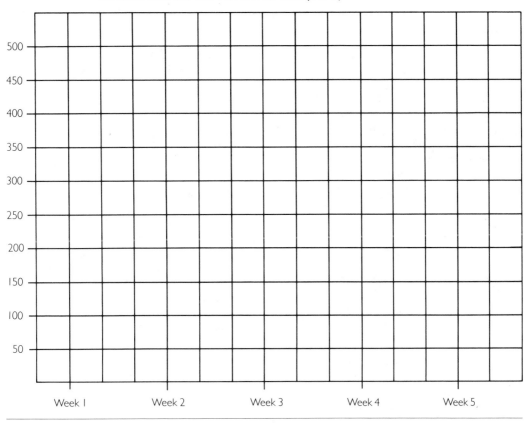

Figure 2.5 Contract management chart (B): points leading to large reward. (From Corry, J. M. *Consumer health: Facts, skills and decisions.* Belmont, CA: Wadsworth, 1983, p. 374.)

establish rules about how many points per day can be used, how many points are awarded for easy versus hard behaviors, and so on.

Many people who experience robust health report feeling closer to their potential and feeling generally superior to their old selves. Maslow, a psychologist who researched motivation, personality, and human potential, would probably describe these people as *self-actualizing personalities* or at least as having the tools to become self-actualizing people.[4] In any case, awareness of these emotional feelings or shifts in consciousness and perception of self seem to be a chief reward for following a wellness plan and seem to reinforce the new healthy behaviors. Combined with the use of a behavior-modification contract, awareness of the delightful emotional states accompanying high-level wellness should result in permanently changed behavior. Even when a person backslides into unhealthy behavior, the guilt about so doing acts as a lever to get him or her back into the wellness plan.

It is a good idea to keep a diary to recognize the benefits of your wellness plan. The advantages of using a diary and sticking to your wellness plan, especially in the difficult early days, are well worth the effort.

Some other things to consider: Can you find someone other than yourself to act as a monitor for your system? Can you keep track of or manage the reward-and-punishment system?

Recognizing Feelings About New Behaviors The payoff for involvement in a wellness program includes many physiological gains that together help you to resist communicable disease, cope better with everyday challenges, and avoid chronic degenerative diseases such as atherosclerosis. These benefits are subtle and may not be apparent to you. Other kinds of experiences and feelings, however, may become apparent to you and may serve as the reinforcers that keep you in the wellness program. Examples of these feelings as reported by people who exercise regularly are: greater confidence, especially in competitive situations; greater "stick-to-it-ness" (greater willpower over a period of time); more energy throughout the day; feeling of self-satisfaction resulting from accomplishing tasks; continual personal and professional growth as goal after goal is accomplished; improved ability to concentrate; psychophysiological feeling of joy (the body feels a delightful sort of tension, as does the mind); play experience wherein the personal ego dissolves and a joyous, carefree feeling ensues; greater ability to focus energy on a task (one-pointed energy), resulting in easier accomplishment of tasks; and a tranquil, peaceful feeling.[19]

TestWell

TestWell (Figure 2.6) is another wellness inventory, developed at the University of Wisconsin's Steven's Point.[20] It asks about health-enhancing behaviors, assigns a value to the amount of times the participant does the behavior, and derives a composite score for the whole instrument that is then labeled as excellent, good, average, fair, or poor.

TestWell is a typical motivational instrument, good for an initial entrée into a program, and can raise the curiosity of the test taker about health. Presumably, the health/fitness professional can capitalize on this curiosity by scheduling the participant in health-education sessions, fitness experiences, and so on.

Other versions of this questionnaire exist; for example, a computer software version allows the participant a great deal of interaction with health information as the test is being taken. This is similar to several other instruments that have been released as computer software packages (Table 2.1 on pages 39–53 lists many of the instruments currently available).

Compute-A-Life II

Compute-A-Life (Figure 2.7) is more typical of the health-hazard appraisal instruments that have proliferated in the last 5 years.[21] This interactive software package derives a risk-factor index for several areas including safety, drugs, diet, lifestyle, physiological data, mental health, and family health, and has a special section for women's health risks. Based on actuarial figures, Compute-A-Life II ultimately provides information on risk factors, appraisal and probable achievable ages if behaviors become healthy, probable life expectancy given current lifestyle, and ways to reduce risk.

This type of approach to health/fitness programming is preferable to one in which participants simply are told what to do. Participants can see quite graphically where they need to improve, what they need to do to reduce risk, and why they must do so. But the choice is theirs, a feature of this type of screening that is in keeping with ethical health/fitness programming.

Selecting and Using Instruments ∎

Table 2.1 lists and briefly describes over 50 health-screening devices currently available; more are being developed every day. The health/fitness professional should consider carefully which, if any, to choose for program participants. Some of these instruments are clearly concerned with uncovering health-risk factors—either immediate ones that threaten health and life in the near future, or long-range ones that might affect a person 10 years or more in the future. Other instruments are designed more as motivators or even ice-breakers to allow the health/fitness professional and participant to begin working on a wellness plan. The health/fitness professional should examine these carefully to see if they can be used ethically, can fit into a wellness program, and are valid and reliable. This last point is important because at least one study has shown that a popular health-hazard instrument not tested for reliability resulted in changed findings of a most curious nature when followup studies were done after a health-education intervention.[22] For example, under the family health history some participants resurrected parents whom they earlier reported had died from heart problems. Others failed to report their hysterectomies when tested a second time. Apparently the instrument caused confusion or fatigue, or both, such that spurious results were recorded. This obviously negated any scientific usefulness of the assessment as a research instrument or even an evaluative instrument for checking the worth of a health/fitness program.

▍ Special Populations

Generally, the mentally, physically, and/or emotionally handicapped individual has disabilities or conditions that place that individual at a disadvantage in fulfilling his or her potential. The handicapped individual may have a congenital condition or may have incurred a disability without warning at some time during life. To define the disabled worker, Burkhauser and Haveman's *Disability and Work: The Economics of American Policy*, use the following: "a limitation of a physical, mental, or emotional sort which reduces, to varying degrees, ones ability to perform the functions required for the job one is, on other grounds qualified to hold."[31]

Naturally, the estimated number of disabled Americans varies depending on the definition of *handicapped*: the range is from 20 to 36 million; from one in seven to one in four people are disabled in some way before they retire.[32] The disabled population in the United States is growing, perhaps in part because lack of social stigma has encouraged better reporting and record keeping.

During the past 15 years, there has been a change in legislative philosophy concerning the handicapped. The 1970s brought acts and amendments aimed at achieving equal opportunities for the handicapped. As corporations develop ways to place the handicapped worker, it is important that these individuals be integrated into company health/fitness programs. Most have the same basic health and fitness needs as does the general work force, but they may have specific needs as well. Moreover, because of their particular disability, the handicapped may find it difficult to participate in group programs. They may need extra reassurance from other participants and the leader. Make sure the handicapped feel welcome and that their involvement is important.

Physical fitness programs are important to all mentally, physically and emotionally handicapped individuals. Such programs can provide the handicapped with independence, as well as a desire to set and the means to achieve personal goals. It may be that some disabled individuals have a greater need to be physically fit than the nondisabled.

The following organizations can provide further information on structuring your program to meet the needs of handicapped participants.

▍ American Alliance for Health, Physical
  Education, Recreation, and Dance
  Units on Programs for the Handicapped
  1900 Association Drive
  Reston, Virginia 22091

▍ American Cancer Society
  Public Information Department
  777 Third Avenue
  New York, New York 10017
  (or local chapter)

▍ American Diabetes Association
  One West 48th Street
  New York, New York 10020   (continued)

Figure 2.6 Sample questions from TestWell: a self-scoring wellness assessment questionnaire. (From Institute for Lifestyle Improvement. *TestWell: A self-scoring wellness assessment questionnaire.* Steven's Point, WI: University of Wisconsin at Steven's Point, 1983. Reprinted by permission of the National Wellness Institute, University of Wisconsin at Stevens Point.)

Physical Fitness

1. I exercise aerobically (continuous, vigorous exercise producing sweat for a minimum of thirty minutes) at least _____ per week.

  1 = five times   2 = four times   3 = three times
  4 = two times   5 = less than twice
  ANSWER = 1   2   3   4   5

2. My resting pulse rate is _____ beats per minute.

  1 = 40 to 55   2 = 56 to 69   3 = 70 to 79
  4 = 80 or above   5 = don't know
  ANSWER = 1   2   3   4   5

3. I avoid the extremes of too much or too little exercise.

  1 = strongly agree   2 = agree   3 = neutral/not sure
  4 = disagree   5 = strongly disagree
  ANSWER = 1   2   3   4   5

4. I approach exercise in a relaxed manner.

  1 = almost always   2 = very frequently   3 = frequently
  4 = occasionally   5 = almost never
  ANSWER = 1   2   3   4   5

5. I stretch before exercising.

  1 = almost always   2 = very frequently   3 = frequently
  4 = occasionally   5 = almost never
  ANSWER = 1   2   3   4   5

Nutrition

  Check.

  1 = almost always   2 = very frequently   3 = frequently
  4 = occasionally   5 = almost never
  ANSWER = 1   2   3   4   5

1. When choosing non-vegetable protein, I select lean cuts of meat, poultry, and fish.

  ANSWER = 1   2   3   4   5

2. I minimize salt intake.

  ANSWER = 1   2   3   4   5

3. I eat fruit and vegetables fresh and uncooked.

  ANSWER = 1   2   3   4   5

4. I eat breakfast.

  ANSWER = 1   2   3   4   5

5. I intentionally include fiber in my diet on a daily basis.

  ANSWER = 1   2   3   4   5

6. I drink enough fluid to keep my urine light yellow.

  ANSWER = 1   2   3   4   5

7. I plan my diet to insure an adequate amount of vitamins and minerals.

  ANSWER = 1   2   3   4   5

6. I stretch after exercising.
   1 = almost always   2 = very frequently   3 = frequently
   4 = occasionally   5 = almost never
   ANSWER = 1   2   3   4   5

7. I increase my exercise by walking or biking whenever possible.
   1 = strongly agree   2 = agree   3 = neutral/not sure
   4 = disagree   5 = strongly disagree
   ANSWER = 1   2   3   4   5

8. I get an adequate amount of sleep.
   1 = almost always   2 = very frequently   3 = frequently
   4 = occasionally   5 = almost never
   ANSWER = 1   2   3   4   5

9. My exercise program includes an adequate amount of each of the three major fitness components—endurance, strength, and flexibility.
   1 = almost always   2 = very frequently   3 = frequently
   4 = occasionally   5 = almost never
   ANSWER = 1   2   3   4   5

10. If I am not in shape, I avoid sporadic (once a week or less) strenuous exercise.
   1 = almost always   2 = very frequently   3 = frequently
   4 = occasionally   5 = almost never
   ANSWER = 1   2   3   4   5

TOTAL =   1   2   3   4   5

8. I minimize foods in my diet that contain large amounts of refined flour (bleached white flour, typical store bread, cakes, etc.)
   ANSWER = 1   2   3   4   5

9. I minimize my intake of fats and oils including margarine and animal fats.
   ANSWER = 1   2   3   4   5

10. I avoid adding sugar to my food and I minimize my intake of presweetened foods such as sugar-coated cereals, syrups, chocolate milk, and most processed and fast foods.
   ANSWER = 1   2   3   4   5

TOTAL =   1   2   3   4   5

■ **Figure 2.7**   Sample questions from Compute-A-Life II. (From Institute for ■
Lifestyle Improvement. *Compute-A-Life.* Steven's Point, WI: University of
Wisconsin at Steven's Point, 1985. Reprinted by permission of the National
Wellness Institute, University of Wisconsin at Stevens Point.)

1. WHICH CATEGORY DESCRIBES YOUR PRESENT WEIGHT (CHART??)
   ( ) 1) MORE THAN 50% OVERWEIGHT
   ( ) 2) 21%-50% OVERWEIGHT
   ( ) 3) 6%-20% OVERWEIGHT
   ( ) 4) AVERAGE . . . + OR - 5%

2. IN TERMS OF ALCOHOL CONSUMPTION, HOW WOULD
   YOU DESCRIBE YOURSELF? LEAVE BLANK IF YOU
   CONSUME NO ALCOHOL.   DRINKS PER WEEK
   ( ) 1) ALCOHOLIC   40+
   ( ) 2) HEAVY DRINKER   25-39
   ( ) 3) MILD EXCESS   7-24
   ( ) 4) MODERATE   2-7
   ( ) 5) USED TO DRINK, BUT STOPPED, OR
            INFREQUENT SOCIAL DRINKER

3. A HIGH CHOLESTEROL LEVEL IS ASSOCIATED WITH
   INCREASED RISK FOR CARDIOVASCULAR DISEASE.
   WHAT IS YOUR CHOLESTEROL LEVEL? IF YOU DON'T
   KNOW, LEAVE BLANK. AN AVERAGE NUMBER FOR AGE,
   RACE, AND SEX WILL BE USED.
   ( ) 1) LESS THAN 180
   ( ) 2) 180-200
   ( ) 3) 201-220
   ( ) 4) 221-250
   ( ) 5) ABOVE 250

4. HOW MANY MILES DO YOU DRIVE/RIDE A YEAR? (THE
   AVERAGE DRIVER/RIDER TRAVELS 10,000 MILES PER
   YEAR.)
   ( ) 1) 3000-5000
   ( ) 2) 5000-10,000
   ( ) 3) 10,000-20,000
   ( ) 4) 20,000-30,000
   ( ) 5) OVER 30,000

5. OF THE TIME SPENT IN A VEHICLE, WHAT
   PERCENT DO YOU WEAR A SEAT BELT?
   ( ) 1) 0% OF THE TIME
   ( ) 2) 1%-33%
   ( ) 3) 34%-66%
   ( ) 4) 67%-99%
   ( ) 5) 100% OF THE TIME

6. WHICH CATEGORY BEST DESCRIBES THE
   DRINKING HABITS OF PEOPLE YOU NOR-
   MALLY DRIVE WITH?   DRINKS PER WK.
   ( ) 1) HEAVY DRINKER   25+
   ( ) 2) MILD EXCESS   7-24
   ( ) 3) MODERATE   1-6
   ( ) 4) NON DRINKER
   ( ) 5) NEVER RIDE WITH A DRINKING
            DRIVER

7. FOR WHATEVER REASONS, DO YOU CARRY
   A WEAPON?
   ( ) 1) YES
   ( ) 2) NO

■ American Heart Association
  Inquiries Section
  7320 Greenville Avenue
  Dallas, Texas 75231
  (or local chapter)

■ The National Association of Sports for
  Cerebral Palsy
  66 East 34th Street
  New York, New York 10016

■ National Clearinghouse for Mental Health
  Information
  Room 11A21, Parklawn Building
  5600 Fishers Lane
  Rockville, Maryland 20857

■ National Council on Alcoholism
  733 Third Avenue
  New York, New York 10017

■ National Handicapped Sports and
  Recreation Associates
  Rod Hernley, President
  1200 15th N.W., Suite 205
  Washington, D.C. 20005

■ National Heart, Lung, and Blood Institute
  Public Inquiries Office
  Room 4A21, Building 31
  National Institute of Health
  Bethesda, Maryland 20205   (*continued*)

■ T A B L E 2 . 1 ■
Health-Risk Appraisal (HRA) Instruments

Name	Cost	Method of Analysis	Comments	Target Group	Ordering Information
Compute-A-Life software package	$400 per program	A microcomputer-based HRA. This package is an interactive program that uses the CDC's HRA as its base	Color graphics; risk-factor appraisal; health information, achievable age, life expectancy, health tips	N.S.*	Institute for Lifestyle Improvement University of Wisconsin, Steven's Point Dolzell Hall Steven's Point, WI 34481
Confidential Health Profile for adults/teens	$5.00	Computer-scored	Asks about values and health attitudes and derives a health-risk score; printout is in narrative form	Adults and teens	University of Florida c/o Linda Moody 3041 McCarty Hall Gainesville, FL 32611
Determine Your Medical Age	$.10	Self-scored	Brief questionnaire on lifestyle, physical health, family and women's health; allows calculation of medical age vs. actual age	Healthy adults over 25 years	The Health Education Center Blue Cross/Blue Shield of Greater NY 3 Park Avenue New York, NY 10016
General Well-Being Questionnaire	Free to qualified users; write for more information	Scoring key	Participants respond to statements about health; an index is derived for general well-being as well as specific scores for physical, mental, emotional, ideological, behavioral, environmental, and experimental areas of well-being	Healthy Adults	St. Louis University, Medical Center c/o Robert Wheeler Department of Health Promotion 1325 S. Grand Blvd. St. Louis, MO 63104

*N.S.: not specified

Name	Cost	Method of Analysis	Comments	Target Group	Ordering Information
Go To Health	First 25 copies free	Self-scored	Adapted from a test produced by the Canadian government; asks 35 questions to derive one's level of health risk; information as well as a behavioral contract are provided to help participants change their lifestyles	N.S.	Public Relations Department Blue Cross/Blue Shield of Michigan 600 East Lafayette Detroit, MI 48226
Health Action Plan	$1.00	Self-analyzed	Asks questions about career, heart disease, and stroke; no score devised; "yes" answers signal a concern area; health information is provided throughout	N.S.	Preventive Medicine Institute—Strang Clinic 55 East 34 Street New York, NY 10016
Health Age	$200	Software for Apple II, Nos. 3.3; IBM PC; Commodore 64; Osb TRS 80, Model III	Computes health age vs. actual age; also gives achievable age	N.S.	Computerized Health Appraisals 13705 Southeast 142 Street Clarkamas, OR 97015
Health & Lifestyle Questionnaire	$7.50	Computer-scored	Focuses on lifestyle and quality of life; asks about psychological and job attitudes and gives a profile ranging from excellent to immediate attention; not based on statistical analysis	N.S.	Health Enhancement Systems 9 Mercer Street Princeton, NJ 08540
Health Awareness Games	$99.00	Software for Apple II, II plus II's. Dos 3.3.	Five microcomputer programs use statistics about lifestyles	JHS through college; also for home use	HRM Software 175 Tompkins Ave. Pleasantville, NY 10570

Instrument	Cost	Scoring	Description	Audience	Source
Health Education Action Plan	Single copies free with stamped, self-addressed envelope	Self-scored	and health as they relate to life expectancy / Derived from several other health risk appraisals, asks 74 questions regarding personal health, exercise, diet, safety, dental health, and tobacco, alcohol, and drug use	N.S.	Erie County H.E. Council P.O. Box 872 Erie, PA 16512
Health 80's Questionnaire	$5–$14	Computer-scored	Several versions available for specific groups; different lengths for each group; asks questions on illness and medical problems, feelings, nutritional and exercise habits, family medical history, smoking, self-care, and others; a health-risk appraisal instrument	General, college students, employees	Medical Data Motion Southwest and Harrison Bellevue, OH 44811
Health Graph	$50 per copy	Self-scored	Used to help college students evaluate the effects of their lifestyles on their health and to teach health-promoting habits; 50 questions, health tips; no numerical score; participant learns the areas where his or her greatest strengths and weaknesses lie	17–26 years	University of Rhode Island Health Services Health Education Department 4th Floor Roosevelt Kingston, RI 02881

Name	Cost	Method of Analysis	Comments	Target Group	Ordering Information
Health Hazard Appraisal: Auto-mated Personal Risk Registry	$4–$12	Computer-scored	The prototypical NHA instrument; asks 55 questions of the usual variety; a personalized risk analysis is prepared giving participants appraisal age, methods to reduce appraisal age (i.e., live longer), levels of stress and a bar graph of health risks in descending order of priority, and ac-tions needed to re-duce appraisal age to achievable age	N.S.	Methodist Hospital Prospective Medicine Department 1604 North Capital Indianapolis, IN 46202
Health Hazard Appraisal: Clues for a Healthier Lifestyle	$.50 for 1–9 copies	Self-scored	Adapted from the Canadian test Your Lifestyle Profile; 35 questions assess the typical risk areas; gives limited health information	N.S.	Public Affairs Pamphlets 381 Park Avenue South New York, NY 10016
Health Hazard Questionnaire	$25–$40	Computer-scored	99 questions on the standard risk factors plus specific labora-tory tests such as blood chemistries and urinalysis; print-out lists present, risk, and achievable ages; ranked listing of most likely causes of death in next 10 years, physical measure-ments, health information, and a summary	Adults over 18 years	Well Aware About Health University of Arizona P. O. Box 43338 Tucson, AZ 85733

Name	Price	Description	Format	Audience	Source
Health Maintenance Vol. II	$36	Health-risk appraisal—computer mortality risk	Computer software for Apple II	High school students	MECC Distribution Center 2530 Broadway Drive St. Paul, MN 55113-5199
Health Rap	$5.50	Uses CDE's health risk appraisal plus 45 more questions on wellness; gives a risk profile and a wellness index	Computer-scored	College students	Health Enhancement & Promotion Co. P. O. Box 546 Ames, IA 50010
Health Risk Appraisal	See ordering information	Adapted from the Canadian government appraisal instrument; developed for internal CDC use; contact CDC for further information	Computer-scored	N.S.	C.A. Althafer Director Special Projects Center for Health Promotion & Education Centers for Disease Control Atlanta, GA 30333
Health Risk Appraisal	$97	Interactive—asks questions then gives participants risks for 10 leading causes of death	Computer software for Apple II plus or II	N.S.	David Garloff Director University of Minnesota Biomedical Graphics/Field Services Program B-192 Phillips Wangensteen Building 516 Delaware Street S.E. Minneapolis, MN 55455
Health Risk Appraisal	$40	Based on CDC software for mainframe computers; designed for batch processing of questionnaires	Computer software for IBM-PC with 128 K memory	N.S.	HRA Microcomputer Software Building 3, Room 108 Center for Health Promotion and Education Centers for Disease Control Atlanta, GA 30333

Name	Cost	Method of Analysis	Comments	Target Group	Ordering Information
Health Risk Appraisal	$4–$5	Computer-scored	Covers health-related behaviors and personal medical status; reports a narrative interpretation of the tabulated risk data and a summary profile	N.S.	University of Michigan Fitness Research Center Department of Physical Education 401 Washenow Ave. Ann Arbor, MI 48109
Health Risk Appraisal Questionnaire	$5	Computer-scored	Based on the *Methodist Hospital Health Hazard Appraisal Instrument*; covers personal and family medical history, health habits, and women's health; gives participants risk factors for 12 leading causes of death as percentages by which they deviate from the norm; gives appraisal age, achievable age, and steps to reduce risk	N.S.	St. Louis County Health Department 504 East Second Street Duluth, MN 55805
Health Risk Assessment	$3	Computer-scored	Asks 43 standard risk questions plus 15 for women only; printout compares participant to others with similar demographic profile; provides health tips	N.S.	Department of Epidemiology and International Health c/o Betty Matnigali University of California at San Francisco Room 1699, H5W San Francisco, CA 94543

Name	Cost	Type	Description		Source
Health Risk Assessment Questionnaire	$5 each for orders of 99 or less, $1 extra per assessment for a detailed statistical analysis	Computer-scored	58 questions, 8 for women only; risk questions plus physical measurements; 2-page printout lists most likely causes of death in next 10 years for persons with same demographics as participant	N.S.	Wisconsin Center for Health and Risk Research University of Wisconsin Center for Health Science 600 Highland Avenue Room 84/414 Madison, WI 53792
Health Risk Profile	$12 per evaluation; $18.50 with blood work	Computer-scored	Uses HRA data plus physiological measurements to give participants risk of dying from 10 leading causes of death for age group	N.S.	Steve Ruff Life Extension Division Control Data Corporation P. O. Box O 8100 34th Avenue S. Minneapolis, MN 55440
Health Risk Questionnaire	$5–$6	Computer-scored	Asks about lifestyle, medical history, and some physical and laboratory measurements; a numerical narrative report describes risk factors for 15 major diseases	N.S.	Health Enhancement Systems 9 Mercer Street Princeton, NJ 08540
Health Status Profile	$13	Computer-scored	23 pages; collects information on current symptoms, medications used, and medical history; asks about nutrition, stress, and exercise habits in detail; gives appraisal age and discusses individual findings in detail; allows participant to write questions that are then answered by letter	N.S.	Health Enhancement Systems 9 Mercer Street Princeton, NJ 08540

T A B L E   2 . 1
(CONTINUED)

Name	Cost	Method of Analysis	Comments	Target Group	Ordering Information
Health Style: A Self-Test	Single copies free	Self-scored	By Department of Health and Human Services, Public Health Services; 24 questions on risk in certain areas; scores for each area; health tips	N.S.	National Health Information Clearing House P. O. Box 1133 Washington, DC 20013
Health Style	$100	Computer software for Apple II; Dos 3.3; TRS 80. Model III	Based on Healthstyle, A Self-Test; asks about health and safety habits, then calculates scores for each area and displays as bar graphs	N.S.	Computerized Health Appraisals 13705 Southeast 42nd St. Clackamas, OR 97015
Health Style	$20	Computer software for Apple II, III; IBM PC; TRS 80 Model III or IV; Commodore 64	Based on Health style, A Self-Test	N.S.	Birdprints P. O. Box 5053 Vancouver, WA 98668
Healthwise	$10 per individual; $8.50 for groups of 5 or more	Computer-scored	Comprehensive; 192 questions on behavior plus blood test results; gives a health age and longevity appraisal listing personal test results and recommended values; gives 10–12 leading causes of death for age and sex and individual recommendations to reduce risk	N.S.	Computerized Health Appraisals c/o Donald Hall Health Services Department Upper Columbia Conference P. O. Box 19039 Spokane, WA 99219

Title	Cost	Method	Description	Population	Source
How Do Your Habits Affect Your Health?	Free	Self-scored	Based on the Canadian *Your Lifestyle Profile*; includes unique questions on motorcycle helmet use and television watching	N.S.	Idaho Health Systems Agency 306 N. 5th Street P. O. Box 8868 Boise, ID 83707
I'm a Health Nut	$20	Computer software for Apple II	Interactive HRA; questions on family and personal health, lifestyle, feelings, and locus of control; gives appraisal age and health tips; also, projected appraisal age at age 40 years	Adolescents	Health Education Section St. Paul Division of Public Health 555 Cedar Street St. Paul, MN 55101
Is Your Body Older Than You Are?	$.15	Self-scored	Same as *Determine Your Medical Age*	N.S.	Blue Cross of Oregon Department YYC 100 Southwest Market Portland, OR 97201
Life	$10	Computer-scored	Questions about biographical data, personal and family medical histories, habits and lifestyle, and physical measurements; printout lists 20 major risk indicators, participants' values for these, and recommended values; gives 20 leading causes of death in age group and health tips; gives nutritional profile, stress profile, appraisal age, and achievable age	N.S.	Computerized Health Appraisals 13705 Southeast 142 St. Clackamas, OR 97015

Name	Cost	Method of Analysis	Comments	Target Group	Ordering Information
Life Score for Your Health	Single copies free with stamped, self-addressed envelope	Self-scored	Questions on various risk factors; positive or negative point values awarded depending on answers; higher scores preferable; *Holmes Stress Scale* included; final scores compared against a chart for health level and life expectancy	Healthy adults	The Center for Consumer Health Education 380 West Maple Ave. Vienna, VA 22180
Lifestyle Assessment Questionnaire	$6 per copy for orders of less than 100; $5 per copy for 100 or more	Computer-scored	286 questions on 4 areas: wellness, opportunities for learning, risk of death, medical/behavioral/emotional alert; gives participant scores and average scores for all others who have taken the test; provides a probable life expectancy, leading causes of death, and behaviors client can change (health tips)	N.S.	Institute for Lifestyle Improvement University of Wisconsin Stevens Point Foundation 2100 Main Street Stevens Point, WI 54481
The Longevity Game	$.50 for pamphlet, $7.00 for poster set	Self-scored	Board game with questions and answers based on medical underwriting policies of Northwestern Mutual Life; a token is placed on age 74 (current average life expectancy in U.S.) and moved up or down depending on answers to health-risk questions	N.S.	Northwestern Mutual Life Advertising and Corporate Information 720 East Wisconsin Ave. Milwaukee, WI 53202

Name	Price	Format	Description	Age	Source
Nutrition, Health and Activity Profile	$11.75	Computer-scored	Assesses risk in nutrition and lifestyle as they affect cancer and heart disease risks; requires charting of dietary consumption of 151 different foods on daily, weekly, monthly basis; printout compares participant to RDAs, and gives information about implications of participant's habits, health tips	N.S.	Pacific Research Systems P. O. Box 64218 Los Angeles, CA 90064
Personal Health Appraisal Questionnaire	$26	Computer-scored	260 questions about risk; 45-page printout with participant's health age, attainable age, and life expectancy; lists personal risk factors and information to improve risks; summary includes recommended behaviors	Adults 21–85 years	The Institute for Personal Health 2100 M Street, N.W. Suite 316 Washington, DC 20063
Personal Health Inventory	$200 for corporate version; $34.95 for personal version	Computer software for Apple II	Interactive appraisal; covers health habits and lifestyle, some psychological measurements, medical care, and women's health; results are shown in 5-minute color graphic analysis of the participant's health; gives narrative and tabulated data on participant's risk of dying from the 10 most prevalent causes of death; appraisal age, achievable age, health tips	N.S.	American Health Management and Consulting Corporation 85 Old Eagle School Rd. Strafford, PA 19087

Name	Cost	Method of Analysis	Comments	Target Group	Ordering Information
Personal Health Profile	$25; $15 for groups of college students	Computer-scored	247 questions including attitudes toward health; yields 48-page printout with personalized health analysis of corresponding background information to help participant change behavior	Adults 20–74 years	General Health 1046 Potomac Street, N.W. Washington, DC 20007
Personal Medical History (Female/Male)	$1 plus $19 for processing	Computer-scored	Two versions, designed for physicians to use with patients; questions about body systems as well as health behaviors and risk factors; printout includes findings about body systems	General, but under supervision of physician or other health professional	Life Extension Institute c/o Cindy Molinari 2970 Fifth Avenue San Diego, CA 92103
Personal Stress Assessment Test	$1	Self-scored	Evaluates physical, chemical, emotional, and social factors related to health; the larger the score, the greater the risk	N.S.	The Pain and Rehabilitation Center c/o C. Norman Shealy, M.D. Route 2—Welsh Coulee La Crosse, WI 54601
Pulse	$24.50	Computer-scored	Gathers information on personal and family medical history, lifestyle, women's health, and health knowledge; 20-page narrative report gives personal health status,	N.S.	Shawn M. Connors International Health Awareness Center 148 East Michigan Ave. Kalamazoo, MI 49007

Name	Cost	Description	Method	Availability	Source
Regional Health Resource Center Health Hazard Appraisal	$4–$10	compares mortality index to that of others, and evaluates nutrition, exercise, weight, stress, dental status, and health knowledge; appraisal and achievable ages and risk-reduction information. Covers lifestyle, medical history, frequency of medical screening, women's health, and laboratory findings; gives 5-page report; 10-year mortality estimates for the 12 leading causes of death for demographic category; health advice	Computer-scored	N.S.	Regional Health Resource Center Medical Information Laboratory 1408 West University Ave. Urbana, IL 61810
Risco: A Heart Hazard Appraisal	Free	Gives risk of developing heart disease based on weight, blood pressure, cholesterol level, smoking, and—for women—estrogen use	Self-scored	N.S.	American Heart Association 7320 Greenville Ave. Dallas, TX 75231
SHAPE Lifestyle Questionnaire	$6	Asks about behavior and physical assessment; a health quality profile is calculated; 86–100 points is excellent	Manual performance by SHAPE staff	General but especially for employees; sold through employers	SHAPE 10700 Meridian Avenue N. Seattle, WA 98133 (a subsidiary of Health Care Corporation, Safeco Corporation)

Name	Cost	Method of Analysis	Comments	Target Group	Ordering Information
Sphere	$295	Computer software in English or French versions for IBM-PC and Apple II	Based on Canadian statistics (a second English version is based on U.S. statistics); international program covers medical and lifestyle characteristics; gives graphic displays and narrative to explain risks, appraisal age, achievable age	N.S.	Division of Health Systems Office of the Coordinator of Health Sciences University of British Columbia No. 400 2194 Health Science Mall Vancouver, BC VGT 1Z6 Canada
TestWell	Single copies free	Self-scored	Assesses 10 areas such as fitness, self-care, nutrition, drugs and drinking; derives scores for each area and an overall composite score then categorized as excellent, good, average, fair, or poor	N.S.	Institute for Lifestyle Improvement Delzell Hall University of Wisconsin—Stevens Point Stevens Point, WI 54481
Total Life Stress Test and Symptom Index	$1	Self-scored	Emphasis on stress; also evaluates sugar, salt, alcohol, tobacco, and drug use; scores indicate need to reduce risks	N.S.	Self-Health Systems Route 1 P. O. Box 127 Fair Grove, MO 65648
Wellness Check	$250	Computer software for Apple II or IIe; TRS-801 Model II, 12 or 16; IBM-PC or PC-XT	Gathers data on health habits, family medical history, occupational risks, and women's health; gives health-producing and health-destroying habits and ways to reduce risk	General as well as adolescent and Spanish versions	Chief of Health Promotion Rhode Island Department of Health 75 Davis Street Providence, RI 02908

Name	Cost	Scoring	Description	Audience	Source
Wellness Inventory	$1	Self-scored	Helps client assess position on an illness—wellness continuum; at one end is premature death, at the other is high-level wellness; 100 questions on 10 areas; health tips; average scores of other test-takers given	N.S.	Wellness Associates 42 Miller Avenue Mill Valley, CA 94941
Your Health Profile	$.50	Self-scored	Evaluates the client's level of health by examining standard risk areas	Teen, adult, or senior adult versions	Health Education Center 200 Ross Street Pittsburgh, PA 15219
Your Health Risk Profile	$1 plus $10 for processing	Computer-scored	70 questions (11 for women only) plus information on medical findings; yields information on current and achievable health ages, 10-year death risk, ways to reduce risk	General by individuals alone or in a group setting	Life Extension Institute c/o Cindy Molinari 2970 Fifth Avenue San Diego, CA 92103
Your Lifestyle Profile	Single copies free	Self-scored	Developed by the Canadian government; 35 questions on standard risk areas; health tips booklet	Employees; general public	Bureau of Health Education Kansas Department of Health and Environment Building 321 Forbes Field Topeka, KS 66620

- The National Wheelchair Athletic
  Association
  Andrew Fleming, Executive Director
  2107 Templeton Gap Road, Suite C
  Colorado Springs, Colorado 80907
- Special Olympics, Inc.
  Thomas B. Songster, Director
  1701 K Street, N.W., Suite 203
  Washington, D.C. 20006–1581
- United States Amputee Athletic Association
  Dick Bryant, President
  Rt. 2 Country Line Road
  Fairview, Tennessee 37062
- U.S. Association for Blind Athletes
  David P. Beaver, V.P.
  Western Illinois University
  Macomb, Illinois 61455
- World Games for the Deaf Committee
  c/o Donalda Kay Ammons, V.P.
  Gallaudet College
  Washington, D.C. 20002

▮ Summary

Goldbeck, executive director of the Washington Business Group on Health (WBGH), and Kiefhauber, manager of Wellness and Cost Management Information for WBGH, have written: "Wellness programs are not a fad. They are increasingly part of the American culture and have earned support from employers because the concept makes sense, meets definable goals, and is good for business."[23]

Goldbeck and Kiefhauber state that *wellness* is deliberately used to convey the message of a shift of values away from the crisis-oriented reactionary programs, which deal with only disease, to goal-oriented, forward-looking programs, which seek to enhance human excellence, foster actualization of human potential, and prevent disease. Such programs meet the standards for ethical health/fitness programs; thus, wellness as a philosophical approach to programming is warranted.

As mentioned in Chapter 1, there is a strong social and economic impetus for wellness programs in our communities and corporations; according to Naisbitt, this trend will gain greater importance as people come to rely more on themselves, rather than on institutions, to safeguard their health.[24] Over 3000 companies or organizations have inhouse, comprehensive health/fitness programs. Many others contract with consulting companies to offer services, or pay for their employees to join health/fitness centers.

The experiences of the participants in these programs generally have been very positive. Growing evidence of the positive changes in personality, assertiveness, capability, self-confidence, and autonomy as a result of regular exercise is impressive.[25-30] Health/fitness directors can make a contribution to other facets of their clients' lives by offering comprehensive programs in meditation, biofeedback, hypnosis, relaxation, values clarification, problem solving, time management, and other subjects to develop the clients' total wellness. Wellness inventories are promising tools that make many of these programs "client-driven." These instruments help programs meet the ethical criteria of voluntary change on the part of participants and allow participants to customize a behavioral-change strategy that should lead to personal growth.

References   ▮

1. Sackett, D., and Haynes, R. (eds). *Compliance with therapeutic regimens*. Baltimore, MD: Johns Hopkins University Press, 1976.

2. Allegrante, J. Ethical dilemmas in workplace health promotion. *Health Promotion Technical Reports* 1:2, 1984.

3. Dunn, H. *High level wellness*. Arlington, VA: R. W. Beatty, 1961, p. 5.

4. Maslow, A. *Motivation and personality*. New York: Harper & Row, 1970.

5. Ardell, D. High level wellness strategies. *Health Education* 8(4):2, 1977.

6. Peters, T., and Waterman, R. *In search of excellence: Lessons from America's best run companies*. New York: Harper & Row, 1982.

7. Blumenthal, J., et al. Psychological changes accompanying aerobic exercise in healthy middle-aged adults. *Psychosomatic Medicine* 44(6):529–536, 1982.

8. Barnard, R., et al. Effects of exercise on skeletal muscle, I: Biochemical and histochemical properties. *Journal of Applied Physiology* 28(6):762–766, 1970.

9. Barnard, R., et al. Cardiovascular response to sudden strenuous exercise—heart rate, blood pressure, and ECG. *Journal of Applied Physiology* 34(6):833–837, 1973.

10. Barnard, R. Long-term effects of exercise on cardiac function. In *Exercise and sport sciences reviews*, vol. III, Wilmore, J., and Keogh, J. (eds). New York: Academic Press, 1975.

11. Stamler, J. Scientific evidence for health promotion and disease prevention. In *Marketing and managing health care: Health promotion and disease prevention*. Hamner, J., and Jacobs, B. S. (eds). Memphis: TN: The University of Tennessee, 1983.

12. Trevisan, M., et al. Nervous tension and serum cholesterol: Findings from the Chicago coronary prevention evaluation program. *Journal of Human Stress* 9(1):12–16, 1983.

13. Girdano, D., and Everly, G. *Controlling stress and tension*. Englewood Cliffs, NJ: Prentice-Hall, 1979.

14. Johnson, R. *Reaching out*. Englewood Cliffs, NJ: Prentice-Hall, 1974.

15. Kamiya, J. Conscious control of brain waves. *Psychology Today* I:57, 1968.

16. Zimbardo, P., and Ebbeson, E. *Influencing attitudes and changing behavior*. Reading, MA: Addison-Wesley, 1970.

17. Becker, M., et al. Patient perceptions and compliance: Recent studies of the health belief model. In *Compliance in health care*. Haynes, et al. (eds). Baltimore, MD: Johns Hopkins Press, 1979.

18. Dunbar, J., et al. Behavioral strategies for improving compliance. In *Compliance in health care*, Haynes, et al. (eds). Baltimore, MD: Johns Hopkins Press, 1979.

19. Glasser, W. *Positive addictions*. New York: Harper & Row, 1976.

20. Institute for Lifestyle Improvement. *Test-Well: A self-scoring wellness assessment questionnaire*. Steven's Point, WI: University of Wisconsin at Steven's Point, 1983.

21. Institute for Lifestyle Improvement. *Compute-A-Life*. Steven's Point, WI: University of Wisconsin at Steven's Point, 1985.

22. Sacks, J., et al. Reliability of the health hazard appraisal. *American journal of public health* 70(7):730–732, 1980.

23. Goldbeck, W., and Kiefhauber, A. Wellness: The new employee benefit. *Group Practice Journal* :20, 1981.

24. Naisbitt, J. *Megatrends: Ten new directions transforming our lives*. New York: Warner, 1982.

25. Gettman, L. *Testimony on HR 3525 "Permanent Tax Treatment on Fringe Benefits Act of 1983."* Ways and Means Select Revenues Subcommittee, August 1, 1983. *Employee Benefits Plan Review*, November 1983.

26. Belloc, N. B., and Breslow, L. The relation of physical health status and health practices. *Preventive Medicine* 1:409, 1972.

27. Paffenbarger, R., et al. A natural history of athleticism and cardiovascular health. *Journal of the American Medical Association* 252: 491, 1984.

28. Blumenthal, J., et al. Psychological changes accompanying aerobic exercise in healthy middle-aged adults. *Psychosomatic Medicine* 44(6) 529–536, 1982.

29. Wear, R. F. *Health promotion programs in Campbell Soup Co.* Presented at "Health Education and Promotion for the Eighties," Atlanta, GA, March 16–18, 1980.

30. Friedman, N. Alterations of type A behavior and reduction in cardiac recurrences in post myocardial infarction patients. *American Heart Journal* 108: 237, 1984.

31. Burkhauser, R. V., and Haveman, R. H. *Disability and work: The economics of American policy*, Baltimore and London: The John Hopkins University Press, 1982, p. 8.

32. Pati, G. C., and Morrison G. Enabling the disabled, *Harvard Business Review* 60:152, July–Aug 1982.

TYPES OF HEALTH/FITNESS PROGRAMMING

This chapter provides an overview of the health/fitness field within the corporate, community, and commercial settings. A typical health/fitness program within any of these settings is difficult to describe because:

■ Organizations differ in size, business objectives, management preferences, number of participants, funding, and available resources, equipment, and facilities

■ Organizations differ in their approach to delivering exercise, nutrition, weight control, smoking and substance-abuse elimination, stress management, and low-back pain control

This unique combination of factors customizes any given program within a specific setting. Another reason why it is difficult to describe a typical program is that functional differences traditionally have existed in the three settings. For example, the program aspects of health/fitness such as medical and fitness testing, exercise prescription, offered activities, and scheduling have been emphasized in the corporate and community settings, whereas the promotion and management aspects have been emphasized in the commercial setting (Table 3.1).

Corporations usually have not been concerned in the past with promoting their programs to their employees, but have provided extensive program opportunities and, in some cases, elaborate fitness facilities. On the other hand, commercial health clubs have promoted their facilities by selling memberships without providing qualified health/fitness professionals to design and conduct proper programs. Community-based health/fitness programs usually have recognized the importance of both promoting their programs through good public relations and providing good programs and staff to back the promotion.

At present, the emphasis rankings have changed somewhat in the corporate and commercial settings. Corporations realize now that promotion of the programs is important in getting a high percentage of employees to participate. Commercial health/fitness owners realize that good programs and qualified staff are needed to back up the promotional efforts of the front office. The present contrasts in health/fitness programs in the three settings also are presented in Table 3.1. Emphasis on promotion has increased in the corporate setting and emphasis on program has increased in the commercial setting. The community setting has remained about the same, with high emphasis on both program and promotion.

Another functional contrast in the three settings is that the community agencies and commercial enterprises often provide programs for the corporate organizations. A survey of program providers is presented in the appendix to illustrate the wide range of available services. This survey by Howard is not an endorsement of such programs; it does provide illustration of what is available to organizations that decide that outside program providers are most appropriate.[1]

It would be impossible to describe all existing health/fitness programs in the three settings. It is risky to mention a few programs within each setting, because some excellent health/fitness programs certainly will be omitted. We attempt to give an overview of the health/fitness field in the three settings and present a few organizations, agencies, and commercial enterprises as resource material. More accurate and updated information about the health/fitness programs mentioned here may be obtained by contacting the specific organizations mentioned.

▮ Corporate Setting

Health/fitness program components offered to employees by various companies in the corporate setting may include one, several, or all of the following:

▮ Evaluation: health hazard appraisals, medical examinations, fitness tests, nutrition evaluations

▮ Exercise prescription and counseling: specific recommendations on the type, frequency, intensity, and duration of exercise

▮ Nutrition and weight control: formal programs including educational material, diets, calorie-counting methods, and individual and group counseling sessions

▮ Smoking and substance-abuse elimination: individual counseling and/or referral to community agencies

▮ Stress management: formal courses and individual counseling

▮ T A B L E 3 . 1 ▮

Functional Contrasts in Health/Fitness Programs

| | Component* | | |
| | | | |
Setting	Program (testing, activities, scheduling)	Management (personnel, budgeting, maintenance)	Promotion (advertising, memberships, sales, public relations)
Past:			
Corporate	3	2	1
Community	3	2	3
Commercial	1	2	3
Present:			
Corporate	3	3	2
Community	3	2	3
Commercial	2	2	3

*3: highest emphasis; 1: lowest emphasis.

▮ Low-back pain control: screening tests, flexibility, exercises, proper lifting techniques

▮ Health education: materials, books, pamphlets, newsletters, magazines, and individual and group counseling

We selected 12 organizations in the corporate setting to serve as resources offering these health/fitness program components. Some of the companies offer inhouse programs with paid staff, whereas others contract with outside agencies to deliver various parts of the program. You can contact the companies to obtain current information about the programs.

You can also contact the Association for Fitness in Business (AFB, formerly known as AAFDBI), 1312 Washington Blvd., Stamford, CT 06902, for more information about programs in the corporate setting. AFB was formed in 1975 to promote health/fitness in the corporate sector, and the membership of AFB has now soared to 3000+. A recent survey by the National Heart, Lung, and Blood Institute indicated that 31% of companies surveyed had some form of health/fitness program. Small companies tend to contract with outside agencies for existing services, whereas medium and large companies tend to seek corporate identity through the development of their own inhouse programs.

Table 3.2 is a summary of the program components offered by the 12 sample organizations in the corporate setting. This information is not complete; programs change rapidly, and some of the companies may offer more or less than is described.

Brief summaries of each organization's program, with emphasis on its uniqueness, follow. Descriptions were obtained from four sources: (1) our personal knowledge of the programs; (2) *An Approach to Good Health for Employees and Reduced Health Care Costs for Industry* by Charles A. Berry;[2] (3) *Managing Health Promotion in the Workplace: Guidelines for Implementing and Evaluation* by Rebecca S. Parkinson;[3] and (4) the National Chamber Foundation.[4]

Campbell Soup—Camden, New Jersey

One of the most comprehensive health/fitness programs is offered by Campbell Soup. The medical department initiated a formal cardiovascular disease–prevention program in 1968. Screening for hypertension has been given highest priority. Employees record their blood pressure in booklets at each visit to the medical department. Other parts of the program include medical screening tests, diet and weight-reduction counseling, serum-lipid modification, smoking cessation, and exercise.

Approximately $100 per participant has been spent by the company on the inhouse diagnostic and treatment services. A small fee is charged for some of the behavior-modification programs.

High-visibility campaigns have been used to communicate health-promotion information through Campbell's Institute for Health and Fitness. The Institute publishes a newsletter providing information on the latest nutrition, psychology, and fitness findings. The Institute is dedicated to the belief that regular exercise,

sound nutrition, and other sensible lifestyle habits can enhance the quality of life and the vigor of the employees.

Control Data—Minneapolis, Minnesota

Control Data has implemented a *Stay Well* program to identify disease risks and teach preventive medicine. Stay Well is available to 57,000 employees and their spouses. Education courses are offered in fitness, weight control, nutrition, stress, and smoking cessation. Stay Well is marketed to other organizations through the Life Extension Institute, a subsidiary of Control Data. The costs of this program are approximately $15 to $18 per month per employee.

The program consists of an orientation session, health screening for disease risk, group interpretation session, and courses to teach behavior change. Employees can join support groups and participate in task forces aimed at planning worksite activities related to health.

Forney Engineering—Dallas, Texas

Forney Engineering has instituted a good example of a health/fitness program started and conducted without inhouse professional staff. One interested and concerned vice-president initiated the program using health/fitness professionals as consultants.

In the mid-1970s, this company offered monetary incentives to its employees for losing weight and participating in jogging programs. A 14 foot by 14 foot office area was converted to "fitness central" where weight scales, blood-pressure equipment, and a computer terminal for logging fitness activities were located. Shower and locker space was already available in the company's production area, so walking and jogging trails were designed in and around the plant to promote those activities. Volleyball courts were constructed in an unused open area near one of the parking lots. Minimal expenditure was needed to start the program, and creative ideas have expanded its success. Over 60% of all employees have participated in at least one program.

■ T A B L E 3 . 2 ■
Checklist of Health/Fitness Programs

Company	Evaluation	Exercise prescription	Nutrition and weight control	Smoking cessation	Stress management	Health education
			Program Components*			
Campbell Soup	+	+	+	+	+	+
Control Data	+	+	+	+	+	+
Forney Engineering	–	+	+	–	–	–
Hudson-Shatz	–	+	–	–	–	–
IBM	+	+	+	+	+	+
Johnson & Johnson	+	+	+	+	–	+
Kimberly-Clark	+	+	+	+	–	+
Mesa Petroleum	+	+	+	+	–	+
Pepsico	+	+	+	+	+	+
Tenneco	+	+	+	+	–	+
Texas Instruments	–	+	–	–	–	+
Xerox	+	+	+	+	+	+

* + : present; – : not present.

Hudson-Shatz Painting—New York, New York

Hudson-Shatz Painting also converted existing space for a health/fitness program. A large storage room was remodeled into a 645-square-foot exercise area. Weight equipment, treadmills, stationary bicycles, punching bags, and stall bars were installed to provide a variety of choices for exercise. One professional and staff member was hired to maintain the facility and consult with all employees on exercise programs.

IBM Corporation—Multiple Locations

IBM has a comprehensive health-education program called *A Plan for Life*. The three main objectives of the program are to encourage individuals to take personal responsibility for their health, to offer health-education programs, and to encourage employees to become members of health maintenance organizations (HMOs). Voluntary health screening is offered to employees aged 35 years and older. In 10 years, more than 190,000 employees had health examinations and 41% of them were found to have unsuspected medical problems.

An extensive medical staff of 50 physicians and 150 nurses at a number of sites around the country delivers the medical examinations and health-education programs. Courses are offered in exercise, weight control, nutrition, risk-factor management, smoking cessation, stress management, prevention of back problems, first aid, and cardiopulmonary resuscitation (CPR). No fees are charged when the courses are taught by IBM staff, and tuition assistance is available when outside agencies conduct a program for IBM.

Johnson & Johnson—New Brunswick, New Jersey

Johnson & Johnson's health/fitness program is delivered to a group of decentralized companies, each of which operates independently within the corporation. The program is called

Live for Life and functions as a service organization for the participating companies. It supplies the consulting expertise, program components, services, and promotional materials. Volunteer employee leaders assume responsibility for promoting good health practices among the employees at the branch locations. Examples of implementing the programs at the worksite include development of exercise facilities, improvement of food service in the company cafeteria, and establishment of a no-smoking policy.

The Live for Life program objectives are to improve fitness, nutrition, weight control, stress management, smoking cessation, and health knowledge. Proper use of the blood pressure–control and employee-assistance programs is strongly encouraged. The company anticipates that healthier lifestyles will lead to positive changes in employee morale, relations with fellow employees, perception of the company, job satisfaction, and productivity as well as reductions in medical costs, accidents, and absenteeism. An epidemiological study is in progress to evaluate the program's effectiveness on individual health and on health-care costs.

Kimberly-Clark—Neenah, Wisconsin

Kimberly-Clark delivers health/fitness programs through the company's medical department, which has developed a *Health Management Program* that includes assessment, intervention, and education components. Assessment procedures involve physical examination, health-hazard appraisals, and cardiovascular stress testing. Intervention and education programs involve inhouse exercise, nutrition counseling, smoking cessation, blood-pressure control, and weight reduction.

A $2.5 million physical fitness center contains a jogging track, a swimming pool, exercise rooms with weight-training equipment, and extensive locker and shower areas.

The program staff consists of 25 full- and part-time personnel including medical, exercise, and swimming specialists. Cardiac rehabilitation programs are monitored by the medical department. Consulting cardiologists, radiologists, dieticians, and family practitioners help with exercise testing, medical examinations, and individual counseling.

Newsletters and brochures have been used to communicate information on health management, fitness tips, classes, and program results. A travel diary has been developed to encourage employees to stay fit while on the road.

Annual cost of the program is approximately $260 per employee, all of which is covered by the company.

Mesa Petroleum—Amarillo, Texas

Mesa Petroleum is a midsize company that has a strong commitment to delivering a comprehensive health/fitness program to its approximately 700 employees, as evidenced by the $450 per employee ($600 per participant) annual cost paid entirely by the company.

The company provides a well-organized health/fitness program that includes fitness evaluations; prescription plans for exercise, weight control, nutrition, and smoking cessation; followup fitness testing and personal counseling; educational strategies such as newsletters, booklets, and seminars; motivational techniques such as rewards and incentives; and research documentation of the program's effectiveness.

A $2.5 million exercise facility is provided at the corporate headquarters for 300 employees, and $300 to $700 health-club memberships are available to 400 employees in division offices.

Pepsico—Purchase, New York

Pepsico is one of the few corporations that offers every aspect of a health/fitness program listed in Table 3.2. The company offers programs at two levels. The executive program provides rigorous screening for disease and advanced coronary problems and exercise prescriptions on an individual basis. The employee program is designed as a high-risk intervention process. It offers regular exercise, recreation, and rehabilitation classes at corporate headquarter facilities. The employee program also provides large group orientations, with discussions about risk factors and the value of exercise.

Flex time is available to employees to enable them to exercise at the company's facilities any time. The exercise session, however, is not considered part of the workday.

Tenneco—Houston, Texas

Tenneco's management has a high-level commitment to offering comprehensive health/fitness programs to 3700 employees located at the downtown corporate headquarters. A multimillion-dollar employee fitness center houses elaborate facilities including a 5-lap-per-mile indoor jogging track, four racquetball courts, strength-training equipment with separate areas for men and women, saunas, and a computerized exercise record system. A large employee cafeteria serves a variety of nutritious foods, the calorie content of which is labeled.

Seminars and courses are provided on fitness, nutrition, weight control, and smoking cessation. Inhouse medical personnel administer health-screening tests before employees initiate their personalized exercise programs. Professionally trained health/fitness specialists prescribe and supervise the exercise programs.

Texas Instruments—Dallas, Texas

Texas Instruments supports a strong recreation program for its employees. Employees organized a recreation association called the *Texins* to meet their activity needs and recreation interests. A physical fitness club with the specific purpose of promoting employee health and fitness grew out of the recreation association. Members of PATH (positive approach to total health) keep records of their physical activity, body weight, and resting pulse. Awards are used to reinforce different levels of exercise

accomplishment. Regular meetings are held to discuss the effects of exercise on blood pressure, cardiovascular disease, body composition, and stress. Organized exercise classes such as aerobic shapeup (dance) also are offered to members.

Xerox—Leesburg, Virginia

Xerox takes two unique approaches to health/fitness programs. First, self-help educational materials called the *Health Management Program (HMP)* were developed to increase employees' awareness of health and exercise principles, to help them administer their own fitness tests, and to enable them to design their own activity programs. A thorough *Fitbook* manual is provided to employees who express interest in learning more about cardiovascular fitness and aerobic exercise, flexibility, muscle strength and endurance, diet and nutrition guidelines, relaxation techniques, back exercises, smoking cessation, or substance-abuse elimination. The self-help materials were needed because of the enormous size of the company (more than 40,000 employees): an unrealistically large health/fitness staff would be needed to instruct that many employees personally.

The second approach is to send all managers to employee-training sessions at the Center for Training and Management Development in Leesburg, Virginia. The training center is an extensive physical fitness and recreation complex where employees and their family members participate in a variety of fitness activities. This type of setting can have a positive influence on employees and their family members by encouraging a lifetime of good health and fitness.

Community Setting: Social Service Agencies

There are many health/fitness education and service programs available in most large communities from social service agencies. Also, several schools and medical centers now offer health/fitness programs to the general public. We will describe selected health/fitness education and service programs as examples of resources available in the community setting. You can contact the agencies for more information.

Because social-service agencies usually are nonprofit organizations, they can provide various aspects of a health/fitness program at no cost or very low cost to individuals and groups in the community. The agencies listed in this section have health/fitness professionals and paid staff available to consult with individuals or groups interested in implementing specialized parts of a health/fitness program.

American Cancer Society

A simple self-testing method has been designed by the American Cancer Society to help an individual assess personal risk factors for common types of cancer. The self-administered questionnaire includes screening questions for lung, colon, skin, breast, cervical, and endometrial cancer. The Society also provides curricula materials for schools.

American Heart Association

A variety of educational materials, such as literature, films, and exhibits on all aspects of cardiovascular disease, is available to organizations from the American Heart Association (AHA), which also has produced guidelines on how to implement health/fitness programs in the workplace. The guidelines are called *Heart at Work*, and they consist of five modules: exercise, blood-pressure control, nutrition, stop smoking, and signals and actions for survival (CPR and first aid). To help organizations reduce needless deaths, lost work hours, unnecessary costs, and disability, the AHA provides programs in CPR training, blood pressure education, and risk-factor awareness.

The AHA's Committee on Exercise prepared *Exercise Testing and Training of Apparently Healthy Individuals: A Handbook for Physicians* with the purpose of providing guidelines to physicians whose patients ask for medical advice before beginning a regular program of exercise. The recommendations were made in response to numerous inquiries from the medical profession, which reflects the mounting public interest in physical fitness.

American Lung Association

A 20-day self-help stop-smoking program is available for a nominal fee from the American Lung Association. The program originally was designed for self-implementation, but information on how to conduct group programs has been added recently. The stop-smoking program consists of identifying types of smokers, learning what triggers the smoking urge, and progressively changing behavior to achieve smoking cessation in 20 days.

Also available to organizations (especially schools) are informational materials on occupational lung disease, tuberculosis, and air conservation.

American Red Cross

In addition to emergency services, the American Red Cross provides school-oriented and community-based programs in CPR training, blood-pressure monitoring, learn-to-swim classes, and first-aid instruction. Health-education services are provided for individuals and special groups in the community, such as the elderly.

Department of Parks and Recreation

Several large communities and some states provide recreation programs available through their respective departments of parks and recreation. Walking/jogging paths in parks and around lakes are becoming increasingly popular. Several of these trails include a *parcourse* system in which stretching and calisthenic exercise stations are placed at prescribed points along the path.

These types of services usually are provided by taxpayer money and use fees are not charged. Companies wishing to implement fitness programs at little or no cost would be wise to investigate nearby parks and recreation services.

Government of Canada

The Government of Canada, Fitness and Amateur Sport, and the Ontario Ministry of Culture and Recreation, Sports and Fitness Branch, have published several brochures and booklets on various health and fitness topics including:

■ *Aerobic Fitness*

■ *Employee Fitness*

■ *Exercise at the Office*

■ *Fit-Kit*

■ *FITNEWS*

■ *Fitness and Nutrition*

■ *Fitness Questions and Answers*

■ *Health and Fitness*

■ *Lunch on the Run*

■ *Physical Activity and Weight Control*

■ *Prescription for Physical Activity*

A cooperative project involving the Canada Life Assurance Company, the YMCA of Metropolitan Toronto, and the Fitness and Amateur Sport Branch of the Department of National Health and Welfare resulted in a report on the employee fitness and lifestyle project of Toronto, 1977–78.[5] The intent in publishing the report was to help companies implement their own employee fitness programs. The report includes a description of the recruitment and training program, an explanation of how health-related lifestyle components were integrated into the physical fitness program, a listing of available brochures and pamphlets, and a description of special motivation techniques, such as music for group exercise classes, special events, and theme weeks. The project resulted in improved fitness levels and less absenteeism for volunteer participants from Canada Life. In addition, the control company, North American Life, developed an employee-fitness program as a result of the study experience.

Public Health Department

Public health departments offer extensive health-education programs including support group services in smoking cessation and alcoholism. Education classes also are provided in risk-factor identification and promotion of healthy lifestyles to prevent health problems. The U.S. Government Printing Office is a good source for free material on health education and promotion.

The U.S. Public Health Service has recommended that all branches and departments of the federal government provide their employees with time and facilities for regular, vigorous physical activities.

YMCA

One of the major goals of the YMCA is to improve the health and well-being of the people served. YMCAs are the largest deliverers of health-enhancement programs in the United States. Over 12 million men and women are serviced by 2200 YMCAs. Small-to-medium businesses or branch offices of major companies are the primary corporate users of YMCA programs.

YMCAs deliver their health/fitness services in two ways: (1) YMCA staff will help an organization provide the programs at the company's location, and (2) an organization may send participants to the YMCA for program delivery. Downtown YMCA programs usually are employee fitness–oriented, whereas programs in the suburban branches of YMCAs usually are family fitness– and recreation-oriented.

Most YMCAs offer risk-factor screening, health-hazard appraisal, fitness testing, beginning exercise, aerobic dance, and weight-management, nutrition, healthy-back, stress-management, and smoking-cessation programs. Many corporations use the YMCA to deliver complete programs, individual classes, or corporate memberships in the fitness centers. The space and equipment necessary for complete fitness programs are available in most YMCAs. Facilities usually include gymnasiums, weight-training rooms, dance studios, fitness-testing rooms, running tracks, swimming pools, racquet-ball courts, classrooms, and locker rooms.

YMCA professional staff are college graduates with degrees in physical education, exercise physiology, exercise science, or related areas. An extensive training network provides additional knowledge in healthy-back, weight-management, and general-administration programs. The professional staff have the expertise and willingness to consult with individuals and corporations to help meet health-enhancement needs.

In addition to providing courses in health and fitness to adults, many YMCAs offer complete child-care programs. Physical and educational activities are presented to children, and parents participate in their respective classes.

Community Setting: Schools

Secondary Schools

The health services, health education, and physical education programs offered within secondary schools have served as prototypes since the early 1900s. In addition to these curricula, some secondary schools open their facilities for use by the community population. In areas of declining student enrollment, unused classrooms and vacant buildings may be dedicated to *wellness centers*. Gymnasium facilities can be used for fitness programs, and the physical and health education staff may conduct the programs. This can provide an opportunity for a company to offer a no-cost fitness program to its employees.

Some school districts offer health/fitness programs to their employees—the teachers. The Dallas Independent School District (DISD) in Texas serves as a model program for such an endeavor. With the aid of consultation services from the Institute for Aerobics Research in Dallas, Texas, the DISD provides an employee-fitness program for its public school teachers. The program was funded by tax revenues, grants, and participant fees as a benefit process to counteract stress and absenteeism. Three wellness centers were established to provide medical screening, fitness assessment, goal set-ting, exercise, education, and motivation. The program has improved fitness levels and morale among the teachers. Continued research is being conducted.

Colleges and Universities

Institutions of higher learning now offer health/fitness courses as extensions of their continuing education or health and physical education departments. Many programs offer health-hazard appraisals, fitness evaluations, exercise classes, diet and nutrition counseling, stress management, hypertension screening, and low-back–pain rehabilitation to the individuals and corporate organizations in the community.

The fees for these services vary but usually are nominal at the schools that are able to provide these programs as a part of their commitment to community service.

Community Setting: Medical Agencies

Medical agencies currently are taking a three-fold approach to providing health/fitness programs. First, hospitals often provide cardiac and pulmonary rehabilitation programs on both inpatient and outpatient bases. Second, many hospitals provide inhouse health/fitness programs for their employees. Third, *wellness programs* are offered to individuals and groups in the community as profit-making health-promotion services.

The wellness programs offered by hospitals usually are comprehensive and have holistic philosophies. In other words, the wellness programs are designed to influence the whole individual in preventing health problems by addressing the physical, mental, and spiritual concerns of each participant.

American Hospital Association— Chicago, Illinois

The goals of the *Well Aware About Health* program offered by the American Hospital Association are to help hospital employees identify disease risk factors and provide educational programs to prevent health problems. Health questionnaires and physical examinations are used in the screening process.

Local health professionals teach health-promotion seminars and classes on fitness, weight control, nutrition, stress management, and smoking cessation. A fee is charged to each employee for the classes, but a portion is refunded if a certain number of classes is attended.

In 1981, 48% of the total workforce participated in the Well Aware About Health program. Survey data indicated a high degree of satisfaction with the program content and structure.

The American Hospital Association also facilitates the implementation of exercise and health-promotion programs for its patients and for individuals in the community. A book entitled *Planning Hospital Health Promotion Services for Business and Industry* was prepared in 1982 and is available to members for a nominal fee.

American Medical Association

Anticipating the need for health/fitness programs in business and industry, the American Medical Association (AMA) Committee on Exercise and Physical Fitness, in cooperation with the President's Council on Physical Fitness, produced a monograph entitled *Guidelines for Physical Fitness Programs in Business and Industry*.[6] Essentially, the monograph states that the AMA supports company physical-fitness programs that are developed in accordance with current scientific and medical knowledge. Company-sponsored physical-fitness programs should be conducted as an adjunct to the company's medical program and should receive medical endorsement. Companies that do not have their own medical departments should develop their programs in consultation with medical and physical-fitness authorities. Consideration should be given to physical-fitness education, rehabilitation, training, and maintenance. A qualified physical education instructor and an exercise physiologist should supervise the exercise program under the direction of the company's medical services. Health-education programs such as seminars on smoking cessation, obesity, and alcoholism should be included where appropriate. All participants should understand the specific benefits of the program that is prescribed for them.

Blue Cross/Blue Shield Associations

A booklet entitled "Building a Healthier Company" is available from the Blue Cross/Blue Shield Associations, 676 St. Clair, Chicago, Illinois 60611. It is provided to companies as an attempt to help defray high medical-insurance costs by encouraging the companies to offer health/fitness programs to their employees. A brief overview of the benefits of having healthy employees is given along with points on how to get the program going. Two necessary ingredients are emphasized for making the program successful: (1) get management behind the program, and (2) find the right leader.

Commercial Setting

Most communities now have businesses that sell specific services for health/fitness programs. Comprehensive services usually are available from exercise studios, health clubs, or profit-making fitness centers. Several private health-care facilities have been built to provide services within areas that have large populations. More specific exercise or recreation activity memberships are sold by dance studios, racquet clubs, aquatic clubs, and martial-arts studios. Hotels also provide health/fitness centers as a service to their clientele.

The purchase of outside services or prepackaged health/fitness programs usually involves minimal expenditure on the part of the company, especially when compared to the construction and operation of inhouse facilities. The scope of packaged programs available today varies as widely as does the number of providers.

Private Health-Care Facilities

The unique private health/fitness centers provide services in these areas: (1) health evaluations through preventive medicine centers; (2) elaborate exercise facilities for jogging, swimming, tennis, racquetball, handball, basketball, exercise classes, and weight training; (3) injury rehabilitation services through a sports medicine clinic; (4) professional expertise in preventive cardiology, nutrition, and exercise counseling; (5) consultation and education workshops on implementing health/fitness programs; (6) computerized exercise logging service; and (7) outreach programs on health/fitness education and implementation procedures. Health/fitness specialists from private health-care facilities often are available to provide the professional services necessary to implement a health/fitness program, thus possibly eliminating the need for full-time, inhouse staff to start a program.

Exercise Studios/Health Clubs/ Fitness Centers

The commercial health clubs grew out of the professional gyms, which were primarily associated with training boxers and body builders. The primary emphasis has been on the use of machines, supposedly to bring about the spot reduction of fat, contour the body, and develop strength. Relaxation services include saunas, steam baths, and massage. Figure salons for both women and men now include exercise classes to supplement the machinery.

In the past, the instructors and managers in these studios usually were not fitness professionals but rather were salespersons trained to recruit new members. Few precautions, if any, were taken when prescribing exercise for the physically unfit. However, the recent trend by health club conglomerates has been to improve the quality of staff by requiring training and certification programs in physical fitness.

Dance Studios

In addition to traditional dance programs, several dance studios now offer a form of *aerobic dance*, which appears under a variety of names such as *dancercise*, *jazzercise*, and *aerobicise*. In the past, exercise has not been individualized or carefully prescribed and monitored. The intensity of dance is often too high for the capabilities of beginning exercisers. However, this continuous and rhythmical vigorous exercise can provide excellent total body conditioning. Coed classes are becoming increasingly popular. Dance classes led by professional fitness instructors, who allow for the individual approach to exercise intensity and duration, may be a viable way to offer a core or supplemental exercise program.

Racquet Clubs

In recent years, numerous racquetball and tennis clubs have been designed to include weight-training rooms, jogging tracks, and exercise classes to meet the needs of a comprehensive fitness program. Racquet sports alone offer good recreational activity, but the inclusion of other exercise facilities moves the racquet club a step closer to being a total fitness center.

Aquatic Clubs

Most aquatic clubs offer family memberships and a few accommodate corporate memberships. Aquatic clubs provide swimming lessons and a few clubs conduct water exercise classes. Like the racquet clubs, some aquatic clubs are adding weight-training rooms to supplement their exercise facilities.

Martial Arts Studios

The strength of a martial arts program usually is the highly personalized instruction. Regular classes are held with well-designed, regimented training programs. Most martial arts programs involve self-discipline and control in addition to the vigorous, calisthenic exercise. These classes may serve as a valuable supplement to an exercise program.

Hotels and Health/Fitness Resort Spas

Some hotels have developed fitness centers to complement the variety of services available to guests. Weight-training rooms including stationary bicycles and treadmills, swimming pools, tennis courts, racquetball courts, and jogging tracks or trails are provided in the most extensive centers.

Health/fitness resort spas have been created in recent years to provide contemporary programs in health care, proper nutrition, weight control, exercise, and productivity. Several resorts now schedule retreats for groups wishing to combine wellness with business meetings. Nutritionists, physical therapists, exercise specialists, psychologists, and health educators provide wellness programs within the business meeting's agenda.

■ Summary

Health/fitness education and service programs exist in three settings: corporate, community, and commercial. The unique combination of an organization's objectives and the selection of specific health/fitness program components customize a given program. In other words, no typical program exists.

The program aspects of health/fitness, such as medical and fitness testing, exercise prescription, and scheduling, traditionally have been emphasized in the corporate and community settings, whereas membership promotion and management aspects have been emphasized in the commercial setting. Recently, emphasis has increased for promotion in the corporate setting and for programs in the commercial setting. Examples of programs in the three settings were described to illustrate available resources.

This chapter gave an overview of the types of health/fitness programs available; the next chapter gives an overview of the professional practitioner roles in the health/fitness field.

References ■

1. Howard, B. Fitness for Sale. *Corporate Fitness & Recreation* 2:18, 1983.

2. Berry, C. A. *An approach to good health for employees and reduced health care costs for industry.* Washington, DC: Health Insurance Association of America, 1981.

3. Parkinson, R. S., et al. *Managing health promotion in the workplace: Guidelines for implementing and evaluation.* Palo Alto, CA: Mayfield, 1982.

4. National Chamber Foundation. *A national health care strategy: How business can promote good health for employees and their families.* Excelsior, MN: Interstudy, 1978.

5. Peepre, M. (ed). *Employee fitness and lifestyle project.* Toronto, Canada: Minister of State, Fitness and Amateur Sport, Government of Canada, 1980.

6. Wilson, P. K. (ed). *Adult fitness and cardiac rehabilitation.* Baltimore: University Park Press, 1975.

Survey of Program Providers

Company	Employee Fitness Evaluation, Risk Analysis	Fitness Program Design	Healthy-Back Classes	Nutrition Counseling	Smoking Cessation	Stress Management	Alcohol, Drug Abuse Prevention	Weight Management	Recreation Programming	Facility Design	Onsite Supervision	Comprehensive Fitness/Health Promotion Package Available	Computerized Fitness Program	Audiovisual Materials
Alive Institute, Inc. 2757 NW 42nd Ave Coconut Creek, FL 33066 (305) 972-1914		■				■		■						■
American Corporate Health Programs Personal Health Inventory 85 Old Eagle School Rd Strafford, PA 19087 (215) 293-9367	■	■								■	■		■	
American Hospital Association 840 N Lakeshore Dr Chicago, IL 60611 (312) 280-6000						■						■		■
American Leisure Facilities Management Corp 119 W 58th St New York, NY 10019 (212) 245-1144	■	■								■	■	■		
Battle of the Corporate Stars 2209 N St NW Washington, DC 20037 (202) 223-5400									■					
Business Health Education Programs Division of Northern California Research 965 Mission St, Suite 750 San Francisco, CA 94103 (415) 777-0611	■	■	■	■	■	■	■	■	■			■	■	
Cardio-Fitness Center 345 Park Ave New York, NY 10022 (212) 838-4570	■	■	■	■				■		■	■	■	■	■
Center for Health Promotion Health Central Inc 2810 57th Ave N Minneapolis, MN 55430 (612) 574-7800	■	■	■	■	■	■	■	■				■		■

Source: Howard, B. Fitness for Sale. *Corporate Fitness & Recreation* 2:18, 1983. Used by permission.

Company	Employee Fitness Evaluation, Risk Analysis	Fitness Program Design	Healthy-Back Classes	Nutrition Counseling	Smoking Cessation	Stress Management	Alcohol, Drug Abuse Prevention	Weight Management	Recreation Programming	Facility Design	Onsite Supervision	Comprehensive Fitness/Health Promotion Package Available	Computerized Fitness Program	Audiovisual Materials
Club Management Systems 7250 S Ivy Ct Englewood, CO 80112 (303) 773-2212												■	■	
Control Data Corporation Stay Well Employee Assistance Program 8100 34th Ave S Minneapolis, MN 55440 (612) 853-7777	■		■	■	■	■	■	■	■		■	■	■	■
Data-Pep Associates, Inc 1355 15th St Fort Lee, NJ 07024 (202) 592-8701	■	■		■						■	■		■	■
Executive Fitness Center 3 World Trade Center New York, NY 10048 (212) 466-9266	■		■	■				■	■	■				
Fitness Systems, Inc. PO Box 71606 Arco Plaza Los Angeles, CA 90071 (213) 488-9949	■	■								■	■		■	
Health & Human Resources Group PO Box 426 Mill Valley, CA 94941 (415) 845-4519 922 Pennsylvania Ave SE Washington, DC 20003 (202) 547-6644	■	■	■	■	■	■	■	■		■		■		■
Health Management Associates 2120 S Ash St Denver, CO 80222 (303) 692-0767	■	■	■	■	■	■	■	■		■	■	■		■
Health Marketing Systems, Inc. 18 E 48th St New York, NY 10017 (212) 753-4545												■		

Company	Employee Fitness Evaluation, Risk Analysis	Fitness Program Design	Healthy-Back Classes	Nutrition Counseling	Smoking Cessation	Stress Management	Alcohol, Drug Abuse Prevention	Weight Management	Recreation Programming	Facility Design	Onsite Supervision	Comprehensive Fitness/Health Promotion Package Available	Computerized Fitness Program	Audiovisual Materials
The Health Works 808 Busse Hwy Park Ridge, IL 60068 (312) 696-3037	■	■		■	■	■	■	■			■			■
Human Resources Institute Tempe Wick Rd Morristown, NJ 07960 (201) 267-1496				■	■	■		■				■	■	
The Institute for Aerobics Research 12200 Preston Rd Dallas, TX 75230 (214) 661-3374	■	■				■				■	■	■	■	■
Institute of Lifestyle Improvement University of Wisconsin–Stevens Point Delzell Hall Stevens Point, WI 54481 (715) 346-4646	■	■		■	■	■	■	■	■	■	■	■		■
Jacki Sorenson's Aerobic Dancing 87 Main St Millburn, NY 07041 (201) 379-6313											■			■
Living Well 111 N Post Oak Lane Houston, TX 77024 (713) 680-3330	■			■		■	■	■		■		■	■	■
Mindbody Inc 50 Maple Pl Manhasset, NY 11030 (516) 365-7722	■	■	■	■	■	■	■	■		■	■		■	■
National Athletic Health Institute 575 E Hardy St, Suite 104 Inglewood, CA 90301 (213) 674-1600	■	■		■						■		■		■
Northwestern National Life Insurance Co 20 Washington Ave S Minneapolis, MN 55440 (612) 372-5432	■	■		■	■	■	■	■				■		■

Company	Employee Fitness Evaluation, Risk Analysis	Fitness Program Design	Healthy-Back Classes	Nutrition Counseling	Smoking Cessation	Stress Management	Alcohol, Drug Abuse Prevention	Weight Management	Recreation Programming	Facility Design	Onsite Supervision	Comprehensive Fitness/Health Promotion Package Available	Computerized Fitness Program	Audiovisual Materials
Pacific Fitness Systems 507 Third Ave, Suite 300 Seattle, WA 98104 (604) 383-9508		■												■
Participaction* 80 Richmond St W, Suite 805 Toronto, Ontario, Canada M5H 2A4 (416) 361-0514												■		
Perfect Fitness PO Box 178622 San Diego, CA 92117 (714) 277-3065	■	■	■	■	■	■	■	■						
Self-Development Associates 1381 Church St Ventura, CA 93001 (805) 648-4055		■							■	■			■	■
Smokenders Lifeline Foods 800 Roosevelt Rd PO Box 3146 Glen Ellyn, IL 60137 (312) 790-3328				■	■	■						■		
Sun Valley Health Institute PO Box 1025 Green Bay, WI 54305 (414) 433-5100	■	■		■	■	■	■	■				■		
Upjohn Health Care Services Upjohn Health Programs 270 Madison Ave New York, NY 10016 (212) 696-4170				■	■	■		■						■
Wilson Learning 6950 Washington Ave S Minneapolis, MN 55544 (612) 944-2880						■								
YMCA USA 101 N Wacker Dr Chicago, IL 60606 (312) 269-0500	■	■	■	■	■	■	■	■	■		■	■		■

*Services only in Canada.

CHAPTER 4

OVERVIEW OF
PROFESSIONAL ROLES

This chapter describes the types of practitioner roles that the health/fitness professional plays in the corporate, community, and commercial settings.

The characteristic staffing structures differ considerably among the corporate, community, and commercial settings. As we saw in the last chapter, corporations may employ inhouse staff to deliver health/fitness programs or they may use resources within the community and commercial settings. Community and commercial health/fitness programs offer a variety of staffing expertise to deliver their programs to individuals and organizations contracting their services.

In the past, this variety of staffing expertise included physicians, nurses, health educators, exercise physiologists, recreation directors, physical education teachers, coaches, and dance instructors. In some cases, especially in the corporate setting, a balance in the health/fitness program was lacking. For example, a corporation may have provided an excellent recreation program of bowling, softball, and basketball leagues for its employees, but lacked a fitness evaluation and exercise prescription component. The recreation director may not have had the background in exercise physiology to provide this kind of expertise. Another corporation may have offered an excellent fitness-testing program conducted by a well-trained exercise

physiologist, but not have provided organized activity programs because the exercise physiologist did not have a solid recreation background.

In addition, both the recreation director and the exercise physiologist may have lacked preparation in management and supervisory skills. At present, colleges and universities in this country are endeavoring to prepare a more balanced individual for the health/fitness field. Health/fitness professionals play many roles simultaneously, including manager, planner, supervisor, educator, exercise leader, motivator, counselor, promoter, assessor, and evaluator, regardless of the setting. Therefore, a new academic field is being formed, mainly within the physical education departments of colleges and universities, to prepare individuals as health/fitness professionals. In addition, several academic institutions are offering workshops and seminars to individuals in the health/fitness field as "refresher courses" or as adjunct preparation for the advancing field.

The American College of Sports Medicine* and the Association for Fitness in Business**

---

*American College of Sports Medicine, 1 Virginia Ave., P. O. Box 1440, Indianapolis, IN 46206.
**Association for Fitness in Business, 1312 Washington Blvd., Stamford, CT 06902.

offer certification programs at various levels within the health/fitness field. These classifications are described in Chapter 15.

The best health/fitness preparation programs are designed to prepare individuals in all of the roles. To aid in the development of such programs, some characteristic duties are described in Table 4.1.

▌ Delineating the Different Roles

With so many roles to consider, how do health/fitness professionals establish priorities? The primary answer to this question lies with the purpose of the health/fitness program within the organization. For example, in the corporate setting the purpose is to help employees with their personal health/fitness programs. Therefore, the health/fitness professional is primarily a motivator of individuals and a manager and planner of programs to deliver to the employees. This concept was confirmed in a survey of corporate fitness directors conducted by Breuleux in 1982.[1] He asked them to rank their job duties in order of importance and their worktime by percentage. He found the following ranking for duties:

1. Communication
2. Program development
3. Motivation
4. Counseling
5. Management interface
6. Supervision
7. Public relations
8. Program evaluation
9. Budgeting
10. Purchasing

The percentage of time devoted to different activities was:

- Administration: 28%
- Supervision: 16%
- Teaching: 14%
- Public relations: 14%
- Testing: 11%

- Consulting: 8%
- Research: 6%

It is interesting that communication was listed first in job duty importance. The health/fitness professional must use active listening and genuine understanding to be able to motivate and counsel participants effectively. Communication with management is important to interface the goals of the health/fitness program with the goals of the company. These communication skills are elaborated in Chapter 15.

If we merge the rankings from the job duties and the percentage of worktime, it seems that administration involves mainly communication and program development. Supervision and teaching involve motivation and counseling of participants. The corporate fitness directors in this survey verified the emphasis placed on programs and management illustrated in Table 3.1, page 57.

In community and commercial settings, health/fitness professionals' aim is to market programs to individuals and organizations within the corporate setting; therefore, their primary role may be that of promoter and planner of programs. Based on the inherent characteristics and purposes of health/fitness programs in the three settings, priorities may be assigned to the professionals' roles as suggested in Table 4.2.

Descriptions of the ten roles that a health/fitness professional plays in a program are presented in the following sections. These roles are delineated on an arbitrary basis; in reality, there is much overlap. For example, an exercise leader is also an educator who is also a planner, motivator, and assessor.

Manager

Health/fitness program directors are managers of people and of programs. Expertise is required for handling all staff answering to the director and for handling participants in the program. Managers must be able to administer a budget, know how to purchase and maintain equipment and supplies, and make wise decisions on expenditure of funds.

■ T A B L E 4 . 1 ■
Some Characteristic Duties of the Health/Fitness Practitioner

Manager
Administer daily operation
Design program activities
Control program
Guide and direct staff
Purchase equipment
Maintain facilities
Regulate budget
Schedule activities
Communicate with staff and participants
Cooperate with other departments

Planner
Assess organization needs
Establish goals for program
Design program
Organize resources
Arrange schedule

Supervisor
Hire and dismiss staff
Oversee program and staff
Coordinate staff and program
Motivate staff
Evaluate staff

Educator
Train staff
Instruct participants
Evaluate learning
Develop curricula

Exercise Leader
Guide participants
Conduct classes
Use safe techniques
Provide a role model

Motivator
Give impetus to program
Persuade participants
Influence participants
Induce changes in participants
Incite action

Counselor
Advise participants
Suggest changes
Express opinions
Judge effectiveness of actions
Recommend action
Consult with participants

Promoter
Design marketing techniques
Encourage participation
Use sales techniques
Advance program advantages

Assessor
Conduct participant tests
Interpret test results
Follow safe procedures

Evaluator
Design program-evaluation procedures
Perform statistical analyses
Interpret results
Analyze program trends
Convey reports to management

Managers often are required to design facilities for the exercise program. They construct the program components to blend with the facilities. They design the schedule when the program components are delivered to the participants.

Good managers communicate effectively with other managers in the organization. This boosts the cooperative effort of the entire organization in providing a meaningful health/fitness benefit to the employees.

Planner

Good program planners learn the vision and philosophy of the organization, assess the needs of the organization, establish the goals and objectives for the program, and then design the programs, activities, and services to meet the objectives. Health/fitness professionals must have a vision for the overall program that is consistent with that of the organization. As organizers, health/fitness professionals decide

∎ T A B L E 4 . 2 ∎
Some Practitioner Roles in Health/Fitness Settings

Role	Setting*		
	Corporate	Community	Commercial
Manager	5	3	2
Planner	5	5	4
Supervisor	4	1	1
Educator	4	4	1
Exercise leader	4	5	3
Motivator	5	5	4
Counselor	3	3	2
Promoter	2	4	5
Assessor	2	3	1
Evaluator	2	1	1

*5: highest emphasis; 1: lowest emphasis.

how the plans will be carried out, how the work will be divided among the staff, and what relationships will exist among different units of operation.

For a program to be implemented successfully, it must be well-planned and well-organized. The planner must pay attention to details and strive for an efficient operation to stimulate participant confidence in the staff and program.

Supervisor

Health/fitness professionals supervise staff and participants. To be good supervisors they must be attentive to the needs and interest of both. Supervisors are responsible for hiring staff, developing their potential, directing and coordinating their responsibilities, motivating them, evaluating their performance, and promoting or dismissing them if necessary. Supervisors must use good judgment in making decisions because, in a sense, staff morale hinges on the supervisor's influence in this area.

In supervising participants, health/fitness professionals need to be sensitive to the needs and interests of their clients, giving individual health and safety top priority.

Educator

Health/fitness professionals need expertise in educating and training the program staff to implement effective programs. In-service training and weekly staff meetings are needed for several reasons: to keep the staff abreast of current health/fitness knowledge, to increase staff confidence, and to boost staff interest in their jobs and in the program.

Educators also must have the expertise to educate participants about proper use of health/fitness principles. They must possess good communication skills and be able to explain the rationale for and positive outcomes of health/fitness programs.

Exercise Leader

Health/fitness professionals should have the ability to lead exercise programs, including calisthenic, dance, weight-training, jogging, cycling, swimming, and various sports activities. They must be able to organize different classes and must understand the dynamics of group leadership. Because of the recent popularity of exercise to music, exercise leaders must have the ability to choreograph routines.

Exercise leaders must be enthusiastic motivators of participants; they should encourage an enjoyable, informal atmosphere. Good exercise leaders are sensitive to individual needs in the midst of group activities. They should be consistent, dependable, and professional in supervising exercise. Because exercise leaders are extremely visible to the participants, they should be excellent role models. That is, they should exemplify good physical-fitness characteristics such as good cardiovascular endurance, average-to-low body fat, and good muscular strength and flexibility. They should also practice and demonstrate good health and living habits, including good nutrition and smoking and substance-abuse abstinence.

Motivator

Health/fitness professionals should be able to encourage participants to begin health/fitness programs and to participate regularly. This usually requires an extroverted personality, a positive attitude, persistent enthusiasm, and an extraordinary amount of energy.

Being a good motivator requires some hidden talents. The communication skills and the techniques of motivation differ with the participants' job status, personality, age, sex, and many other factors. Different people respond to different approaches; therefore, health/fitness professionals should have the talent to provide a wide variety of motivational strategies. This requires imagination, an understanding of human nature, and a sincere concern for each participant. The best motivators have positive attitudes and convincing commitments to the health/fitness program.

Counselor

In addition to being inspired motivators, health/fitness professionals must counsel individuals, establishing rapport through confidence, personal concern, and confidentiality. An effective counselor is a good listener and a diplomatic advisor: suggestions are better than dictated action plans. A good counselor has a genuine concern for the individual, has a positive attitude, and is sincere, professional, consistent, and authentic.

Promoter

Health/fitness professionals must be able to promote the program to both management and participants. As promoters, health/fitness professionals need an excellent knowledge of the program components and confidence in the program in order to have an effective influence on the target population. A good promoter is an enthusiastic extrovert, a persuader, and a salesperson.

Promoters must have skills in advertising, public relations, special events planning, and production or provision of materials such as newsletters, posters, and brochures.

Assessor

Health/fitness professionals should have the ability to conduct tests assessing various aspects of fitness including cardiovascular function, body composition, flexibility, and muscular strength and endurance. The assessor must be thoroughly competent in conducting fitness tests and be knowledgeable in the signs and symptoms of participant distress so that the health and safety of the individual are protected.

Expertise is required in interpreting results from the fitness tests, health-hazard appraisals, and medical examinations, and for prescribing appropriate and safe health/fitness programs. In their role as assessors, health/fitness professionals must be perceptive to the participant's reaction to the tests and the subsequent results.

Evaluator

Health/fitness professionals evaluate their own programs by documenting participation, fitness levels, and activity patterns. Their findings are then related to the company goals of cost-effectiveness and productivity. Evaluators should keep accurate records and be able to apply ba-

Figure 4.1 Four organization strategies in corporate settings.

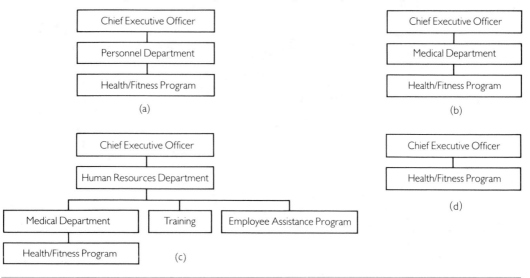

sic statistical techniques for describing results and examining trends in the health/fitness data.

Organization Strategies

The previous section described the various roles that health/fitness professionals play; this section describes various organizational structures in which health/fitness professionals are found. Staff structures of health/fitness professionals differ considerably among the three settings depending on the type of organization and the purpose of the program.

Corporate Settings

Health/fitness staffing in corporations usually is organized under supervision by the personnel, human resource, or medical departments. In rare instances, the health/fitness program is a stand-alone department answering perhaps to the chief executive officer (CEO) of the company. These four strategies are illustrated in Figure 4.1.

The size of any health/fitness staff depends on the size of the company, the number of participants to be serviced, and the available resources of the company. According to a survey conducted by Breuleux,[1] 84% of the corporate fitness directors polled were employed directly by their company and 16% were from private fitness agencies, consulting firms, or YMCAs. The average ratio of inhouse staff to participants was reported to be approximately 1:500 in a survey of 18 corporations that varied in size.[2] This ratio is not necessarily ideal; because most corporate health/fitness programs have been formed within the past 10 years, the ideal ratio has not been determined.

In those corporations that have organized health/fitness programs, medical consultation has been considered to be of prime importance. Some large corporations use medical consultants from the community; others create their own medical departments staffed with physicians, nurses, health educators, nutritionists, and psychologists. Health/fitness programs in this setting may have a program director, one or more exercise specialists, a recreation specialist, and support personnel such as secretaries, clerical workers, and custodians. These medical and

Figure 4.2 Staff organization in a corporation with a medical department and in a corporation that uses medical consultants.

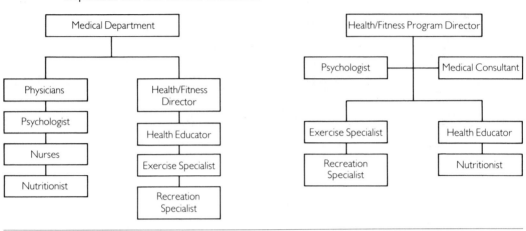

health/fitness specialist positions are defined in Chapter 15. Two examples of staff organizations, one in a corporation with a medical department and one that uses medical consultation, are presented in Figure 4.2.

As mentioned previously, there can be a considerable range in size and composition of health/fitness staff in the corporate setting. Table 4.3 summarizes the selection of health/fitness professionals based on organization and program size.

Community Settings

As in corporate settings, health/fitness staff structures in community programs vary considerably depending on the type of community agency and the purpose of the service provided. Health/fitness professionals in social service agencies such as the American Cancer Society, American Heart Association, American Lung Association, American Red Cross, and public health departments include volunteer physicians, psychologists, nurses, nutritionists, administrative specialists, and health educators. The fees charged for their services usually are nominal.

Other community agencies, such as the YMCA, deliver health/fitness programs to indi-

viduals and corporate organizations for moderate-to-high fees for the purpose of raising money to support ongoing social services. Health/fitness professional staff at YMCAs usually are college graduates with degrees in physical education, exercise physiology, exercise science, or related areas. YMCA professional staff are willing to consult with organizations on how best to meet health/fitness needs (see Chapter 3).

Recreation agencies, such as the local city Parks and Recreation Department, have specialists who can help individuals and corporations with the recreational aspects of health/fitness programs. Colleges and universities have health/fitness professionals such as program directors, exercise specialists, health educators, and recreation specialists who deliver programs to individuals and corporate organizations.

Commercial Settings

Health/fitness professionals in commercial settings deliver their programs to individuals and corporate organizations for the purpose of making a profit. Private health-promotion facilities usually have available well-qualified physicians, psychologists, nutritionists, exercise specialists, and health educators. These professionals act as

▌ T A B L E 4 . 3 ▌
Selection of Health/Fitness Professionals Based on Program Size

Personnel	Organization/Program Size (Based on Number of Employees)		
	Small (50 or less)	Medium (50–1000)	Large (1000 or more)
Program director	+	+	+
Medical consultant	+	+	+
Exercise specialist	–	+	+
Health educator	–	–	+
Recreation specialist	–	–	+
Support personnel	–	–	+

Source: American Heart Association (AHA)—Texas Affiliate. *Employee fitness programs: Guidelines for implementation.* Austin, TX: AHA, 1983. Used by permission.

paid consultants or part-time staff and deliver their contract services to individuals and corporate organizations.

Dance studios, racquet clubs, aquatic clubs, and martial arts studios have health/fitness personnel trained to provide services within their respective specialties.

Health spas and health studios historically have not employed well-qualified health/fitness professionals. The instructors and managers in these studios usually are salespersons trained to recruit new members. Few precautions, if any, are taken in prescribing exercise for the unfit. However, the rapid expansion of health clubs will dictate improved programs once competition for consumers becomes critical; trained professionals and quality programming eventually will distinguish the surviving clubs from those that fail.

▌ Summary

This chapter has presented an overview of the practitioner roles played by health/fitness professionals and the organizational structures found within the corporate, community, and commercial settings. Regardless of the setting, health/fitness professionals play many roles including manager, planner, supervisor, educator, exercise leader, motivator, counselor, promoter, assessor, and evaluator.

It is apparent from our experiences in the health/fitness field that the cornerstone of a successful program is the staff's ability to communicate not only with the participants but with management and other staff members. Next in importance is a well-planned program. Third is that the health/fitness staff be enthusiastic motivators. We mentioned other job duties that cannot be neglected.

References ▌

1. Breuleux, C. E. *A profile of corporate fitness directors*, Ph.D. dissertation. Columbus, Ohio: Ohio State University, 1982.

2. *Survey of corporate fitness and recreation programs.* Mt. Kisco, New York: Fitness Systems, 1983.

A GENERIC HEALTH/FITNESS DELIVERY MODEL

There are many approaches to delivering health/fitness programs and, as innovations are introduced during the current fitness boom in America, programs probably will be in a state of constant change. Some of the approaches to delivery involve "packaged programs" that are implemented directly into existing programs. The YMCA programs, for example, have a traditional approach used by many programs; a number of consulting groups, such as the Institute for Aerobics Research, Dallas, Texas, provide programming models in their services to programs. This is popular among embryonic programs that lack experienced personnel and leadership but have access to facilities for implementing the packaged programs. Another approach to implementing programs is to pay for the participants' membership in a local health club or Y. This is popular when neither experienced leadership nor facilities are available within the organization. Another approach is to offer inhouse programs with a core service of exercise and to bring in consultants to complement the exercise program by expanding services to include weight-control, stress-management, and other wellness-oriented activities.

These approaches vary in expense and are dependent on the program goals and resources available. It is often necessary to start small, with cost-containment being a constant limitation to program breadth and depth. The major distinction commonly observed between small, new programs and large, well-established programs is in the area of assessment and evaluation. Although much of the programming of services can be accomplished with limited personnel and resources, participant assessment and program evaluation require equipment and expertise that often is unavailable to the director of a small, unestablished program. This limits the program in attempts to screen, monitor the progress of, and motivate program participants, and to evaluate the effectiveness of the program in costs and benefits.

We believe that a comprehensive health/fitness program must have certain elements of participant assessment prior to implementation. Goal-setting and planning strategies to counteract indicators of poor health and fitness also must be accomplished prior to starting the delivery of exercise and other programming. Reassessment of participants is essential to (1) establish a baseline starting point; (2) monitor participant progress; and (3) provide motivation to continue adherence. A comprehensive health/fitness program must have both education and service components for participants to maximize the benefits afforded by participation in the program. This chapter presents a generic health/fitness delivery model that can maximize successful implementation of a comprehensive program.

■ The Generic Health/Fitness Model

The steps involved in the health/fitness delivery model are not unlike those any manager would use in running a program in a modern organization. For example, the techniques called MBO (management by objectives), PERT (planning and evaluative review technique) charting, and the PRECEDE (predisposing, reinforcing, and enabling causes in educational diagnosis and evaluation) model all attempt to harness limited resources to move energetically toward some measurable goal. Also, each system builds in continuous evaluation to allow refinement of the strategies or actions originally chosen to achieve the goals. Thus, all of these systems can be considered "generic" because they are similar and can be applied to many disparate settings.

Our system is not unlike the ones we mentioned and therefore should be familiar to managers, directors, and educators who have attempted goal-oriented planning. The steps in our suggested model include: (1) needs assessment, (2) goal setting, (3) planning or choosing strategies to meet goals, (4) delivery of program, and (5) evaluation (see Figure 5.1).

The delivery model begins with a needs assessment to determine the program participants' interests, behaviors, and attitudes about the program as well as their medical and health/fitness status. Once this information is obtained, health/fitness goals can be set and planning regarding the subsequent program implementation can occur. The evaluation is performed to determine the change in status of the participants following the program implementation. This approach is dynamic and interactive; it provides insight and feedback at all stages to better meet the needs of the participants. Input from a previous stage in the model modifies the program-delivery approach in subsequent stages of the model. Moreover, feedback from later stages becomes an important modifier of the program delivery. A quarterly fitness evaluation, for example, can assist the participant in setting new exercise goals. The interaction of education and service also is an important feature. We believe that a mind–body approach is essential to effective program delivery: a well-informed and knowledgeable participant will be more effective in changing health/fitness behaviors. This interaction, frequently overlooked in many program-delivery approaches, serves as the basis for ultimately altering the lifestyles of program participants.

Our model focuses on the individual rather than a group. It should help tailor any health/fitness program to the needs of the individual because he or she is intimately involved in planning and selection of strategies for his or her program. We recognize that an individualized approach to implementing a health/fitness program is expensive and time-consuming. Many organizations will need to use group approaches to implementing the education and service components of core programs. However, we believe that an individualized approach to implementation should be the primary goal of the program.

Another major consideration is the delivery of the education aspects of the program. The education and service components of a health/fitness program most often are implemented as a single unit. The exercise services, for example, would have elements of education introduced concurrently with the exercise classes. The physiological importance of warmup could be explained during a stretching session before an exercise class. Other services, such as stress management, nutrition, or low-back–pain management, can be logically divided into separate education and service elements. We have chosen for the sake of clarity to separate these discussions in this chapter. Figure 5.2 provides an example of the program delivery model.

▮ Figure 5.1   A generic health/fitness delivery model. ▮

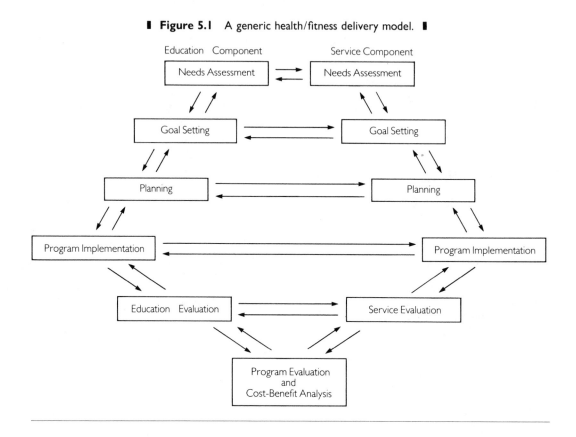

The generic model of implementation, however, will be followed in both the education and service sections of the discussion.

The integration of individual- and group-oriented programming that incorporates separate and concurrent educational and service aspects will be discussed in Part 3 of the book.

▮ Education Component

There is no single best way to assist program participants in changing lifestyles to promote enhanced health/fitness. Research indicates that a variety of educational and behavioral methods may be necessary in separate or combined implementation approaches. Individual counseling may prove effective for one person, whereas group instruction might be best for another participant. A combination of approaches may be necessary to maximize health/fitness compliance in a third person.

Table 5.1 illustrates the types of participant groupings that can be used effectively in implementing educational programs. Outcomes of these approaches also are indicated.

Note that the key to program success remains at the individual level. Personal contacts between program staff and each participant are a signal feature of most successful programs. We will examine the steps of our generic model as it focuses on the individual program participant.

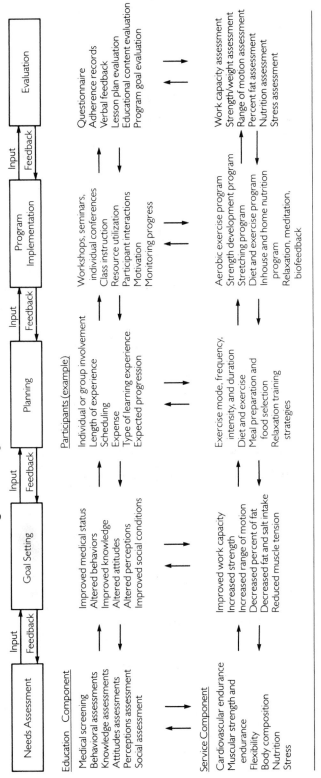

Figure 5.2 A generic health/fitness delivery system.

The figure depicts a flow from left to right through the following stages, each connected by "Input" and "Feedback" arrows:

Needs Assessment → Goal Setting → Planning → Program Implementation → Evaluation

Education Component

Needs Assessment:
Medical screening
Behavioral assessments
Knowledge assessments
Attitudes assessments
Perceptions assessment
Social assessment

Goal Setting:
Improved medical status
Altered behaviors
Improved knowledge
Altered attitudes
Altered perceptions
Improved social conditions

Planning (Participants example):
Individual or group involvement
Length of experience
Scheduling
Expense
Type of learning experience
Expected progression

Program Implementation:
Workshops, seminars, individual conferences
Class instruction
Resource utilization
Participant interactions
Motivation
Monitoring progress

Evaluation:
Questionnaire
Adherence records
Verbal feedback
Lesson plan evaluation
Educational content evaluation
Program goal evaluation

Service Component

Needs Assessment:
Cardiovascular endurance
Muscular strength and endurance
Flexibility
Body composition
Nutrition
Stress

Goal Setting:
Improved work capacity
Increased strength
Increased range of motion
Decreased percent of fat
Decreased fat and salt intake
Reduced muscle tension

Planning (Participants example):
Exercise mode, frequency, intensity, and duration
Diet and exercise
Meal preparation and food selection
Relaxation training strategies

Program Implementation:
Aerobic exercise program
Strength development program
Stretching program
Diet and exercise program
Inhouse and home nutrition program
Relaxation, meditation, biofeedback

Evaluation:
Work capacity assessment
Strength/weight assessment
Range of motion assessment
Percent fat assessment
Nutrition assessment
Stress assessment

■ T A B L E 5 . 1 ■
The Educational Program

Approach*	Delivery Capability	Materials	Outcomes
All participants	Media campaign	Audiovisuals: film, TV, videotape, slide/sound; visuals: exhibit, poster; print: bulletin, brochure, pamphlet, newsletter	Increase in awareness
Large group	Program introduction	Audiovisuals: film, TV, videotape, slide/sound; visuals: slide, chart, bulletin, newsletter; print: brochure, pamphlet	Increase in awareness; increase in knowledge; change in attitudes
Small group	Skill training Self-help Behavior modification	Print: self-instruction kits, workbook; audiovisuals: videotape, slide/sound, filmstrip, film; visuals: transparency, slide, flip chart, chart pad, video disc, audio disc, games	Change in behavior; reduction in risk; reduction in cost, morbidity, and mortality
	Learning seminars	Same as for skill training	Increase in knowledge; change in attitudes
Individual	Person to person Computer teaching	Interactive: computer, teaching machine; print: self-instruction kit, programmed instruction, pamphlet	Increase in knowledge; change in attitudes; change in behavior; reduction in risk; reduction in cost, morbidity, and mortality

Source: Adapted from Parkinson, R., et al. *Managing health promotion in the workplace.* Palo Alto, CA: Mayfield, 1982, p. 38. Used by permission.
*Imaginative programs are created through use of more than one approach, combined with well designed and tested materials.

Needs Assessment

Perhaps the most widely adopted means of assessing participants is through a survey determining program offering and scheduling interests. There are many indicators available to help the health/fitness professional customize an education offering for program participants. These indicators can be based on both clinically developed data and questionnaire-generated information. Table 5.2 illustrates the type of information that can be gathered and the method of data collection frequently used to assess the needs of participants.

The medical assessment normally should include a comprehensive examination compris-

ing a medical history, physical examination, and laboratory evaluation of blood and urine chemistries. Frequently, a graded exercise test is indicated. These assessments could serve as the basis for goal setting in both education and service components and can be beneficial to each aspect of the delivery model.

The remaining indicators can be assessed by a variety of paper-and-pencil instruments. The "LifeStyle Assessment Questionnaire" is an excellent instrument that includes a variety of different categories related to health/fitness.[1] Other instruments also are available to assess nonmedical factors related to wellness.

Once the health/fitness professional has uncovered the various indicators related to a

▌T A B L E 5 . 2▐
Types and Methods of Educational Needs Assessment

Type of Assessment	Method of Assessment
Medical	Medical history
	Physical examination
	Laboratory
	Graded exercise test
Behavioral	Questionnaire, health risk
Knowledge	appraisals, or content-
Attitudes	specific instruments
Perceptions	
Social	

person's level of wellness (good or bad), a plan can be created to *reinforce* or *increase* already existing wellness-enhancing behaviors, and to *reduce* or *change* wellness-destroying behaviors. This includes an educational effort combined with a comprehensive service component. The intervention must be planned in consultation with the participant to set goals and strategies necessary to increase wellness. Committed participants with high self-motivation might accomplish the necessary interventions through group orientations; this is more cost-effective than individual counseling.

A negative change in wellness status may stem from many things, such as personal tragedy, financial ruin, or health problems. Our educational model can be applied to any or all of these events, but we will focus on health problems, which include obesity, high blood pressure, atherosclerosis, diabetes, myocardial infarction, stroke, cancer, or traumatic injury. Some of these problems are functions of behavior, others of genetic or situational variables.

To track one set of possibilities, let us assume that a fictitious Mr. Jones has had several medical insurance claims recently, that his wellness status seems poor as indicated by low energy, mediocre performance at work, and a short temper, and that he recently has been diagnosed as having high blood pressure. It may be possible to determine some behaviors Mr. Jones has (or does not have) that are causing his

blood pressure to remain high. Assume Mr. Jones's pattern includes the following behaviors that probably exacerbate his condition: uses excess salt; eats too much, and food contains a high percentage of fat; does not take his hypertension medication; does not exercise; and smokes cigarettes.

In the educational component of a health/fitness program, needs assessment focuses on learning what Mr. Jones knows about his condition, his values that may relate to the condition, his skill level regarding techniques necessary to reverse his health problem, and the factors in his day-to-day living that tend to contribute to his health-destroying behaviors.

Goal Setting with the Participant

Goal setting usually should occur during a consultation with the participant before he or she starts a program. Using the information from the needs assessment, the health/fitness professional can develop a program. The first thing is to establish *goals*, so that progress toward these goals is observable and measurable. For example, a goal might be that by the end of the first month in the program Mr. Jones will have the knowledge to begin making the necessary changes in his life to improve his wellness. He should attempt to change only one behavior at a time, recognize the importance and success associated with each change, and realize he will have occasional setbacks as he progresses toward a healthier lifestyle. Specifically, he might aim to learn how to take his blood pressure and to change systematically the behaviors known to exacerbate his condition, for example, by reducing his salt intake, stopping his smoking, and beginning an exercise program. His program and those of two other participants are shown in Table 5.3.

Another approach is to examine the participant population and determine the group trends in needs. For example, in a corporate setting in which a similar population of employees has similar work habits and lifestyles, it is reasonable to assume many of them have

▌ T A B L E   5 . 3 ▌
Goal Setting for Three Participants

Participant	Needs Assessment: Problems Identified	Goal Setting: Behaviors Changed
Mr. Jones	Mediocre work performance	Time management
	Short temper	Stress management
	Hypertension	Diet and exercise
	Low energy level	Aerobic exercise
Ms. Smith	Low-back pain	Specialized exercises
	Obesity	Walking/swimming; low-calorie diet
	High-fat diet	Increased-carbohydrate diet
	Excessive smoking	Smoking cessation
Mr. Johnson	Alcohol excess	Substance-abuse management
	Antidepressant medication abuse	Substance-abuse management
	Low energy level	Aerobic exercise
	Poor diet	Nutrition enhancement

common program needs. A group approach might be an effective strategy in setting companywide goals. The industrial setting, for example, tends to emphasize recreational activities in its programming because of the tedium of production-line work—intramural and club sports activities often are popular. The goals of a corporate home office health/fitness program, however, tend to be more wellness-oriented. A group approach in a homogeneous population usually is the best way to set program goals. An example of this approach might be the administration of a health-risk appraisal and an interest survey. Central tendencies regarding both the needs and the interests of the participants then can be determined by data analysis, and effective programming can be implemented.

Planning the Education Intervention

Planning education components in a health/fitness program necessarily involves both group and individual approaches. The group approach to participant education requires the selecting of education offerings; formatting, scheduling, and promoting classes; projecting expenses; seeking guest speakers; and arranging facilities, to mention a few steps in the process. Using external resources, such as local university personnel, medical societies and associations, and community agencies, can enrich the program with little additional cost. The education component can be related to any number of aspects in the program—exercise, hypertension, weight control, stress management, and so on. Ideally, the planning also should be individualized as much as possible, involving the participant and permitting co-ownership of the plan. The planning usually is accomplished at the same meeting during which the health/fitness professional and participant determine goals.

Several aspects of the education intervention can be accomplished with Mr. Jones at this point. If Mr. Jones believes he learns best by watching a film, a film should be provided. If Mr. Jones can benefit from skill work (for example, learning to take his blood pressure), and

▮ T A B L E 5 . 4 ▮

Educational Strategies According to Characteristics of the Program Participant

Participant	Characteristic	Audiovisual aids	Lecture	Individual instruction	Mass media	Programmed learning	Peer-group discussion	Modeling	Behavior modification	Social action	Social planning and organizational change
		Recommended Educational Strategies									
High adherers	Fit / High wellness level / High self-motivation		■		■	■		■	■	■	
Moderate adherers	Moderately fit / Moderate wellness level / Moderate self-motivation	■		■			■				■
Low adherers	Not fit / Poor wellness level / Low self-motivation	■		■			■				■

Source: Adapted from Green, L. W., et al. *Health education planning: A diagnostic approach.* Palo Alto, CA: Mayfield, 1980, pp. 107–112. Used by permission.

wishes to try his hand at this, then this should be included.

The health/fitness professional has an incredible variety of learning techniques at her or his disposal, but none of them are "magic" in the sense that 100% of the participants will respond to a particular technique. The strategies must be chosen to complement the style of learning to which the participant responds best. Some participants learn visually, some aurally, some tactually. Most respond to all three. Some participants detest group work, others hate researching a problem. Therefore, the professional must ask each participant what is the best way he or she learns.

In practical terms, there are three distinct types of individuals involved in a health/fitness program. Table 5.4 illustrates educational approaches for each. The *high adherers* are highly self-disciplined and require little motivation and education. They are already sold on the program and simply need to be exposed to a well-organized, well-staffed, and well-operated service program; the long-term compliers to the program will come from this group. The *moderate adherers* can go either way with regard to programming compliance. They require a great deal of motivational support and benefit greatly from educational programming, especially individualized approaches. The *low adherers* have tried everything at least once, but rarely endure. They could benefit greatly from an individualized approach to the educational planning. It is in this group that we have cast Mr. Jones.

In individualized instruction, the professional's main concern is motivation. Monitoring and reinforcing progress are key elements in this approach, as is demonstrating a concerned interest in the participant.

If classes are the education strategy, then each class requires planning. Examples of specific behavioral objectives for a particular lesson might include that by the end of the session, the participant (1) will be able to repeat three or four facts about low-fat diets and their relationship to hypertension; (2) will be able to demonstrate the correct position and breathing rhythm for the relaxation response to occur; (3) will describe three techniques for managing time effectively in the office and in the home; and (4) will make a values choice concerning the use of medication to control hypertension, and describe this choice.

Lesson planning should be participant-centered. Consult participants about what they need to learn and how they learn best. This avoids the difficult issue of the professional being a manipulator, propagandist, or coercer; the health/fitness director should try to maintain a role of *motivator*.

Implementing the Education Plan

When you implement the education plan, you should consider several questions: Who is best skilled at delivering a particular learning strategy? An inhouse staff member? A community resource person? What are the resources available to implement the plan? A seminar room? An audiovisual system? How will you know the learning strategies should be altered for better effect? Participant feedback? Intuition? How is progress to be monitored? Formal evaluation? Participant feedback? What is the least expensive, yet still effective, way of reaching the learning goals? Group classes with an instructor? Individual conferences? What format should the educational component

adopt? Instructional packages? Classes and conferences? What motivation techniques are to be used for best effect? Awards? Incentives? How will the education and service components be delivered? Combined? Separated?

Efficient implementation of the learning programs must include the committed participants. If the participants are fighting the program, there is little chance for success. If they are involved, and if the program runs smoothly, is active, is exciting, contains a variety of learning strategies, and builds in regular successful experiences for the participants, then chances are good the educational intervention will achieve its goals.

Evaluation of the Learning Plan

An evaluation of the education component can be performed at two levels: (1) lesson plan level—evaluation of specific objectives, or (2) education plan level—evaluation of long-range goals.

Lesson Plan Evaluation Periodic evaluation of daily learning sessions helps to determine if progress is being made toward ultimate goals. The evaluation can be done on a preclass, post-class basis to determine increase in knowledge, change in attitude, and increase in skill. Evaluation can employ various instruments such as Likert scales (to determine shifts in attitude) and checklists for observing skills. Of course, the type of instrument would depend on the lesson objective and, in many instances, an instrument may not even be used. For example, if a lesson objective is for the participant to be able to verbalize an opinion about medication, it would suffice for the health/fitness professional simply to hear the values expressed. The more experienced the professional, the less reliance on formal lesson plans.

Education Plan Evaluation of Goals Evaluation of longer-range goals may be somewhat more difficult than evaluation of daily lesson plans because the uncontrolled variables occurring over a month-long or year-long period may cloud the results. Therefore, in addition to selecting proper instruments and criteria values (for example, adherence, program offering, attendance, fitness improvements, weight loss), the health/fitness professional may design a study using matched cohorts to offset the problem of uncontrolled variables.

∎ Service Component

The service component of program implementation is both a logical followup to the education components and an integral part of the participants' educational programming. Thus, these elements rarely are separated completely. Indeed, most program directors choose to integrate these concurrently so one can feed on the other to maximize program effectiveness.

Needs Assessment

Assuming the programmatic organization and planning has been achieved, the first step in implementing a service component is to assess the participants' interests and needs. Interests can be evaluated by questionnaire and will provide direction for the core program services. The needs of the participants usually are determined through health/fitness status assessments that might include a wellness inventory, medical screening, and fitness evaluation.

Wellness Inventory The wellness inventory, or health hazard appraisal (Chapter 2), usually includes participant information regarding such areas as: (1) physical exercise habits, (2) physical self-care habits, (3) safety practice, (4) drug usage, (5) social–environmental concerns, (6) emotional awareness and acceptance, (7) emotional management, (8) intellectual abilities and interests, (9) occupational considerations, and (10) spiritual beliefs. Information obtained from such questionnaires can give the health/fitness

director insight into the participants' needs for wellness-oriented services. Medical information about the client also should be assessed.

Medical Screening Medical screening can be accomplished through inhouse procedures as well as through referrals. Regardless of who conducts it, the medical screening should include a complete medical history and a physical examination including blood pressure measurement, blood and urine chemistries, and an electrocardiogram. The results provide information regarding participants' health problems in terms of type, severity, and probable duration, as well as regarding risk factors needing intervention. Individuals with health problems can then be referred to secondary prevention programs. Those participants who have no contraindications can be directed to higher-level health-promotion and wellness programs.

Fitness Evaluation The assessments for each service program component will be different; the specific instruments will be discussed and illustrated in Chapters 6 through 11. These assessments should include exercise ability, nutrition, weight control, stress level, substance abuse, and low-back flexibility. We will give a brief description of each assessment area.

Exercise testing usually requires an evaluation of cardiovascular endurance, muscular strength and endurance, and flexibility. The cardiovascular endurance assessments can be accomplished in either the clinical laboratory or a field setting. The age and health status of the participants, equipment available, and training of the evaluators dictate the type of tests performed. The laboratory setting usually is used for older, symptomatic participants and the test is performed on a treadmill or bicycle ergometer under physical or trained technician supervision. Various protocols are available for different populations of individuals and should be selected on the basis of appropriate need. The field tests most commonly used to evaluate cardiovascular endurance in young, asymptomatic individuals are the bench-stepping test and the run–walk test. Either can provide a direct or an indirect assessment of cardiovascular function.

Muscular strength and endurance usually are assessed by using weight-lifting equipment. Hydraulic and electronic equipment presently on the market provides readouts of muscular strength and endurance, but these may be prohibitively expensive. The most common approach to assessing muscular strength and endurance involves using free weights or a rack-mounted exercise apparatus such as the Universal Gym. Frequently, a single measure of upper-extremity (bench press) and lower-extremity (leg press) muscular strength and endurance is used. Strength is assessed by determining the maximal amount of weight that can be lifted in a single effort; muscular endurance is assessed by determining the maximal number of repetitions that can be performed until a failing effort at a predetermined percentage of the strength measurements occurs.

The assessments of the weight-control service program require evaluation of body composition, and eating and exercise behaviors. Body composition can be assessed either through hydrostatic weighing or through skinfold or anthropometric measures (such as body segment girths) to estimate body density. Body density is converted to percentage body fat, which is then used to calculate a target body weight. Eating and physical activity behaviors can be assessed through a paper-and-pencil or computerized approach.

Nutritional status can be assessed using a variety of techniques. A blood chemistry analysis is one indicator. A trained clinician also can tell a great deal about the nutritional status merely by scrutinizing the participants' hair, skin, nails, eyes, and other features. Body composition measures also are markers for nutritional needs, especially with regard to body-fat percentage. Finally, a dietary intake history is a common method to assess the nutritional status of a participant.

Assessment of stress level is not as straightforward. Stress is a manifestation of the difference between one's coping resources and the stress-producing environments. A single test usually is inadequate to appraise accurately a person's stress level. A variety of paper-and-pencil tests usually are administered to assess recent life events in the work and home environments and other stress measures.

Once the baseline measures are obtained, the health/fitness professional begins goal setting. We now know where the participant is and we need to find out where she or he needs and wants to go with the health-enhancement program.

Goal Setting

Goal setting is highly individualized. Each participant should be consulted, and the baseline data should be used to establish goals.

Remember Mr. Jones, who was asymptomatic on his medical screening and graded exercise test, but was unfit, overfat, and used too much salt. The educational components of the program provided a statement of behavioral objectives for Mr. Jones. However, several of these specific objectives relate to the service program, because this is where the action occurs. Mr. Jones and the health/fitness professional might determine these objectives: at the end of 1 month, Mr. Jones will be able to complete a 1-mile walk–jog without stopping; at the end of 1 month, Mr. Jones will have lost 4 pounds of body weight; and at the end of 1 month, Mr. Jones will average less than 5 grams of daily salt intake.

Similar goal statements could be developed for any of the areas of assessment made at the start of the health/fitness program. The key to success is the integration of the education and service components of the program and active involvement of the participant in the process.

Planning

Failure to plan destines a program to failure. The planning stage of the service program must be individualized. The health/fitness professional explains and negotiates the education and service components to encourage an informed, motivated participant who understands his or her own objectives and also knows how to go about accomplishing them. This process requires that the health/fitness specialist provide enough educational information about the health-promotion program that the participant will be able to function effectively in the various experiences. The service program should be the source of specific and detailed information.

In Mr. Jones's case, the planning stage of the component would provide him with ideas about exercises, such as: what equipment to purchase for the exercise selected, for instance, the type of shoes best suited to his specific needs in aerobic exercise; when facilities and classes are available and convenient; what services are available, including locker space, towel service, and equipment; and how exercise records and information will be kept.

Similar examples could be illustrated for any other service program area Mr. Jones might need or want. The planning stage should optimize his readiness for the various programs and maximize the potential for his adherence to the program involved.

Implementation

The implementation stage can occur in either an individual or a group setting. It should be well organized and have built-in progressions for implementing the various component services. Each stage of the implementation process should be developed accommodate the needs and abilities of the participants. Perhaps most important are the motivational strategies used to reinforce progress of the various participants. Participants all should have ongoing feedback about their progress and should feel they are an important part of the program. Mr. Jones, for example, should know that when he attends the exercise program trained personnel will be available to monitor and supervise his activity. He should be informed of all aspects of program promotion, such as upcoming special events, and be confident that he is in good hands.

Evaluation

Evaluation of the service program component is based largely on the changes in the program participants and on their adherence to the program. Therefore, a reevaluation by retesting on the appropriate assessments made at the outset of the program is necessary to determine progress. Changes seen in each participant on every assessment should be discussed in a followup session. This posttesting can be used as an entry measurement into any subsequent programming for the participant. Mr. Jones, for example, could have a second evaluation on his blood pressure, fitness level, and dietary patterns to note progress and provide data for goal setting and subsequent programming.

It is important to link the educational and service components of each individual's program and the overall health/fitness program. One place this occurs is in the area of evaluation. We will briefly examine two other levels of evaluation to show the way the participant's evaluation ties into the overall evaluation of any organization's health-promotion endeavor. These levels are an evaluation of program goals and cost–benefit analysis.

Program Evaluation
Health/Fitness Program Goals

The implementation of the overall program and the many aspects of this process will be discussed in Part 3. Here we will discuss briefly the evaluation of the overall program. The health/fitness program goals normally will be written in the same way as described for the education and service components. Overall program evaluation is distinguished from individual evaluation in that the program goals probably are to reduce morbidity and stop the rise in health-care–related expenditures, such as loss of money due to costs of absenteeism, employee recruitment, insurance premiums, medical care and counseling, disability payments, and disability insurance premiums.

To differentiate the true effects from the changes due to uncontrolled variables, it is important for the health/fitness professional to design a study using matched cohorts to see if significant differences exist between experimental and control groups. A large company with several different programming sites could determine experimentally the direct effects of a new approach using this method. Later, when a program is shown to contribute to reduced costs, the professional can redesign the evaluation to ascertain the total economic benefits and costs of the health/fitness program.

Cost–Benefit Analysis

Several authors, including Philips and Hughes,[2] have presented useful models for showing relationships between various parts of occupational-health programs and their ultimate costs and benefits. These will be examined in greater detail in Chapter 13, but it is worthwhile to note here the vital importance of these models and the process of cost–benefit analysis of health/fitness programs. Without these evaluations, directors are limited to platitudes and statements of principle when defining their programs in the inevitable budget battles. By acquiring objective indicators of the cost–benefit ratio and the cost-effectiveness of their programs, directors can fine tune their offerings to increase efficiency, thus building an economic argument for continuing and perhaps expanding their programs. Given the cyclic economic expansion and contraction that seem to predominate today, this form of evaluation must be viewed as a survival skill for health/fitness professionals.

Summary

The model we have proposed to implement health/fitness programs is widely adaptable to any programming area. It can be used for exercise, nutrition, weight control, and any other program deemed necessary for a particular setting. It allows the professional to emphasize individuals or groups in the implementation process. The education component, which focuses on attitudinal change, can be integrated with the service component, which focuses on behavioral change. The education and service components also can be separated when dictated by necessity or programming appropriateness.

The model also is an ongoing process that can be employed for a single instructional or activity unit, or it can be used to evaluate participants at the end of a programming period to provide a needs assessment for subsequent instruction or activity.

Part 2 will illustrate the utility of our generic model by describing the most common forms of health/fitness programming.

References

1. Hettler, B., et al. *LifeStyle Assessment Questionnaire*, 2d ed. Stevens Point, WI: The University of Wisconsin-Stevens Point, Institute for Lifestyle Improvement, 1980.

2. Philips, R., and Hughes, J. Cost–Benefit analysis of the occupational health programs: A generic model. *Journal of Occupational Medicine* 16:158, 1981.

PART 2
IMPLEMENTATION OF
HEALTH/FITNESS PROGRAMS

EXERCISE

Fitness development is the most popular service offered in health/fitness programs. Exercise and fitness programs can have a significant effect on wellness. A skeletal discussion on exercise programming is presented here; most discussions in Part 3 of the book speak to the detailed aspects of exercise program implementation.

We will use the generic implementation model of core programs in this and subsequent chapters. Although the education and service components are separated in this chapter, remember that these can be blended into a single approach.

■ Education Component

The education component helps participants learn about exercise and its role in enhancing wellness. This is useful because it enables participants to understand more precisely what their test results mean in norm-referenced terms, it provides information about available exercise programs, and ultimately it helps participants achieve greater fitness levels.

Needs Assessment

During needs assessment, data about the participant are obtained and then discussed. These data are gathered from medical screening, exercise testing, behavioral information, and paper-and-pencil tests of knowledge, attitudes, perceptions, and social factors. This process is best accomplished in individual consultations. Explain the nature of the tests and their importance in determining present health/fitness status. Translate test results into norm-referenced terminology.

The evaluation itself should use objective and subjective measures to provide sound objective data. The objective data are combined with subjective data obtained from a physical activity history record (Figure 6.1). Several lifestyle assessments should be included—nutrition, drug use, stress, and emotional, occupational, intellectual, and spiritual information.

After this information is clearly explained to the participant, make a general assessment of the participant's overall health/fitness status. This must be clearly communicated to each participant: if participants do not recognize weak areas in their needs assessment, they will not be motivated to improve.

Also educate participants about the nature of fitness in general, and the various components that make up a total fitness program. Participants should be able to discriminate among cardiovascular endurance, muscular strength, muscular endurance, flexibility, and other components of fitness. They should have a clear understanding of the role that each of these fitness components plays in remediating the weak points in their health/fitness profile.

▮ Figure 6.1 Exercise history questionnaire. ▮

Name _____

Are you currently involved in a regular exercise program? Yes _____ No _____

Do you regularly walk or run 1 or more miles continuously? Yes _____ No _____
Don't know _____
  If yes, average number of miles you cover per workout or day: _____ miles
  What is your average time per mile? _____ minutes:seconds Don't know _____

Do you practice weight lifting or home calisthenics? Yes _____ No _____

Are you now involved in an aerobics program? Yes _____ No _____
  If yes, your average aerobics points per week: _____

Have you taken in the past 6 months: 12 minute test _____ 1.5 mile _____ neither _____
  If yes, your miles in 12 minutes: _____ or your time for 1.5 miles: _____ minutes:seconds

Do you frequently participate in competitive sports? Yes _____ No _____
  If yes, which one or ones? Golf _____ Bowling _____ Tennis _____ Handball _____
  Soccer _____ Basketball _____ Volleyball _____ Football _____ Baseball _____
  Track _____ Other _____
  Average number of times per week _____

In which of the following high school or college athletics did you participate?
None _____ Football _____ Basketball _____ Baseball _____ Soccer _____ Track _____
Swimming _____ Tennis _____ Wrestling _____ Golf _____ Other _____

What activity or activities would you prefer in a regular exercise program for yourself?
Walking and/or running _____ Bicycling (outdoors) _____ Swimming _____ Stationary
running _____ Stationary bicycling _____ Tennis _____ Jumping rope _____ Handball,
basketball, or squash _____ Other _____

Comments: _____
_____
_____

Goal Setting

Goal setting can be accomplished during the same conference in which the test results are discussed with the participant. In fact, this is an ideal time to discuss exercise goals. Set safe, reasonable expectations for the participant's exercise program, providing tangible goals.

To be effective, goal setting must be appropriate, measurable, and renewable. The *appropriateness* of participants' goals is determined largely by their present fitness needs and interests, and by the rate of progress that can be expected with regular participation in the exercise program. Generally speaking, a person can expect to gain about 1% to 10% improvement each week during the initial months of a fitness program. The extent of gain depends on several factors—age, sex, level of fitness, amount of exercise, and whether the participant is genetically predisposed to be a "hard gainer" or an "easy gainer."

Measurable short- and long-term goals should be set. In assessing short-term goals, emphasize that progress during initial stages of exercise often results in performance *decreases*. Muscular soreness, as well as loss of motivation due to self-imposed comparisons with more fit companions, often leads to setbacks for novice exercisers. The short-term goals should focus on orientation to and familiarization with the equipment, facilities, staff, and individual exercise prescriptions. Other short-term goals include obtaining target heart rates and levels of perceived exertion associated with aerobic exercise. Another short-term goal might be to determine the amount of resistance the participant can handle for the desired repetitions in a strength-development program. A short-term goal for a flexibility program might include determining the range of motion necessary to produce a good stretch.

Measurable long-term goals might be to jog a mile without stopping, successfully complete a local fun run with a spouse or friend, perform a pull-up or 50 sit-ups, or touch one's toes and hold this position.

All of these goals are not only measurable but also *renewable*: new goals can be set as the old ones are achieved, and old goals can be re-evaluated if they are not achieved.

Planning

Planning can be approached from both the group and individual level. Most often, the health/fitness specialist is forced to use a group approach for economic reasons. At this level, planning is mostly a management process. Prepare education materials describing the exercise program benefits and scope. You might develop a clinic for runners or weight trainers; guidelines for selecting exercise equipment (such as jogging shoes); record keeping and progress monitoring; newsletters; guidelines for each exercise program; and motivational materials to promote adherence to programs.

Planning can be accomplished on an individual level as well. Establish periods when participants can come by the health/fitness offices for individual conferences to clear up any questions arising from testing or consultation sessions. Encourage the staff to be available on a casual basis. Implementing the program is easier when participants feel they are in good hands, and when they have available a knowledgeable and competent staff.

Implementation

The implementation of the education component is the nuts and bolts of the program. It usually is accomplished by working with groups of participants in a structured setting. For example, you can provide a training clinic for a 10K or marathon race; a workshop in selected racquet sports; speakers on topics such as sports medicine or the heart and cardiovascular system; classes on how to use new equipment; regular exercise class instruction; or classes for special populations (individuals with cardiac disease, or the elderly).

Education programming does not always require staff involvement. Interactions among participants are essential in establishing an *esprit de corps*; program members often educate one another through shared information. Simply creating a place where participants can chat, such as a lounge, allows many education experiences.

Individual counseling is the essence of the education component. Conferences provide awareness of progress via updated record keeping and personal involvement.

Evaluation

The education component can be evaluated by obtaining feedback from the participants through questionnaires regarding the program's effectiveness. Another source of feedback is the adherence and progress records of the participants. Records of traffic through the facility, attendance at special events, and so on provide indirect data about the effectiveness of the program.

Lesson-plan evaluations of each exercise class can serve as another source of information. The content must be reevaluated constantly, and development sessions should be conducted to keep staff abreast of up-to-date practices.

Most important, participant posttesting provides an overall estimate of the worth of the education process. Posttesting should use those instruments used to obtain baseline data. Informal feedback from participants also is invaluable in modifying and restructuring the program.

Service Component

The service component consists of implementing the exercise program and is influenced by many factors. One significant consideration is the location of the program; onsite programs differ from offsite ones. In the latter case, the program director probably will not tailor exercises for the participants.

The facilities also influence the type of exercise programs that can be implemented. A residential Y, for example, may offer programs focused on family recreation and thus may be inappropriate as a health/fitness program site. The organizational structure of the setting also influences the nature and quality of the program. The organization of a health club, which may be heavily vested in membership sales rather than programming, may influence the exercise services. The size of the program—that is, number of participants and staff—also determines to some extent the nature of the exercise programs. Scheduling, finances, proximity of facilities, climate, type of program participants, program objectives, and medical considerations also influence the exercise programs.

We will assume that an onsite facility is being used, and that services are not limited significantly by cost-containment considerations. We will also assume that there is adequate staffing for a large corporate or community-based program.

Needs Assessment

Needs assessment for exercise and fitness service involves three distinct phases: *promotion, screening,* and *testing.*

Promotion The *promotion* is designed to acquaint the program participants with the assessment process. The health/fitness specialist can develop newsletters, demonstrations, promotional releases to local media, promotional films, slide demonstrations, and testimonials.

Screening The screening of program participants should involve a medical evaluation. The American College of Sports Medicine (ACSM) has published guidelines for such medical screening.[1] The two basic elements are a medical history and an examination. A physical activity readiness questionnaire is an excellent initial screening tool to identify individuals that

might be placed at risk by beginning exercise. Figure 6.2 is a self-administered questionnaire consisting of a few simple questions; positive response to any item indicates a need for medical clearance prior to exercise testing or prescription.

Second-level screening consists of a physical activity readiness examination. Individuals who require more extensive screening or testing should be referred to a physician. Prior to starting an exercise program or undergoing a graded exercise test, an individual should be informed of the inherent risks and benefits of these procedures and should sign a consent form.

It is important that the health/fitness specialist remain available to participants during this screening period. Participants who are at risk in exercise programs are likely to drop out at this stage, and may need extra encouragement.

Test Protocols Several factors affect the selection of testing protocols, such as the training and expertise of those administering the test, equipment and facilities available at the testing site, availability of medical support, types of exercise programs being offered, and individuals being tested.

The health status and needs of the participants dictate the level of sophistication that is employed in the exercise testing. Ideally, the testing staff should include a physician and ACSM-certified exercise-test technicians, especially if symptomatic individuals are tested. However, if asymptomatic young adults comprise the primary test populations, well-trained and uncertified staff are adequate if submaximal testing is employed. A minimal requirement, however, is that all personnel involved with testing be trained in CPR.

Most exercise testing laboratories have equipment for functional capacity testing, strength assessment, flexibility testing, and body composition evaluation. After you have completed all testing, develop a fitness profile for each participant. Pinpoint areas that need improvement, and use the profile for setting exercise goals.

■ **Figure 6.2** Screening questionnaire. (From O'Donnell, M. P., and
Ainsworth, T. H. *Health promotion in the workplace*. New York: Wiley,
1984, p. 116. Used by permission.)   ■

		No	*Yes*
1. Has a doctor ever said you have heart trouble?		___	___
2. Have you ever had angina pectoris or sharp pain or heavy pressure in your chest as a result of exercise, walking, or other physical activity, such as climbing a flight of stairs (Note: this does not include the normal out-of-breath feeling that results from vigorous activity)?		___	___
3. Do you experience any sharp pain or extreme tightness in your chest when you are hit by a cold blast of air?		___	___
4. Have you ever experienced rapid heart action or palpitations?		___	___
5. Have you ever had a real or suspected heart attack, coronary occlusion, myocardial infarction, coronary insufficiency, or thrombosis?		___	___
6. Have you ever had rheumatic fever?		___	___
7. Do you have diabetes, high blood pressure, or sugar in your urine?		___	.
8. Do you have or does any one in your family have high blood pressure or hypertension?		___	___
9. Has more than one blood relative (parent, brother, sister, first cousin) had a heart attack or coronary artery disease before the age of 60?		___	___
10. Have you ever taken any medication to lower your blood pressure?		___	___
11. Have you ever taken medication or been on a special diet to lower your cholesterol level?		___	___
12. Have you ever taken digitalis, quinine, or any other drug for your heart?		___	___
13. Have you ever taken nitroglycerin or any other tablets for chest pain—tablets that you take by placing them under the tongue?		___	___
14. Have you ever had a resting or stress electrocardiogram that was not normal?		___	___
15. Are you overweight?		___	___
16. Are you under a lot of stress?		___	___
17. Do you drink excessively?		___	___
18. Do you smoke cigarettes?		___	___
19. Do you have any physical condition, impairment, or disability, including any joint or muscle problem, that should be considered before you undertake an exercise program?		___	___
20. Are you more than 65 years old?		___	___
21. Are you more than 35 years old?		___	___
22. Do you exercise fewer than three times per week?		___	___

▌ T A B L E 6 . 1 ▌

Comparisons of Laboratory and Field Tests for Cardiovascular Function

Type of Assessment	Advantages	Disadvantages
Laboratory tests	Greater diagnostic capability	Expensive equipment required
	Direct VO_2 max capability	Complicated procedures
	More data collected	More staff required
	Medical supervision	Single-subject testing
	Safer	Time consuming
Field tests	Less expensive equipment	Less diagnostic capability
	Simple procedures	Indirect VO_2 max estimates
	Fewer staff required	Less data collected
	Mass testing possible	No medical supervision
	Rapid testing possible	Less safe

CARDIOVASCULAR TESTS. Cardiovascular tests can be administered in laboratory or field settings. The laboratory tests commonly use treadmills or bicycle ergometers to examine the subjects' heart rate and electrocardiogram (ECG) during and after a standardized graded exercise test. These are functional capacity tests that may be diagnostic if overt or latent disease is evidenced by ECG abnormalities.

The best indicator for cardiovascular fitness is maximal oxygen uptake (VO_2 max), which reflects the collective adaptations of both central and peripheral circulation in oxygen transport and utilization. Direct assessment of VO_2 max requires gas-analysis equipment; most laboratories resort to indirect estimates of VO_2 max from known work responses to the graded exercise test. The estimation of VO_2 max from various modes of exercise is possible through calculation of the greatest workload achieved during the exercise test using formulas provided by ACSM.[1]

Many health/fitness programs use submaximal exercise tests to estimate participants' functional capacity: VO_2 max is estimated from submaximal work, which is usually performed on a bicycle ergometer. The VO_2 max can also be predicted from field tests such as the 1.5 mile run.

Select tests by considering the purpose of the testing. If the testing is done for diagnostic purposes, then laboratory tests should be performed and medical personnel should be available. If the tests are being conducted for functional capacity assessments of healthy, young adults, then field tests can be used. Table 6.1 outlines the advantages and disadvantages of each.

MUSCULAR-STRENGTH TESTS. Like cardiovascular tests, muscular-strength tests can be performed in both laboratory and field settings. The most sophisticated strength-testing equipment uses computerized interfaces to provide torque curves throughout the range of motion for attempts made at different velocities. Such equipment can be used to generate exercise prescriptions for strength-development programs, but is found in only the most sophisticated laboratories; it is most useful for special populations such as athletes and rehabilitation patients.

The most common equipment used to assess strength is the rack-mounted machine, such as those made by Nautilus or Universal Gym. Although pneumatic and hydraulic systems also are useful, we will describe how muscular strength can be tested using the traditional rack-mounted equipment.

The most common, practical method of testing for muscular strength is to determine the maximal amount of weight one can lift in a single effort, the *one repetition maximum* (1RM).

■ T A B L E 6 . 2 ■
Strength-to–Body-Weight Ratios for Selected Dynamic Strength Tests

Men

Bench Press	Arm Curl	Lateral Pull-Down	Leg Press	Leg Extension	Leg Curl	Points
1.50	0.70	1.20	3.00	0.80	0.70	10
1.40	0.65	1.15	2.80	0.75	0.65	9
1.30	0.60	1.10	2.60	0.70	0.60	8
1.20	0.55	1.05	2.40	0.65	0.55	7
1.10	0.50	1.00	2.20	0.60	0.50	6
1.00	0.45	0.95	2.00	0.55	0.45	5
0.90	0.40	0.90	1.80	0.50	0.40	4
0.80	0.35	0.85	1.60	0.45	0.35	3
0.70	0.30	0.80	1.40	0.40	0.30	2
0.60	0.25	0.75	1.20	0.35	0.25	1

Women

Bench Press	Arm Curl	Lateral Pull-Down	Leg Press	Leg Extension	Leg Curl	Points
0.90	0.50	0.85	2.70	0.70	0.60	10
0.85	0.45	0.80	2.50	0.65	0.55	9
0.80	0.42	0.75	2.30	0.60	0.52	8
0.70	0.38	0.73	2.10	0.55	0.50	7
0.65	0.35	0.70	2.00	0.52	0.45	6
0.60	0.32	0.65	1.80	0.50	0.40	5
0.55	0.28	0.63	1.60	0.45	0.35	4
0.50	0.25	0.60	1.40	0.40	0.30	3
0.45	0.21	0.55	1.20	0.35	0.25	2
0.35	0.18	0.50	1.00	0.30	0.20	1

Total Points	Strength Fitness Category*
48–60	Excellent
37–47	Good
25–36	Average
13–24	Fair
0–12	Poor

Source: Heyward, V. *Design for fitness.* Minneapolis: Burgess, 1984, p. 25. Used by permission.
*Based on data for 250 college-age men and women.

This is accomplished by selecting a resistance (weight) that can be lifted with moderate difficulty and progressively lifting heavier loads until a failing effort is observed. The maximum value successfully lifted is the 1RM. Ideally, the 1RM values should be ascertained for all major muscle groups.

You can also assess participants' relative strength. Table 6.2 shows strength-to–body-weight ratios for college-age males and females.

The populations in most programs are older and less fit and thus require some downward adjustments of these norms. Recent studies have revealed that measures of bench-press and leg-press strength are the two best indicators of overall dynamic strength. Certainly the use of only two tests is more practical than a battery using all exercise stations.

MUSCULAR-ENDURANCE TESTS. Tests for muscular endurance are frequently used in

▌ T A B L E 6 . 3 ▌
Dynamic Muscular Endurance Test Battery

Exercise	Percent of Body Weight Lifted		Repetitions (max = 15)
	Men	Women	
Arm curl	0.33	0.25	_____
Bench press	0.66	0.50	_____
Lateral pull-down	0.66	0.50	_____
Triceps extension	0.33	0.33	_____
Leg extension	0.50	0.50	_____
Leg curl	0.33	0.33	_____
Bent-knee sit-up			_____
		Total repetitions (max = 105) =	_____

Total Repetitions	Fitness Category*
91–105	Excellent
77–90	Very good
63–76	Good
49–62	Fair
35–48	Poor
<35	Very poor

Source: Heyward, V. *Design for fitness.* Minneapolis: Burgess, 1984, p. 47. Used by permission.
*Based on data for 250 college-age men and women.

health/fitness testing programs. One common approach is to administer a single test of bent-knee sit-ups. The timed sit-up test is a good measure of muscular endurance for the abdominal musculature. However, unlike strength, muscular endurance is specific to each muscle group. Thus, a single measure cannot serve as a predictor for overall muscular endurance.

We recommend a broader testing protocol that supplements the timed sit-up test by using rack-mounted weight machines. Basically, this procedure determines the maximum numbers of repetitions of a percent of body weight that can be lifted (Table 6.3).

FLEXIBILITY TESTS. The most effective determination of flexibility uses a gravity goniometer, an instrument that determines the range of motion of each body part. This approach is the most comprehensive, because flexibility has been shown to be highly specific to each body segment. However, it is highly impractical in most adult fitness programs because of the time and expense it involves. The most widely used measure for flexibility is the sit-and-reach test to assess trunk and hip flexibility (see Chapter 11).

BODY COMPOSITION TESTS. Still another important element in any fitness test battery is the determination of participants' body composition and the calculation of a desirable body weight (see Chapter 7).

Goal Setting

Goal setting is usually accomplished concurrently with any education component and it is best done on an individual basis. Education and service goals are closely related. Within the service component, however, goal setting relates specifically to exercise goals.

Short- and long-term service goals are established by referring to the fitness profile and projecting goals for each fitness area that needs improvement. Short-range goals should build toward the long-term goal.

The participant should be involved in the establishment of both short- and long-term goals. The specialist's role is to assure that these goals are both reasonable and safe. Goals must be realistic or participants may lose their motivation; unrealistic goals also may be unsafe. Goals should be renewable.

Planning

On the program level, planning is a management process; it will be discussed in Chapter 13. In this section, we will discuss group- and individual-level planning.

Using the group planning approach, you should plan facility use. Most programming must be scheduled for early morning, lunch time, and the hours after work.

Plan course length. Exercise classes generally are 8 to 12 weeks. Adherence tends to be better in programs of shorter length. Moreover, participants who must miss several classes tend to wait until the next session to reschedule their exercise. The shorter the course, the shorter the layoff period. Finally, beginning a new course keeps people interested.

Try to group classes by ability. Each new session brings newcomers. If possible, people should be grouped so that beginners and advanced participants are not in the same class.

Seasonal changes influence planning. Structured fitness classes attract large enrollment in the fall and winter months when the weather is unpleasant, holiday foods present temptation, and New Year's resolutions are made. In contrast, spring and summer months are not the best time to plan structured exercise classes; most participants prefer outdoor, individualized activities. Informal club activities such as water skiing, softball, tennis, and SCUBA are more successful during these periods.

Early morning and late afternoon classes can be longer than those at midday. Classes should be scheduled at least three times per week to ensure the potential for a training effect. Intervening days should be scheduled

for activities that are likely to be used as weekend recreational pursuits, such as racquet sports.

The format of a course should provide progression. Early stages in an exercise course should be less strenuous than the latter stages.

Periodic motivational techniques will help maintain participant interest, especially during periods such as holidays, when poor attendance can be anticipated. Awards, incentives, and contests are appropriate techniques to boost motivation. The early enthusiasm for exercise displayed by new participants usually is replaced by boredom if the exercise program is repetitive and uneventful. Creative exercise leaders plan "fun" activities frequently (see Chapter 12).

The program must be convenient for participants. Easy access to the exercise facility is important. The facility itself should have locker room and exercise areas.

You should also plan your record keeping. Good registration forms, exercise record keeping, and progress monitoring are discussed in Chapter 14.

Make sure your activities offer diversity. Not everyone likes to jog! But you can also provide programs in aerobic dancing, aquatics, cycling, and walking. Calisthenics, weight training, and circuit training all develop strength. Flexibility can be improved by stretching, yoga, relaxation training, and low-back exercises. You can also plan a variety of recreational sports, such as racquet sports, aquatics, team sports, or leisure activities (SCUBA, backpacking).

Many participants travel often. Develop an exercise program that they can use while in a motel room or at facilities other than the onsite program. You can also schedule exercise during morning and afternoon breaks.

To promote adherence, plan a program that allows involvement of influential persons such as spouses. Some programs, for example, open their facilities to families on weekends.

Finally, you must not neglect program safety and emergency procedures. Equipment and facilities should be inspected for safety. All personnel should be CPR trained and maintain certification. Emergency procedures should be practiced at regular intervals.

Planning can also take place on an individual level. Although motivated participants do not need an individual counseling session, many participants need more direction and can benefit from planning. Discuss with them: *mode* (What kind of exercise does the individual need and want?); *frequency* (How often will the participant need to and be able to schedule the exercise?); *intensity* (How intense should the exercise be? For example, what exercise heart rates should be achieved during aerobic exercise; what sets and repetitions should be performed in the strength development program?); *duration* (How long will the participant need to and be able to exercise during each exercise session?); *rate of progression* (When should the participant expect to see a change in fitness and how much improvement should be expected?); and *duration of training* (How long should the participant pursue the exercise program prior to a follow-up evaluation?).

Implementation

The successful implementation of an exercise program requires good organization and administration, well-trained personnel, a varied program, and convenient, well-equipped facilities. All of these will be discussed later in the book. This discussion will focus on processing of participants through the program. We assume that management support and facilities are available.

For both practical and economic purposes, the implementation of exercise programs must be viewed as a group process. The health/fitness specialist must create an environment that promotes interest and involvement, yet is accomplished at the least possible cost in terms of personnel time and capital expenditure. The program director's duties are discussed in detail in Chapters 4 and 15. Many are "behind the scenes" tasks that are not readily seen by the participants in their daily exercise programs. More visible is the exercise leadership provided in the classes.

The exercise leader probably has the most influence on the success of the program because she or he provides the interface between the program and its participants. The leader is more important than facilities, types of activities, or any other feature of a program. A good leader can encourage the enthusiasm and vitality necessary to stave off the apathy that so often develops among participants and creates high dropout rates. The exercise leader should possess a number of traits and skills, as discussed in Chapters 4 and 15.

Among the important considerations in the implementation of exercise activities are safety and injury prevention. Safety precautions appropriate to the particular activity should be discussed at the beginning of any exercise class. Assure that proper apparel and equipment are used. Schedule 5- to 10-minute warm-up and cool-down periods. If heat and humidity are oppressive, temper the amount of exercise expected of participants.

You should also adjust activities to the age and sex of the participants. An individual's work capacity generally declines with age, as does the heart rate required to achieve a training effect. Moreover, lean body mass tends to diminish, reducing the amount of muscle tissue available to overcome resistance in weight training. Finally, people tend to become less flexible with advancing age. Women generally have less cardiovascular endurance and muscular strength than do men, but they tend to have greater flexibility. Women tend to enjoy group activities more than do men.

Finally, a few principles serve as guidelines for successful programming:

- Overload: a certain threshold of exertion is necessary for adaptation to exercise training. Too little exertion will produce no results; too much will produce injury.

- Specificity: each exercise is designed to produce a unique result that has little transfer to other areas of performance. One will not, for example, get stronger from a jogging program.

- Use and disuse: the body adapts to exercise only when it is used regularly and in a progressive fashion of overload. Irregular or intermittent exercise will result in little improvement, if any.

■ Individual differences: everyone responds to exercise training in a unique fashion. Program adjustments can accommodate these differences.

Evaluation

Evaluation should be an ongoing facet of the program. A complete evaluation of the test battery can be performed for each participant every year. Retesting shows the progress made during the year and motivates participants to adhere to their exercise program. It also permits new goals, plans, and implementation strategies to be generated.

You can also conduct more frequent, less comprehensive tests that are tailored to the goals and needs of each participant. This can be accomplished at the end of a course or can be scheduled separately. Moreover, there is a critical period, about 3 or 4 months after starting an exercise program, when the participant is getting over the initial aches and pains and needs to see results. In fact, the motivation provided by these tests is probably more important than the data obtained. In addition, the improvements thus documented allow you to evaluate the overall program and the effectiveness of various activities in promoting health and fitness.

Summary

This chapter presented some practical guidelines for implementing an effective exercise program. Needs assessment of the participants is based on both objective and subjective data, which help you to screen participants and set up realistic and appropriate short- and long-term goals. An important aspect of the program is the exercise leader, whose role it is to encourage enthusiasm, prevent injury, and control the exertion level and execution of each exercise. Periodic evaluation of the participants will enable you to make adjustments to the individual's exercise program and to judge the overall effectiveness of the program.

Reference

1.   American College of Sports Medicine. *Guidelines for graded exercise testing and exercise prescription*, 2d ed. Philadelphia: Lea and Febiger, 1980.

WEIGHT CONTROL

Weight control is a core offering in health/fitness programs. In this chapter we will show how to implement this service using our generic implementation model.

Approximately 25% of adult Americans attempt to reduce their body weight each year at a cost of at least $10 billion annually. At least 25% of preadult Americans are obese: about 70 million people.[1] Obesity is associated with level of education, sex, race, and wealth. Men with high incomes tend to be 20% fatter than those who earn less; men with a college education are 10% heavier than those with only high school educations. Women follow almost the reverse pattern: wealthier women are 20% thinner than males with the same incomes, and more-educated women are 20% thinner than less-educated ones. Black American men are thinner than white American men, but black women are heavier than white women. Americans of British descent tend to be thinner than those of Eastern European backgrounds. Yet, as a population we are suffering from creeping obesity. Approximately one-third of the U.S. population is overweight to a degree that diminishes life expectancy.[2]

Being overweight and being obese are not synonymous. *Overweight* usually is defined as body weight in excess of a standard established for one's height and sex. *Obesity* is defined as an excessive accumulation of body fat regardless of body weight. It is possible, therefore, for an individual to be overweight but not overfat or obese, as are virtually all professional football players. Conversely, it is possible to be underweight and yet be obese, as are many diet conscious but sedentary individuals. Notwithstanding the distinction, a person 20% or more above ideal weight is considered to be obese. The normal range of body fat among young adults, however, is 10% to 15% of weight for men and 20% to 25% for women. The aging process generally results in progressively increased percent body fat values.

Etiology of Obesity

The origin of obesity frequently is traced to childhood. Overweight infants tend to become overweight children; more than 80% of overweight children become overweight adults. The odds against an obese child becoming a normal–body-weighted adult are 4:1 at age 12 years and increase to 28:1 if the weight has not been reduced by the end of adolescence. Once an individual becomes obese, there is a high probability that the problem will persist.

Most overweight individuals want to reduce their excess body weight for cosmetic reasons. Although personal motives related to enhancement of physical appearance have merit, there are many physical and psychosocial problems that are caused or exacerbated by obesity. Obesity is associated with increased mortality at all ages, because the risks of cardiovascular disease (hypertension and coronary heart disease), diabetes mellitus, gallbladder disease, and any surgical procedure are increased. Numerous other physical health problems are associated with obesity. The psychological effects of obesity are just as serious: low self-esteem, poor body image, decreased employment opportunities, restricted social development, anxiety, and possibly behavioral immaturity.

The cause of obesity ultimately is consumption of more calories than the body uses. For every 3500 excess calories, 1 pound of body fat is formed and stored (each pound of adipose tissue is 87% fat; because 1 pound equals 454 grams, 0.87×454 g/lb $\times$ 9 kcal/g = 3555 kcal/lb). The manner in which the fat is stored and the point in time when excessive caloric intake occurs affect substantially the control of obesity.

There are two major types of obesity: (1) *hyperplastic*—the formation of *additional fat cells* during critical periods (last trimester of pregnancy, infancy, and adolescence) because of excess caloric intake; and (2) *hypertrophic*—the formation of *excessively large* fat cells (characteristic of adult-onset obesity) because of excess caloric intake. Thus, it appears that once adulthood is achieved a constant number of fat cells, or *adipocytes*, is established. They neither increase nor decrease in number under most conditions—they merely expand or contract. Thus, obese individuals who lose weight tend to gain it back quickly—the abundant adipocytes are available as vacant storage sites.

Animal studies have demonstrated that genetic factors can contribute to obesity. The incidence of obesity in children with two lean parents is about 9%; in those with one obese parent 40%; and in those with two obese parents 80%. Those who support an environmental etiology of obesity, however, would counter the conclusion that obesity is genetically determined by suggesting that if more individuals in a family are obese, it creates an environment conducive to obesity. Further, a study demonstrated that adopted children tend to display a similar incidence of obesity as do other children in obese families.

The quantity and quality of the dietary intake of calories significantly influence the incidence of obesity. Leaner individuals tend to consume more vegetables, fruits, and complex carbohydrates, whereas fatter individuals tend to consume more meats, sweets, and fatty foods. There is a direct relationship between the caloric density of these foods and obesity: the lower the caloric density of commonly eaten foods, the leaner the individual. Table 7.1 illustrates this relationship.

Other support for the environmental etiology of obesity is found in the physical activity patterns of normoweight and obese individuals. Although obese individuals may not eat any more than the nonobese, they have been shown to be far less active and to seek out sedentary situations. This creates a self-perpetuating condition in that the less an obese person moves, the more obese he or she becomes—and thus becomes even less likely to move about, and so on. This cycle of events becomes a trap for many obese people.

Many other environmental factors may contribute to obesity: availability of food, sedentary lifestyle, poor eating habits, stressful occupation, and emotional factors. Researchers generally agree that the obesity syndrome has a multifactorial etiology—physiological, psychological, hereditary, and environmental causes contribute to the problem.

❚ T A B L E 7 . 1 ❚
Caloric Density of Preferred Foods for Lean and Obese Individuals

Weight of Individual	Preferred Foods	Caloric Density (kcal/oz)
Lean	Vegetables	5–10
	Fruits	15
	Complex carbohydrates	50
Obese	Meats	75
	Sweets	150
	Fats/oils	170–270

Starting a Weight-Control Program

The weight-control program can be provided by inhouse or contract services. Depending on the facilities available, an inhouse program may meet the needs of the participants quite adequately. A classroom, cafeteria, exercise equipment, jogging track, racquetball courts, and showers would provide ample facilities for an effective weight-control program. On the other hand, lack of facilities should not be a deterrent to establishing a good weight-control program. Many organizations provide weight-control services on a contractual basis. Table 7.2 lists several services from which you can contract weight-control programs.

Because most health/fitness specialists are not highly trained in weight-control techniques, outside resources may be most effective. Certainly, all participants should be medically screened prior to entering a weight-reduction program. This is especially important when the participants have heart disease, diabetes, or other serious health problems. Also, extremely young or old individuals should be referred to agencies where their special needs can be met. The weight-control program we suggest is most appropriate for individuals whose goal is to lose less than 50 pounds. The very obese often resent attending a program with relatively thin people and should be placed in a separate group or referred to another agency.

A good strategy is a two-program approach. An offsite program may be best for those participants who have been medically screened and have special needs—the very obese, diabetics, and so on. An inhouse program is for those participants who are relatively free of complicating disease and wish to lose 50 pounds or less. This group can be treated within the normal health/fitness program especially if you have a cafeteria and gym. Special exercise classes scheduled at appropriate times in separate facilities as well as menu-planning guides could be blended into a typical program.

Assume that a group of individuals who want to lose weight has been identified. These individuals are not morbidly obese and have come to the health/fitness specialist for help. We will use the combined education and service approach to the generic implementation model. We assume there are available modest facilities including a gym and a cafeteria.

Needs Assessment

The needs assessment should use data from medical screening to eliminate participants with potential health problems, such as diabetics and those needing special care. A medical history and physical examination should be administered prior to admission to a weight-control program. Also, a readiness questionnaire provides a means of selecting participants who are ready to work on their need to lose weight.

The participants selected should be *committed* individuals—those whose attitude is "This time I'm going to give it my best shot." Individuals who give control of their weight top priority will not degrade the program with personal anecdotes and excuses for failure; they will assume responsibility for their weight control and nurture the success of everyone involved. The individual who signs up because of pressure from a spouse or physician is not likely to succeed. A good way to identify individuals who are committed is to administer the checklist in Figure 7.1. A participant who gives positive responses on this instrument probably will demonstrate good adherence to and eventual success in the program. Once a group composed of dedicated weight losers is established, assess their weight-control needs.

Cultural Assessment

There are many negative norms in our culture that predispose people to the problem of obesity. The health/fitness professional must determine the degree to which attitudes regarding eating and exercise behaviors influence an individual's obesity problem. Figure 7.2 provides a checklist of these potentially adverse cultural indicators. Should the participants believe that any of these factors affect their attitudes toward

■ T A B L E 7 . 2 ■
A Sample of Available Weight-Control Services

Name	Treatment Mode	Approximate Cost	Comments
Weight Watchers 800 Community Manhasset, NY 11030 (516) 627-9200	Behavior modification; lectures; regular meetings	$20 to start; $6 per week	Good nutrition; exercise is not emphasized
Nutri-System Weight Loss Medical Centers Old York and Rydall Roads Jenkins, PA 19046 (215) 576-4000	Individual counseling on nutrition and exercise by professionals; planned low-calorie meals; behavior modification	Varies with the individual; based on pounds to lose and how fast lost	Could be quite expensive; aerobic exercise not emphasized
Weight Clinics of America 11520 N. Central Dallas, TX 75243 (214) 340-2222	Hypnosis and behavior modification; optional diets; individual counseling	$15 per session; discounts available	Individuals could become dependent on hypnosis; aerobic exercise not emphasized
Diet Centers Inc. Corporate Headquarters Rexburgh, Idaho 83440 (208) 356-9381	Behavior modification; well-balanced high-nutrient diet plans	$65 registration fee; $38.50 each week	Aerobic exercise not emphasized; good low-calorie nutrition

Norwell Weight Loss Centers 3705 Westheimer Houston, TX 77027 (713) 944-4444	Nutrition programs individually designed by professionals; behavior modification; weekly visits	$95 for maintenance and weekly visits	Exercise not emphasized; costly
Schick Centers for Control of Weight and Smoking 45 E. Alamar Boulevard Santa Barbara, CA 93105 (805) 687-2411	Behavior modification (aversion therapy)	$35 per visit	No individual counseling; no emphasis on nutrition or exercise
Thin For Life Clinics P.O. Box 2894 Durham, NC 27705 (919) 683-5547	Rice diets emphasized; regular exercise	$160–$195 per week	Major impetus is exercise
Pritikin Longevity Center P.O. Box 5335 Santa Barbara, CA 93108 (805) 969-7756	Diet, exercise, medical screening, and counseling	$3400 for 13-day session; $6500 for 26-day session	An effective combination of diet, exercise, and education; quite expensive (may emphasize too low a proportion of dietary fat intake for essential fatty acid intakes)

■ **Figure 7.1** Readiness questionnaire for weight-control program. (Adapted from Nash, J. P., and Ormiston, L. H. *Taking charge of your weight and well being.* Palo Alto, CA: Bull, 1978, pp. 11–12. Used by permission.) ■

1. Are you ready to devote the time and energy necessary to control your weight? Yes __ No __

2. Are you prepared to attend *all* the scheduled meetings we will have in this program? Yes __ No __

3. Will weight reduction and control be your *top* priority during this program? Yes __ No __

4. Is weight loss truly the personal problem you are most concerned about? Yes __ No __

5. Do you have approval from your physician to undertake weight reduction? Yes __ No __

6. Are you willing to schedule regular exercise in your daily life? Yes __ No __

7. Are you entering this weight-control program with a positive attitude and the expectation of reaching a target body weight? Yes __ No __

food or exercise, educational counseling may help. Counseling should be individual.

Knowledge Assessment

The health/fitness professional must understand the knowledge base of the participants before they enter the program. People often have many misconceptions about diet and exercise, and these may contribute to failure. Figure 7.3 is a simple test to assess the knowledge base of participants regarding weight control.

Height and Weight Assessment

The health/fitness professional can make a rough assessment of the participants' need to alter present body weight by using height and

■ **Figure 7.2** Cultural assessment checklist. (Adapted from Allen, R. *Lifegain.* New York: Appleton-Century-Crofts, 1981, p. 113. Used by permission.) ■

Instructions: Check off those items you see as normal for expected, accepted, or supported behaviors.

__ People see children who are slightly overweight as healthier and better cared for than children who are not.

__ Most people are a few pounds overweight.

__ People see desserts such as cake, pie, pudding, and ice cream as a usual part of lunch or dinner.

__ Sweets are thought of as special treats and therefore as more *rewarding* than most nutritious foods.

__ Parents encourage children not to leave food on their plates, even if it is more than they want or need.

__ People associate overindulging in food with relaxation, pleasure, and good social relationships.

__ Hosts and hostesses encourage guests to eat more food than is desirable.

__ People view the offer of large food portions as a sign of generosity.

__ People look at being slightly overweight as natural, particularly among older people.

__ People eat more food than they want or need.

__ People lose weight through dieting but gain it right back again.

__ People find pie-eating, watermelon-eating, and other eating contests to be amusing parts of our culture.

__ People think or say "Everybody loves a fat person."

__ People think it is natural for those in certain ethnic groups to be overweight.

__ People eat when they are lonely or their feelings are hurt.

__ People feed children more than they need for growth and health because it shows love.

__ People think regular exercise is a waste of time.

weight tables. These tables provide only a general indicator. Most of these tables were developed by life insurance companies from data on populations of adult Americans who were already overweight. Table 7.3 has several limitations; however, it does give recommended (rather than average) body weights.

Note that Table 7.3 gives a large weight range for each height. Much depends on an individual's structure. Individuals who are very muscular (such as athletes) may be overweight by the tables but have as little as 5% of their total body weight accounted for by fat tissue. Or people may be well within the limits of the recommended body weight range and have a large percentage of their body weight represented by fat tissue—typical of sedentary but weight-conscious females and most sedentary elderly individuals. Thus, height/weight indices are poor indicators of the makeup of an individual's body weight.

It is also common for individuals who have sedentary lifestyles to have a steady reduction in lean body weight percentage as they age. Reduced physical activity results in atrophy of muscle tissues, which frequently is replaced by fat deposits. Figure 7.4 illustrates the effect of a reduced muscle mass on basal metabolic rate (bmr) and also illustrates the decreased need for calories as a person ages.

Because the energy requirement of lean tissue (especially muscle) is significantly greater than that of fat tissue, retention of muscle mass as a person ages promotes continued BMR

■ T A B L E 7 . 3 ■
Recommended Weight in Relation to Height

Height*	Weight for Men		Weight for Women	
	Recommended	Range	Recommended	Range
4'10"	—	—	102	92–119
4'11"	—	—	104	94–122
5'0"	—	—	107	96–125
5'1"	—	—	110	99–128
5'2"	123	112–141	113	102–131
5'3"	127	115–144	116	105–134
5'4"	130	118–148	120	108–138
5'5"	133	121–152	123	111–142
5'6"	136	124–156	128	114–146
5'7"	140	128–161	132	118–150
5'8"	145	132–166	136	122–154
5'9"	149	136–170	140	126–158
5'10"	153	140–174	144	130–163
5'11"	158	144–179	148	134–168
6'0"	162	148–184	152	138–173
6'1"	166	152–189	—	—
6'2"	171	156–194	—	—
6'3"	176	160–199	—	—
6'4"	181	164–204	—	—

*Height without shoes; weight without clothes.

▌ Figure 7.3 Knowledge assessment for diet and exercise. (Adapted from Allen, R. ▌
Lifegain. New York: Appleton-Century-Crofts, 1981. Used by permission.)

Questions:

1.	It is natural to get fatter as you get older.	True	False
2.	It makes no difference whether a person eats slowly or quickly.	True	False
3.	Toasting reduces the calories in bread.	True	False
4.	Alcohol furnishes calories to the body.	True	False
5.	People who overeat are simply hungrier than those who eat less.	True	False
6.	Although exercise is a good thing, it cannot contribute much toward helping us reduce our weight and maintain our proper weight level.	True	False
7.	The best way to lose weight is to cut back all your food intake drastically.	True	False
8.	The most important factor in weight control for most people is not hormonal but the individual's handling of food.	True	False
9.	If you do not succeed in reaching the weight indicated for you on the standard weight chart, you have failed.	True	False
10.	If you are embarking on a program of extensive weight reduction, the first thing to do is skip at least one of the three meals you ordinarily eat each day.	True	False
11.	Being overweight can be a contributing factor to such problems as heart disease, diabetes, and hypertension.	True	False
12.	Exercise will only make me eat more.	True	False
13.	A person who eats too much is more likely to be getting the vitamins and minerals she or he needs than someone who eats less.	True	False
14.	If you can lose those extra pounds just once, you can go back to eating the way you do now because you are not gaining weight now.	True	False
15.	Most people gain weight when they stop smoking, so it is better to go on smoking rather than get fat.	True	False

Answers:

1. FALSE. Many people do grow fatter as they get older, but it is not natural or necessary. As a person grows older, metabolism and physical activity often decrease. Fat begins to accumulate as the person takes in, day after day, more food than his or her body uses. The answer: eat less and exercise more.

2. FALSE. Most overweight people eat quickly. They consume large amounts of food without even realizing it. One should always eat slowly and chew food well. This gives the sugar-regulatory mechanisms of the body a chance to act on our appetite-regulating centers to allow us to be satisfied.

▮ Figure 7.3 Continued **▮**

3. FALSE. Burning the bread destroys some nutritive value but does not burn away the calories.

4. TRUE. A whiskey or a pint of beer is the caloric equivalent of a slice of bread and butter or an average portion of potatoes.

5. Only sometimes. Actually, many people who overeat do a lot of eating after their hunger is already satisfied.

6. FALSE. It *can* contribute a good deal, but it takes time. To work off 1 pound of fat takes 7.5 hours of bicycling, but the effects are cumulative. A 1-hour bike ride each day means 1 pound per week. The best combination is exercise *plus* lower calorie intake.

7. FALSE. It is not how much you eat, it is *what* you eat. In addition, a drastic reduction in intake is rarely effective in long-range weight control, as it cannot be maintained; it is often unhealthy, because you do not get proper nutrients.

8. TRUE. Although there are isolated cases of persons whose weight control is seriously affected by heredity or disease, for most people the control of their weight is in their own hands.

9. FALSE. First, the ideal weight for you may be somewhat higher or lower than that on the chart. Second, if you are 40 pounds overweight and manage to get down to 20 pounds overweight, you are that much better off. Fifty percent success may not be as good as 100%, but it is certainly better than nothing.

10. FALSE. Usually, skipping meals is not a good idea. It is better to cut down on high-calorie, high-carbohydrate foods. Actually, the first thing you should do is consult your physician.

11. TRUE. Overweight can contribute to the onset of these and other illnesses or exacerbate and magnify their effects.

12. FALSE. Studies have shown that, if anything, regular exercise tends to reduce excess food intake. One study reported that a little exercise tends to make you eat more, but substantial exercise tends to make you eat less.

13. FALSE. Many of the foods we eat contain "empty calories"—they have virtually no nutritional value. The quantity of food eaten has no necessary relation to the nutritional quality of a diet.

14. FALSE. What is a maintenance diet for your present weight will be a weight-gaining diet when you get to a lower weight. Once you get to your desired weight, the best way to stay there is to eat the maintenance diet for that weight.

15. FALSE. The typical weight gain of a withdrawing smoker totals about 7 pounds, an amount not difficult to lose. It is true that exsmokers have a depressed basal metabolic rate, which exacerbates weight-control problems.

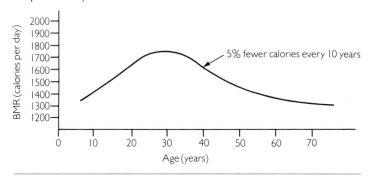

Figure 7.4 Basal metabolic rate (BMR) requirements at different ages. (Adapted from Cundiff, D., and Brynteson, P. *Health fitness: Guide to a life–style.* Dubuque, IO: Kendall/Hunt, 1979, p. 93. Copyright © 1979 by Kendall/Hunt Publishing Company. Used by permission.)

elevation. Appropriate exercise programs for muscular strength development can help older individuals retain muscle mass and thus a high BMR (Figure 7.5).

Body Composition Assessment

The fat and lean components of an individual are best measured by hydrostatic techniques, but these require expensive equipment and considerable time. The most common technique used in health/fitness programs is to estimate body density by evaluating skinfold thickness with calipers. Because approximately 50% of the total fat of a young adult is deposited subcutaneously, skinfold thicknesses at specific sites allow you to estimate overall fat percentage. Different formulas are available; most use several different skinfold sites. The most widely

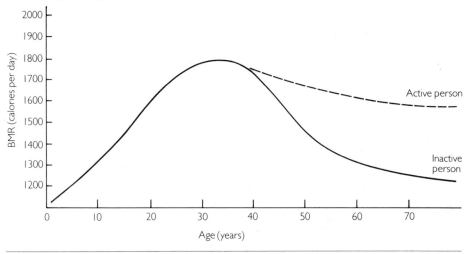

Figure 7.5 Hypothetical comparison of active and sedentary adults in terms of BMR changes with age.

■ **Figure 7.6** Nomogram for estimating percent body fat from skinfold thickness measurements. (From ■ Baun, W., Baun, M., and Raven, P. A monogram for the estimate of percent body fat from generalized equations. *Research Quarterly for Exercise and Sport*, 1981, pp. 52, 380–384. Used by permission of William Baun, Tenneco Health and Fitness Department.)

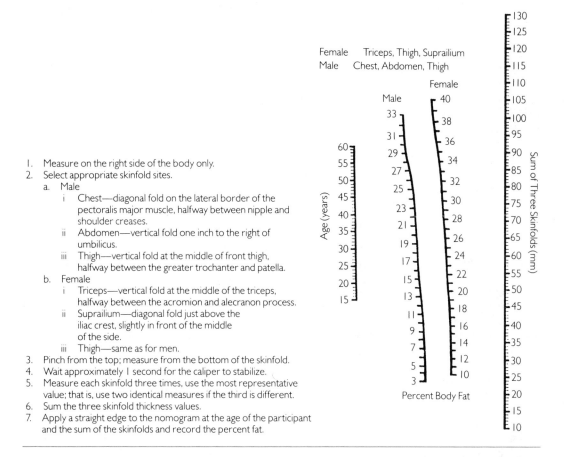

1. Measure on the right side of the body only.
2. Select appropriate skinfold sites.
   a. Male
      i Chest—diagonal fold on the lateral border of the pectoralis major muscle, halfway between nipple and shoulder creases.
      ii Abdomen—vertical fold one inch to the right of umbilicus.
      iii Thigh—vertical fold at the middle of front thigh, halfway between the greater trochanter and patella.
   b. Female
      i Triceps—vertical fold at the middle of the triceps, halfway between the acromion and alecranon process.
      ii Suprailium—diagonal fold just above the iliac crest, slightly in front of the middle of the side.
      iii Thigh—same as for men.
3. Pinch from the top; measure from the bottom of the skinfold.
4. Wait approximately 1 second for the caliper to stabilize.
5. Measure each skinfold three times, use the most representative value; that is, use two identical measures if the third is different.
6. Sum the three skinfold thickness values.
7. Apply a straight edge to the nomogram at the age of the participant and the sum of the skinfolds and record the percent fat.

used skinfold assessment is described in Figure 7.6, a nomogram.

Sample Needs Assessment

To illustrate the needs assessment in action, we will use a fictitious Ms. Jones, an executive who is free of serious disease and wants to lose about 30 pounds. She is committed to losing weight, but has several misconceptions and very little knowledge about nutrition and exercise. Her height-to-weight ratio is below average, and 35% of her body weight is fat. Her medical screening included a physical activity history and nutritional assessment. Ms. Jones has been sedentary for a number of years and eats out most of the time or snacks on the run. Figure 7.7 profiles Ms. Jones's present status. This profile is typical of a person ready to enter a weight-control program with good potential for success. Ms. Jones is aware of her needs and is committed to doing something about her problem.

Figure 7.7 Ms. Jones's weight-control program profile.

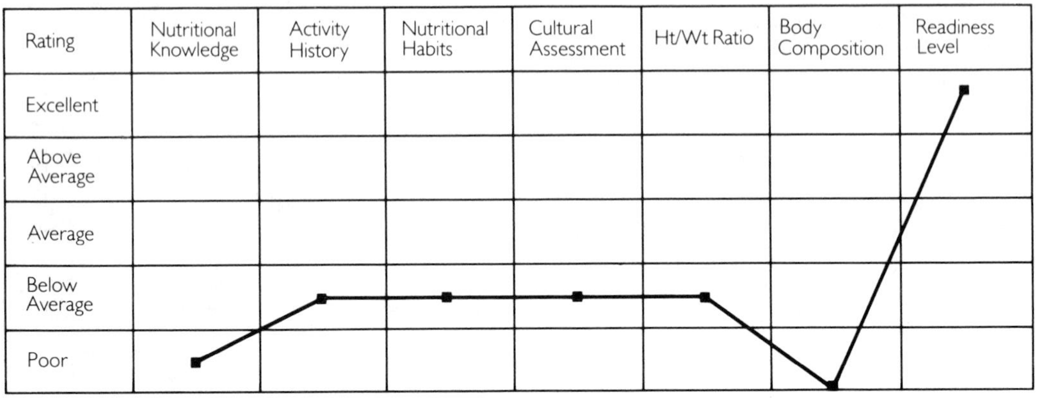

Rating	Nutritional Knowledge	Activity History	Nutritional Habits	Cultural Assessment	Ht/Wt Ratio	Body Composition	Readiness Level
Excellent							■
Above Average							
Average							
Below Average		■	■	■	■		
Poor	■					■	

Goal Setting

Needs assessment can be performed in a group. Goal setting, however, must be done in an individual counseling session: it is a private process. This is also a time when you can discuss candidly the participants' present condition and desired weight loss. The best strategy is first to find out what the participant believes to be his or her desirable body weight. Then, discuss the body composition data and calculation of the desired body weight. Set a target body weight in stages. For example, Ms. Jones presently has 35% fat and is far too heavy for her height. A staged set of goals might be to achieve a body weight of 30% fat, then of 25% fat as a final goal. The calculation of desired body weights at given fat percentages is illustrated in Figure 7.8.

Ms. Jones must lose approximately 10 pounds of body weight to reduce 5% of body fat. The aspiring weight reducer frequently desires a body weight considerably below the level indicated by computing desirable body weight from body composition. Ms. Jones, for example, expressed a desire to lose 30 pounds, whereas her body composition assessments indicated a need for only 20 pounds weight loss. Many obese individuals carry a large lean body mass because of the energy required simply to support their large body weight when they walk and move around. There appears to be an upper limit of about 50% fat, beyond which a person cannot get any fatter and still be able to walk. Because of this, many overweight individuals may be unable to lose a great deal of their unwanted pounds simply because a lot of it is muscle tissue.

Goals set for desirable body weight should be staged in short- and long-term targets. A reasonable expectation of 1 to 2 pounds weight loss each week should be within the reach of most participants. Any loss in excess of this could be deleterious to health and result in lean body weight lose. Moreover, compliance with a reasonable regime is much better than with a starvation-oriented approach.

Lean body mass must be considered in setting a target weight. Most attempts at weight loss involve austere caloric intake, and caution must be exercised to avoid muscle mass loss. Frequent tests of body composition allow you to monitor and develop strategies to avoid wasting away of muscle tissues. Lean body mass preservation should be part of the goal.

To achieve weight reduction, a participant must make behavioral changes. Set behavioral goals that will significantly influence progress toward the long-term goal. Ms. Jones may have discovered from previous nutritional assessments that she overindulges in her evening meal. A short-term goal she might set would be to decrease the portions of food she eats at

Figure 7.8 Calculating Ms. Jones's desirable body weight. ∎

Given: Desirable body weight = DBW = ?
Present body weight = PBW = 150 pounds
Present % fat = % Fat = 35%
Fat body weight = FBW = PBW × % Fat = 150 × .35 = 52.5 pounds
Lean body weight = LBW = PBW − FBW = 150 − 52.5 = 97.49 pounds

Calculation:

$$DBW = \frac{LBW}{1 - \text{desired } \% \text{ Fat}} \quad \text{(Calculating target body weight formula)}$$

$$DBW_{(Stage\ 1)} = \frac{97.5}{1.0 - .30} = \frac{97.5}{.70} = 139 \text{ pounds} \quad \text{(Target body weight at } 30\% \text{ Fat—goal \#1)}$$

$$DBW_{(Stage\ 2)} = \frac{97.5}{1.0 - .25} = \frac{97.5}{.75} = 130 \text{ pounds} \quad \text{(Target body weight at } 25\% \text{ Fat—goal \#2)}$$

night for two nights during the next week. When she has accomplished this goal, she can set a goal for the next week to decrease portions for at least four nights. This process continues until she gains control of her eating and establishes a regular behavior pattern for her evening meal.

The small goals are like stair steps to the top target goal (ideal weight). They must be both challenging and attainable. The following elements of appropriate goal setting may be useful: (1) define behavioral goals, such as I will put my fork down between bites, I will take a walk when I get angry, I won't buy fattening foods; (2) set short-term goals, such as next week I will . . . , tomorrow I will . . . , between now and bedtime I will . . . ; and (3) choose small, realistic goals, such as 4 days of 7 I will . . . , I will plan at least one snack. . . .[3]

Ms. Jones agrees to commit herself to a new lifestyle of weight management. This commitment can be initiated by signing a written agreement (contract) or by simply filling out a goal sheet. Figure 7.9 is such a contract. Notice that rewards and punishments are built into the contract—this is contingency management.

Behavior modification should be included in goal setting and planning. This approach is individualistic because each person's eating habits are unique. Behavior modification begins with detailed data about the participants' dietary behavior, which can be obtained from dietary recall procedures (Chapter 9). Next, the participant records events prior to, during, and after eating that seem to maintain the intake of certain foods. The participant is then taught stimulus-control techniques to help change the events that affect eating.

Planning

∎

Developing a sound blueprint for implementation involves planning both exercise and nutrition (see Chapters 6 and 9). Certain aspects of each of these program elements need special attention.

Exercise Program

Planning exercise requires special attention to facilities. Aerobics exercise facilities are needed. Non–weight-bearing aerobic modalities, such as aquatics, bicycle ergometers, and rowing machines, are particularly useful, especially for older and heavier participants in whom orthopedic injuries are likely. Group activities are

■ **Figure 7.9** Sample weight-control contract. ■

As of _____ at _____ I agree to commit
      date   time
to losing _____ per week for 4 weeks.
         pounds
Accordingly, _____
         health/fitness director
     and I have agreed on the
     following contingencies:
If I lose _____ between _____ and
       pounds   date
_____ I will receive from _____
 date
the following: _____
         specific reward
If I fail to lose _____ during this time,
         pounds
the following will result:

_____
      specific alternative
Signed: _____
         name
Signed: _____
       health/fitness director
Date: _____

best. The participants probably are not habituated to exercise and can benefit from the presence of others who are at the same stage of conditioning. Their exercise program should consist of carefully designed progressions, with gradual increases in work. The transition from walking to jogging, for example, might include weighted belts or "Heavy Hands" with walking. Begin with shorter classes to give the participants a sense of accomplishment when they finish the full period.

Ability grouping is important. Homogeneous groups are best; however, this is not always possible. The health/fitness professional should plan subsets of groups or at least a partner approach to instruction. Moreover, people should move from the weight-control class to the regular exercise program as soon as possible. This can be a big boost to the participants' morale.

Motivational techniques should be employed frequently with the weight-control group (Chapter 15). Incentives could be awarded, for example, for the best attendance, most weight lost, or most miles walked.

Make contingency plans for those who temporarily "fall off the wagon" and fail to exercise for extended periods—develop guidelines for resumption of exercise. Also, make plans for those who must be out of town regularly.

Nutrition Program

Nutrition planning occurs in three broad areas: (1) dietary reductions; (2) group education and support; and (3) behavior modification.

Probably the most important aspect of planning a dietary-reduction program for participants is to have them avoid dangerous diets. Table 7.4 illustrates some of the popular but possibly dangerous diets, briefly describes these diets, and provides reasons for avoiding them.

Dietary reduction will be greatly enhanced by the participants' recognition of safe and healthy ways to limit caloric intake, which requires education. Here are some suggestions: arrange lectures or seminars on topics such as low-density food selection, the Senate Select Committee's nutrition recommendations, or consumer education; teach food preparation, such as low-fat cooking, high-fiber menus, and healthy heart recipes; distribute educational materials, such as those provided by the American Heart Association, the American Dietetic Association, and the American Cancer Society.

Group support can be effective in the weight-reduction program; it can be provided by external resources, such as Weight Watchers, or by an inhouse support group. In an inhouse group: (1) membership should be limited to committed individuals; (2) regular attendance should be required; (3) groups should be small to promote cohesion and interaction; (4) meetings should be scheduled at convenient times; (5) the duration of the meeting should be limited; (6) the group leader should help to make interactions constructive; and (7) the group should provide a forum for failure in which participants can learn to cope with minor setbacks.

▮ T A B L E 7 . 4 ▮
Dangerous Diets: Eaters Beware

Diet Plan	Brief Description	Reasons for Avoiding
Air Force Diet	Low-carbohydrate diet	Unbalanced; causes ketosis and other undesirable side effects; weight loss primarily due to water loss
Beverly Hills Diet	Fruit for 10 days, gradually add other foods but separate foods eaten with "conscious combining"	Unbalanced; based on myths; serious side effects including diarrhea, dehydration, nutrient deficiencies
Cambridge Diet Plan	Very-low-calorie liquid diet formula (330 calories per day)	Dangerously low in calories; serious side effects can damage health
Dr. Atkin's Diet	Low-carbohydrate, high-protein diet	Unbalanced; high in fat/cholesterol; causes ketosis and other serious side effects; weight loss primarily due to water loss
Dr. Stillman's Quick Weight Loss Diet	Low-carbohydrate diet	Unbalanced; causes ketosis and other undesirable side effects; weight loss primarily due to water loss
Fasting	Juices, teas, and/or water only	Dangerous; unbalanced; effective only temporarily
F-Plan Diet	Low-calorie, high-fiber diet	May be deficient in calcium and undesirably high in fiber
Fructose Diet	Low-carbohydrate diet, with relatively large intake of fructose	Fructose does not provide weight-loss benefits claimed
Last Chance Diet	Very-low-calorie liquid-protein diet	Protein of poor quality; side effects include nutrient deficiencies, abnormal heartbeats, death
Liquid Protein Diets	Formula with low-calorie intake plan	Protein may be poor quality; unbalanced; temporary at best; nutrient deficiencies can develop
Mayo Diet	Grapefruit eaten before meals to "burn" fat	Ineffective; based on myth; successful only if calories are reduced
Scarsdale Diet	High-protein diet	Unbalanced; potential for developing ketosis and nutrient deficiencies
Southampton Diet	Low-calorie diet with "mood foods"	Promises unrealistic results; promotes nutrition nonsense
Starch Blocker Diet	Diet supplements supposedly block caloric contributions of starch foods	Ineffective; supplements (now illegal) can cause digestive disturbances

(continued)

Diet Plan	Brief Description	Reasons for Avoiding
University Diet	Liquid-protein diet	Unbalanced; temporary at best; nutrient deficiencies can develop
Any more? Unfortunately, yes.	More of the same nonsense	Most likely unbalanced; dull; dangerous to your health; do not help you to adopt healthful eating patterns for permanent weight control

Source: Adapted from Stare, F., and Aronson, V. *Your Basic Guide to Nutrition.* George F. Stickley, 1983.

▌ Implementation

The implementation of a weight-control program involves reducing caloric intake and/or increasing caloric output: the concept is simple—the successful implementation is not. The success rate in weight-control programs is low—fewer than 10% of participants maintain target body weights achieved during a weight-control program. However, if 10% of a roster of 1000 members in a health/fitness program are successful, 100 people's lives will be immeasurably improved. Moreover, their health-care costs may be reduced, and their work performance may be improved. This type of programming is worth the effort! Implementation can begin with education classes such as those in Figure 7.10.

At the implementation stage of the weight-control program, participants are at risk. They are prone to injury during exercise, they will see few immediate results because they cannot exercise long or strenuously, and they cannot change their eating behaviors overnight and expect such changes to last. Thus, a breaking-in period of educational experiences may prove effective. Classes can be followed up later with formal or informal counseling.

The exercise program may require special planning; label the classes *beginners' rhythmic aquatics* or *starter class in rhythmic aerobics* to avoid stigma. Aside from genuine attempts to be sensitive to the special needs of these participants, few alterations in the regular exercise program need be made. In fact, the more mainstreaming with other program participants, the better. The following precautions are a good idea:

- Participants should wear special footwear to avoid excessive stress due to excess weight; for example, thick soles act as shock absorbers.
- Exercise should be staged in progressions regarding gravity; for example, aquatics, cycle ergometer, walking, and finally jogging.
- Exercise should be substituted for inactive habits; for example, use stairs instead of elevators, park a few blocks from work and walk.
- Overweight persons are more susceptible to heat stress, and therefore should be careful with respect to this matter.
- There is a greater risk of back, ankle, and knee injuries in the obese; thus exercises that stress these areas should be avoided.

The nutrition programming similarly requires little alteration. Some ideas that may prove particularly effective are:

- Remove vending machines with high-caloric-density foods or replace menu selections with lower-caloric-density foods.
- Color-code cafeteria foods.
- List caloric value on menus.

▌ Figure 7.10   Possible weight-control education class topics.   ▌

Exercise Topics

▌ Role of aerobic exercise
▌ Energy cost of various activities
▌ Intensity of exercise
▌ Duration of exercise
▌ Frequency of exercise
▌ Exercise and metabolic rate
▌ Exercise and appetite suppression
▌ Extension exercises while traveling
▌ Exercise log keeping
▌ Exercise and environmental stress—
   heat, humidity, cold
▌ Signs of overdoing it
▌ Exercise injuries when overweight—how
   to avoid
▌ Ingredients of a good workout—
   warmup, exercise, cooldown
▌ Progressions of a normal training
   program
▌ Use of appropriate equipment and
   apparel
▌ What to do when you take a vacation
   from exercise
▌ Spot-reducing misconceptions
▌ Exercise gimmicks
▌ Ways to increase physical activity in
   normal living
▌ Resource materials

Nutrition Topics

▌ Dangers of fad diets
▌ Low-fat diets
▌ High-fiber diets
▌ Dangers of high salt intake
▌ Dangers of high-protein diets
▌ Dangers of fasting
▌ High sugar intake—empty calories, low
   blood sugar
▌ Complex carbohydrates
▌ Caloric density and obesity
▌ Vegetarian diets
▌ Recommended food groups
▌ Vitamin and mineral supplements
▌ Meal planning
▌ How to eat healthy while eating out
▌ What to do when you fall off the wagon
▌ Healthy eating behaviors—how, when,
   where to eat
▌ Behavior substitution—good ones for
   bad ones
▌ Contingency management
▌ Consumer education regarding nutrition
▌ Dangers of diet pills
▌ Fat-burning gimmicks
▌ Resource materials

▌ Post motivational and educational materials
   on the walls of the cafeteria.
▌ Remove salt shakers from tables.
▌ Encourage participants who are cooking
   enthusiasts to bring low-caloric-density
   dishes for others; have contests for best
   casseroles, salads, and so on.

Some other tips for controlling eating behaviors are presented in Table 7.5.

Success in this phase of the weight-control
program depends on staff–participant interaction. Participants should feel that the staff are
concerned and available when needed. The
staff can use several techniques: feedback regarding monthly activity; positive comments regarding progress and efforts; incentives such as
T-shirts for weight loss; general availability to
encourage progress; and home or office calls

when the participant is absent from classes or
fails to attend program.

The recommendations of the American
College of Sports Medicine regarding weight-
loss programs are enumerated in Figure 7.11.

Evaluation   ▌

Evaluation of the participants' progress can
take several forms. Participants can be given the
same tests or assessments that were employed at
the beginning of the program. A log of lifestyle
changes (appendix) might be used for evaluation of progress. Also, reassessment of body
composition certainly provides an indication of
success. Periodic evaluation of the participants'
food and exercise diaries definitely is necessary.

▮ T A B L E 7.5 ▮
Behavior Modification Suggestions for Changing Eating Habits

Cue Elimination and Physical Environment	Manner of Eating	Food Choice	Alternative Activities
Eat only in designated place	Slow rate of eating—chew slowly	Portion control—cut snacks in half	Exercise—walking or jogging, other aerobic activities, recreational activities
Eat only when sitting in designated place	Swallow each bite before taking a second one	Measure foods until portions can be estimated	Relaxation
Set regular eating times	Put utensils down between bites	Serve only amounts planned	Meditation
Plan snacks and meals ahead	Count mouthfuls	Preplan eating when guest or entertaining; set aside portions	Imagery (visualize food to be in an inedible form or think of being in another place)
Determine degree of hunger before eating	Pause in the middle of a meal for a few minutes	Share dessert	Do necessary tasks, errands, yard work, or housework
Dissociate eating from other activities (e.g., reading, watching television)	Relax 60 seconds before eating	Include favorite foods	Write a letter
Plan and order restaurant meals ahead	Savor foods; enjoy each bite	Eat a variety of foods	Call someone
Store all foods; use opaque containers or store in inaccessible places	Eat only until reaching a "satisfied" hunger level (*not* until "stuffed")	Have appropriate snacks planned and "ready to go"	Do problem solving
Use small plates and bowls	Allow at least 20 minutes for eating a meal	Serve "on-the-side" dressings and sauces	Reevaluate goals and priorities
Let others get their snacks	Leave 5% to 20% of meal uneaten	Use spices instead of high-calorie condiments	Practice assertiveness
Record food intake	Push food aside ahead of time	Use garnishes (attractive and take up space on the plate)	Make charts for progress
Shop when *not hungry,* and use a list	Cover plate with napkin when finished eating	Use low-calorie ingredient substitutes	Take up a reward for following plans
Store foods out of sight			Brush teeth
Avoid "problem" places and people			Take a bath or shower
Serve buffets			Go for a drive
Remove plate from eating place after meal			
Clean plates directly into garbage			
Change route of travel to bypass a tempting eating place			
Write notes as reminders or use pictures; put on mirrors or refrigerator			

Source: O'Donnell, M., and Ainsworth, T. *Health promotion in the workplace.* Philadelphia: John Wiley & Sons, 1984, pp. 312–313. Used by permission.

■ **Figure 7.11**   The American College of Sports Medicine guidelines for weight-loss ■
programs.

A good weight-loss program is one that:

1. Provides a caloric intake not lower than 1200 cal per day, and allows
   normal adults to get a proper blend of foods to meet nutritional requirements. (Note: this requirement may be different for children, older
   individuals, athletes, and so on.)

2. Includes foods acceptable to the dieter from viewpoints of sociocultural
   background, usual habits, taste, cost, and ease in acquisition and
   preparation.

3. Provides a negative caloric balance (not to exceed 500 to 1000 cal per day
   lower than recommended), resulting in gradual weight loss without
   metabolic derangements. Maximal weight loss should be 2.2 pounds per
   week.

4. Includes the use of behavior-modification techniques to identify and
   eliminate dieting habits that contribute to improper nutrition.

5. Includes an endurance exercise program of at least 3 days per week, 20
   to 30 minutes in duration, at a minimum intensity of 60% of maximum
   heart rate (refer to: American College of Sports Medicine. Position
   statement on the recommended quantity and quality of exercise for
   developing and maintaining fitness in healthy adults. *Medicine and Science
   in Sports* 10:vii, 1978).

6. Provides new eating and physical activity habits that can be continued for
   life to maintain the achieved lower body weight.

If goals are being achieved and changes in lifestyle behaviors are progressing, detailed record keeping may be discontinued. At this time, the health/fitness specialist should encourage and give positive reinforcement to the participants.

If problems are discovered, reassessment of goals, more detailed counseling, or a different approach to behavioral modification may be indicated. If the specialist discovers that Ms. Jones is attempting to change too many behaviors, he or she must guide Ms. Jones to realize this and help her establish a more reasonable plan, such as eliminating only one or two behaviors each week.

The program evaluation should be based on detailed records of the participants' progress. Evaluation must include data on the number of participants who complete the program, the percent of population of interest who attend, and the percent of participants who lose fat.

To determine long-range results, periodic appointments with former participants should be made 6 to 12 months after completion of the program for weighing or body composition assessments. During the followup session, the assessor should ask about present weight, techniques still being used, lifestyle changes, and other weight-control methods.

Summary   ■

This chapter should provide a guide to establishing a weight-control program. Weight control is a complex process, influenced by biochemical individuality, personal propensities, learned behaviors, and genetic tendencies. The health/fitness specialist must be a Jack of all trades. The extent of his or her creativity, patience, energy, knowledge, and enthusiasm ultimately will determine the success of the program.

▌ References

1. McArdle, W. D., Katch, F. I., and Katch, V. L. *Exercise physiology: Energy, nutrition, and human performance.* Philadelphia: Lea and Febiger, 1981.

2. Winekoff, B. Diet change and public policy. *Conference on future directions in health care: A new public policy.* New York: 1977, p. 7.

3. Nash, J. P., and Ormiston, L. H. *Taking charge of your weight and well-being.* Palo Alto, CA: Bull Publishing, 1978.

A p p e n d i x ■

Log of Lifestyle Changes

Achievements	Mon.	Tues.	Wed.	Thurs.	Fri.	Sat.	Sun.
1. Minutes exercised							
2. Minutes doing relaxation exercises							
3. Did I stick to my high-fiber eating plan?							
4. (List eating goal for the week)							
5. (Goals and strategies I am maintaining)							
6.							
7.							
8.							
9.							
10.							

Source: Edwards, T. *Weight loss to super wellness.* The Mills Medical/Sports Complex, 1983. Used by permission.

SUBSTANCE ABUSE

Smoking, alcoholism, and other substance-abuse cessation courses are core elements of health/fitness programs because use of these drugs can have devastating effects on the participant, his or her employer, and society. People who smoke 1 pack of cigarettes per day have a 50% greater rate of hospitalization and absenteeism from work than do nonsmokers; 2-pack-per-day smokers have double the absenteeism rate. It is estimated that 5% to 10% of the nation's workforce are alcoholics or serious alcohol abusers; alcoholic employees are absent 2.5 times as often as are nonalcoholic employees, and their accident rate on the job is 3.6 times as high. In 1974, alcoholism cost American business $8 billion per year, or $32 million each working day.[1] Eighty-one million working days are lost annually because of smoking.[2] Smoking-related medical care, absenteeism, accidents, and lost work account for $27.5 billion.[3] In 1981, smokers had an unemployment rate of 16.2%, twice the 8.1% rate for nonsmokers.[4]

People abuse a variety of drugs (marijuana, barbiturates, heroin, amphetamines, cocaine, and others) obtained in both legal and illegal ways. Although substance abuse is a significant health and societal problem, drug abusers do not pose as extensive a problem in the workplace as do smokers and alcoholics. Drug abusers have been shown, however, to have a greater absenteeism rate, greater incidence of accidents, and lower productivity than do nonabusers. Because abuse of other drugs is similar to alcohol abuse, all chemical abuse can be treated in the same types of programs.[5]

Substance-abuse programs can be instituted in a health/fitness program with no additional facilities and with minimal cost, and can promote significant improvements in health. Employer-sponsored drug-abuse programs have met with good results when top management supports a written policy statement regarding substance abuse. The health/fitness program serves as a good vehicle for program implementation, both onsite and in conjunction with community agencies such as Alcoholics Anonymous. Actual treatment of substance abusers in the workplace or in commercial programs, however, has been infrequently undertaken; this long-term and costly process usually is best left to the clinical setting. However, the cost−benefit ratios of substance-abuse programs have been shown to be favorable. DuPont Chemical Manufacturing, for example, has indicated that its company-subsidized alcoholism treatment program recovered all costs within 2 years, and averaged a net savings of $419,200 per year through less alcohol-related absenteeism.[1]

Worksite programs and commercial facilities that contract employee programs have the potential to reach 50% of America's blue-collar workers who both smoke and underutilize current smoking-cessation programs. Also, workplace social support can provide nonsmoking norms and reinforcers to help maintain lasting changes in smoking behavior.[3] Almost 50% of U.S. businesses have a policy restricting or prohibiting workplace smoking, and 15% offer some form of smoking-cessation education or promotion programs.[3] Enlightened businesses that prohibit smoking also provide employees access to cessation methods.[2]

Company policy statements forbidding smoking and drinking on the job can provide incentives for employees to resolve their smoking and substance-abuse problems. Between 15% and 19% of American businesses reported nonsmoking employees claiming illnesses related to on-the-job exposure to second-hand smoke. In some cases, nonsmoking employees have resorted to legal action. Such suits will gain momentum from findings that nonsmokers exposed to smoke in the workplace show small-airway dysfunction similar to that of light smokers.[3] In a recent San Francisco election, voters accepted legislation that requires employers to have more designated smoking and nonsmoking areas. If employees disagree about the number and locations of the areas, the nonsmoking faction requests must be followed. In addition, violation is punishable by a $500-per-day fine.

Corporations are not the only segment of the health/fitness arena to conduct smoking-cessation programs. Cessation programs in clinical settings, such as hospital-based wellness programs, can be particularly successful. There is often a ready clientele—patients told by physicians to stop smoking. Hospitals and clinics have established credibility and a wealth of health professionals from which to draw.

Commercial and community health/fitness programs also may include smoking cessation courses. Many such programs compete for contracts and members in industry as well as the private sector, and smoking-cessation programs portray a rounded approach to wellness.

There are many substances that could be targeted for prevention or cessation programs; it would be confusing and difficult to present them all in a single chapter. Therefore, we will limit our discussion to smoking-cessation programs, the most popular. Smoking interventions show the best cost–benefit ranking of the most commonly presented services.

Needs Assessment

Participant Assessment

The initial step in establishing a smoking-cessation program is to determine the status of the participants' smoking behaviors and to determine the number of participants desiring to quit. The need for smoking-cessation programs typically becomes evident from data obtained from medical screening, health hazard appraisals, and past history. Once the smoking population is identified, more assessment is required to decide which, if any, intervention is appropriate. All identified smokers should complete a smoking questionnaire (Figure 8.1) and the "Smokers Self-Testing Kit" (Appendix A). If more in-depth assessments are desired concerning reasons for smoking, other specific questionnaires are available in (Table 8.1).

When the smokers who want to quit are identified, you can assess their probability of success by using such instruments as a motivation grid (Figure 8.2) and life change inventory (Figure 8.3). A subject's score on the latter is the number of all *yes* answers. Low life stress is 2 or less, and high life stress is 3 or more. Participants who score high might be advised to postpone stopping smoking until some stress situations are resolved. If the participant still wants to attempt cessation immediately, you should both be aware of the difficult time he or she may experience.

The motivation grid in Figure 8.2 can be used to predict outcome, particularly when coupled with data about dependence on cigarettes. Degree of dependence is determined by regularity of smoking, amount smoked, and carbon monoxide levels. Motivation can be estimated from the Self-Testing Kit (Appendix A). Plot the variables on the graph. Persons who are not very dependent may need only to be motivated

■ Figure 8.1 Smoking questionnaire. (From Eysenck, H. J. *The causes and effects of* ■ *smoking.* Beverly Hills, CA: Sage Publications, 1980, pp. 327–328. Used by permission.)

Name _____

Please answer each question by putting a circle around the answer with which you agree.

Have you ever smoked? (If your answer is *yes*, answer *all* the following questions.)	YES	NO
At what age did you start smoking?	Before 14 14–15 16–17	18–20 20–25 26 +
Do you smoke now?	YES	NO
How many cigarettes do you smoke each day, on the average?	Less than 1 1–4 5–9 10–14	15–19 20–29 30 +
How many ounces of pipe tobacco do you smoke in 1 week?	Less than ½ ounce ½–1 1½–2 2½–4	4½–6 6½–8
How many cigars do you smoke each day?	____	
How many cigarillos (small cigars) do you smoke each day?	____	
Have you ever tried to give up smoking completely?	YES	NO
Were you successful?	YES	NO
Do you believe that smoking is harmful?	YES	NO
Do you believe that smoking causes lung cancer?	YES	NO
Do you believe that smoking causes coronary and heart disease?	YES	NO
Did you smoke more, less, or about the same in the last year (as compared with before)?	MORE	LESS	SAME
Do you smoke to calm your nerves?	NEVER	SOMETIMES	OFTEN
Do you smoke when you are bored?	NEVER	SOMETIMES	OFTEN
Is smoking simply a habit with you?	YES	PARTLY	NO

■ Figure 8.1 Continued **■**

If you smoke cigarettes, do you inhale (draw on the cigarette, then take a breath in, so that the smoke goes down into your lungs)?	NEVER SOMETIMES OFTEN	USUALLY ALWAYS
Have you ever suffered from any of the following?		
Regular bouts of coughing	YES	NO
Chronic bronchitis	YES	NO
Chest pain	YES	NO
Shortness of breath	YES	NO
Heart disease	YES	NO
Chronic stomach disorder	YES	NO

■ T A B L E 8 . 1 ■
Needs Assessment Instruments

Tools	Description	Time to Administer	Source	Cost
Eysenck Smoking Questionnaire	Specific smoking history	Minimal	Eysenck, H. *The causes and effects of smoking.* Beverly Hills, CA: Sage Publications, 1980, pp. 327–328.	—
Smoker's Self-Testing Kit	Self-administered four-part questionnaire with discussion: (1) do you really want to quit? (2) what do you know about effects of smoking? (3) why do you smoke? (4) would your environment help or hinder your quitting effort?	Minimal	Superintendent of Documents U.S. Government Printing Office Washington, DC 20402 #1701-0180	$2.25
Reasons for Smoking Test	Assesses reasons for smoking; places into 6 categories	Minimal	Leventhal, H., and Avis, N. Reasons for smoking test. *Journal of Abnormal Psychology* 85:478, 1976.	—
The Smoking Patterns Test	Determines importance of various aspects in the individual's motivation to smoke	Minimal	Ashton, H., and Stepney, R. *Smoking—psychology and pharmacology.* London: Tavistock Publications, 1982, pp. 117–119.	—

■ T A B L E 8 . 1 ■
CONTINUED

Tools	Description	Time to Administer	Source	Cost
Smoking Motivation Grid	By plotting motivation and dependence, predicts ability to stop smoking	Minimal	Raw, M. The treatment of cigarette dependence. In *Research advances in alcohol and drug problems*, Israel, Y., et al. (eds). New York: Plenum Press, 1978, p. 476.	—
Life Change Inventory	ssesses current life stress to predict success in cessation	Minimal	Gunn, R. C. Smoking clinic failures and recent life stress. *Addictive Behaviors* 8:85, 1983.	—
Carbon monoxide level determination	Measures CO level of exhaled gas	5–10 minutes	Energetics Science Division of National Draeger 6 Skyline Drive Hawthorne, NY 10532 (914) 592-3010	$1900
Pulmonary function assessment	Simple screening spirometry	10–15 minutes	Breon #2400 90 Park Avenue New York, NY 10016 (212) 907-2731 or	$1000
			Collins Basic Spirometer #06031 Warren E. Collins 220 Wood Road 220 Wood Road Braintree, MA 02184 (617) 843-0610	$995

by health education. People who are both dependent and unmotivated first need to be motivated.

Not all assessment strategies are questionnaires or paper-and-pencil tests. If a test of pulmonary function, such as spirometry, is included in the physical assessment and screening, these data can be assessed. This test should be part of the overall health/fitness program screening; if a participant's values are abnormal, he or she should be informed of the need to stop smoking to avoid further small-airway obstruction. If a smoker's test is normal, encourage him or her to stop now, before pulmonary function becomes affected.

Another physiologic assessment is carbon monoxide content of expired air. Repeat tests give new nonsmokers feedback about the immediate reversible effects of smoking.

Mr. Hacker smokes 2 packs per day. During the first counseling session, he filled out a smoking questionnaire and the Self-Testing Kit. You discussed the results with him and found that he has a high desire to quit, knows smoking is

Figure 8.2 Motivation, dependence, and predicted ability to stop smoking. (From Raw, M. The treatment of cigarette dependence. In *Research advances in alcohol and drug problems*, Israel, Y., et al. (eds). New York: Plenum Press, 1978.)

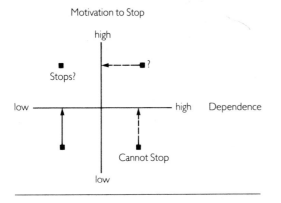

■ T A B L E 8 . 2 ■	
Corporate Costs of Smoking Employees	
Cost Source	Annual Cost per Smoker
Absenteeism	$220
Health care	230
Discounted lost earnings	765
Fire/accident insurance	90
On-the-job time lost	1820
Property damage and depreciation	500
Maintenance	500
Involuntary	486

Source: Weis, W. L. Can you afford to hire smokers? *Personnel Administration* 26:71, 1981.

harmful, has tried to quit two times before, and knows that his smoking is a crutch and a craving; his environment is conducive to quitting, because his wife also wants to stop smoking. He expressed anxiety over repeated failures, so you plotted his motivation grid and he completed a life change inventory. He thought it was too late for him to quit, so you had him take a pulmonary function test and exhaled carbon monoxide analysis. You completed all testing as quickly as possible, to minimize his losing interest.

Corporate Assessment

You must also assess the needs of your company. An analysis of your personnel's benefit records may give evidence of smoking-related insurance claims and sick days. Employees who smoke can cost a company $4600 each (Table 8.2). Determine the total number of smoking employees and multiply by $4600; this is the total cost for your organization. Share this figure with management so it can assess your company's need for a smoking-cessation program. If you have many smokers, the costs of more expensive approaches may be justified.

Goal Setting

Goals must be established such that coownership is maintained between the participant and the health/fitness specialist. Obviously, the main objective of a smoking-cessation program is to quit smoking. Yet several objectives can be established, some short-term, others long-term. Typical short-term objectives developed with Mr. Hacker might be: attend all sessions of onsite 5-day plan, and stop smoking after first night session. Some long-term objectives could be: attend all four followup sessions, and continue as a nonsmoker through the first year. Mr. Hacker agrees to the provisions and then signs a contract (Figure 8.4).

Written contracts are appropriate and effective tool. The participant takes an active role in his or her own cessation efforts; contracts also focus the process and lend an air of "officialness." By having a witness, the participant involves other persons, and perhaps also specific rewards and punishments, and he or she is more likely to follow through.

Goals also need to be set for the overall program. The ultimate objective, of course, is to have a smoking-free population, resulting in lowered health-care costs, reduced absenteeism, and increased productivity. Remember that although 90% of smokers say they would like to

Figure 8.3 Life change inventory. (From Gunn, R. C. Smoking clinic failures and recent life stress. *Addictive Behaviors* 8: 85, 1983. Copyright 1983 Pergamon Press, Ltd. Used by permission.)

1. Has your marital status changed? (for example, married, separated, widowed) YES NO

2. Has your job changed in any way? (for example, new job, new boss, lost job, retired, change in hours) YES NO

3. Have there been any changes in your living arrangements? (for example, moved, new baby, children moved out, new roommate, old friend moved out) YES NO

4. Has anyone close to you had a rather serious illness, an accident, or died? (both family and friends) YES NO

5. Have you been ill or in an accident? YES NO

6. Has your relationship with someone you are close to gone downhill? (for example, more arguments, sex problems, see person less) YES NO

7. Have any financial worries increased for you? (for example, took out a loan, increased spending rapidly, have a lower income) YES NO

8. Were you involved in trouble with the law? (for example, minor violation, in court, jail term) YES NO

9. Have there been any changes in your recreational, social, or church activities? YES NO

10. Have there been any changes in your eating, sleeping, or drinking habits? YES NO

11. Has your spouse started or stopped a job? YES NO

12. Have you or your spouse become pregnant? YES NO

13. Have you experienced any major disappointment or change in life goals? YES NO

14. Has anything else upsetting happened? (for example, robbery, fire, feeling increasingly nervous) YES NO

quit,[6] the success rate of cessation methods is quite low: 1 year after the end of treatment, the cessation rates are between 20% and 30%. In fact, only 5% of smokers who quit use specific cessation methods—the other 95% quit on their own.[7]

Realistic short-term goals for the program are: increased awareness and knowledge, improved morale, and a 3% reduction in the smoking population. Longer-term goals are: reduced health-care costs, increased productivity, and decreased absenteeism.

Planning

The planning for a smoking-cessation program is first accomplished by determining the nature of implementation. Once the target population is determined, the director must decide whether the cessation program is to take place onsite or be contracted to some agency, such as Smok-Enders or the Schick Smoking Control Centers, both of which conduct programs onsite. The costs often are paid partially by the company and partially by the employee. Schick Centers

■ **Figure 8.4** Smoking-cessation contract. (From Nash, J. P. *Taking charge of your smoking.* Palo Alto, CA: Bull, 1981. Used by permission.)

As of _____ at _____ I agree
　　　　(date)　　　　　　(time)
not to smoke any more. Accordingly,
_____ and I have agreed
　　　　(friend)
on the following contingencies:
　　If I do not smoke between _____
　　　　　　　　　　　　　　　　　(date)
　　and _____, I will receive
　　　　　(date)
　　from _____
　　the following:
　　(Specify reward) _____

_____

　　If I do smoke during this time, the following will happen:
　　(Specify alternative) _____

_____

　　　Signed　_____
　　　　　　　　　　　(my name)
　　　Signed　_____
　　　　　　　　　　　(friend's name)
　　　Date　　_____

promises a moneyback guarantee if cessation is not achieved.

Another approach is to use community resources. Table 8.3 lists some resources to supplement inhouse programs.

There are many different methods of smoking cessation. A health/fitness program could not conceivably offer all methods or, realistically, even a variety from which to choose. But a specialist must be acquainted with the wide variety of cessation techniques, not only in deciding which system to implement, but in correctly guiding those who come to him or her for information and advice. There are eight general categories of smoking-cessation methods (Table 8.4). Given such diverse cessation methods, how can a health/fitness specialist decide which plan to implement, or which to recommend to specific individuals? The subject of targeting and self-selection of smoking-modification methods is complex.[8] Remember that 95% of smokers who quit do so without the aid of any structured program. Also, the outcomes of most cessation methods are surprisingly similar. Almost any cessation method (placebo and control groups included) can get people to quit smoking. Initially, there is a 95% cessation rate. At 6 months, this drops to 25% to 30%. At 1 year and after, all cessation methods show cessation rates between 20% and 30%.[9]

Nevertheless, we can make some generalizations. People with a low tolerance for discomfort should be steered away from aversive techniques. Persons who are not self-reliant or self-directed do better with group methods than with self-help methods. Women generally do better in cessation programs with maximum social support, and do poorly when outside factors pressure against quitting. Older male smokers tend to be most successful. Typically, heavy smokers require more intensive treatment, due to their nicotine dependence. Studies show that significant others can greatly help or hinder cessation efforts, so it is wise to include family or friends whenever possible.

Many considerations in the planning process must include the participant, such as:

■ *Scheduling of classes:* cessation classes should be convenient to the work schedule (noon or after work).

■ *Scheduling of facilities:* the participant should have easy access—mark locations clearly and allow adequate time between classes.

■ *Scheduling of resource personnel:* give clear and concise assignments, verify dates and times, have all required materials available and in working order.

■ *Planning education materials:* keep audiovisuals, slides, and handouts simple, direct, and pertinent; begin with topics of most concern.

■ *Planning lessons:* proceed from simple to complex; allow adequate time for discussion and questions; arrange for participants to make up missed classes.

▌T A B L E 8 . 3▐
Community Resources for Smoking-Cessation Programs

Resource	Type of Treatment	Length/Followup	Cost
American Cancer Society	3-step sequence: (1) self-appraisal and insight development, (2) practice in abstinence, (3) maintenance phase; name: *Fresh Start, I Quit Kit*	Variable, usually twice a week for 4 weeks; followup varies	$5–$10
American Lung Association	Self-help manuals in conjunction with education and support groups; name: *Freedom from Smoking in 20 days; Lifetime of Freedom from Smoking*	1½-hour meetings, indefinite	$5–$10
5-Day Plan (Adventist sponsored)	Cold turkey quitting by education, lectures, films, record keeping, buddy system, forced fluids, avoidance of alcohol and caffeine, diet and exercise	5 sequential 2-hour meetings; followup meetings	$30–$50
Hospital-Based	Any combination of above methods	Varies	Varies

▌ *Planning publicity of program*: do not force different programs to compete with one another; make use of bulletin boards, newsletters, and check stuffers; avoid moralizing and threats—portray a helpful and caring approach.

▌ *Planning for evaluation*: use pre- and post-testing when possible to demonstrate changes in behavior; keep careful records of attendance to establish participation trends; verify participants' responses.

▌ *Planning for followup*: publicize ongoing followup sessions; adjust content to needs of participants.

Mr. Hacker and his wife registered for the upcoming 5-day plan, to be held in the staff lounge, Monday through Friday from 7 to 9 P.M. Mr. and Ms. Hacker are both given packets and are asked to complete questionnaires and pretesting. Notices posted in the workplace remind them when and where classes will be held, and what they are to bring the first night.

How do you recruit participants? The optimal manner of announcing or publicizing smoking-cessation programs has not been determined. Campbell Soup held a health fair focusing on many aspects of health. Many smokers feel guilt and self-reproval; announcements that blatantly focus on smoking with disregard to other areas may be threatening.

In planning the staff for cessation programs, you can be both creative and cost-effective. Boeing Aircraft collaborated with the University of Washington; seniors in health studies participated in planning and implementing the cessation program. Graduate students from schools of public health also can be useful, as can local nursing and medical students on public health rotations.

Planning motivation can be of use. To quit smoking, it is not sufficient for people to believe that smoking is a health problem; they must also see themselves as personally susceptible to those adverse effects. The American Cancer Society stages in smoking cessation are: (1) smoker must become *motivated* for change; (2) initial period of *preparation* often is advisable—smokers may need to understand their reasons for smoking and to develop alternative behaviors before quitting; (3) *cessation* period, during which smoker moves from habitual level of smoking to a zero smoking rate; (4) *transition*

▮ T A B L E 8 . 4 ▮
Advantages and Disadvantages of Treatments for Smoking Cessation

Type	Advantages	Disadvantages
1. Self-care books and manuals	Participant not dependent on others; free or minimal expense; can acquire strategies relevant to own lifestyle; can learn stimulus control, eliminate cues, and develop incompatible behaviors	No group support; takes strong self-direction and motivation
2. Behavior modification—aversive therapy	Done in "privacy of own head"	Requires strong self-control
Verbal imagery	Nonnoxious	
Smoke aversion	Attempts to produce aversion to taste of smoke itself	Can cause cardiopulmonary problems; can be expensive
Electric shock	More effective when combined with other techniques	Many find threatening; response often disappears when in own nonshock environment
3. Hypnosis	Attempts to intensify concentration on quitting process	Costly; totally depends on skill of therapist; clinical studies show no better than placebo
4. Medication		
Lobeline (Bantron, Nicoban)	Nicotine substitute	Main result from placebo effect
Nicorette chewing gum	Clinical trials show promising results	
Tranquilizers	To help with withdrawal symptoms	Have own addictive potential
5. Education	Key aspect of all valid treatment methods	Education alone without other cessation method may be counterproductive
6. Individual counseling	Can be effective if counselor seen as authority	Costly; totally dependent on empathy and knowledge of counselor
7. Group counseling	Often uses combination of other methods; group support known to be of value	May not have followup
8. Miscellaneous		
Acupuncture	Could fill need for specific groups displeased with more orthodox methods	Little scientific evaluation, most in form of testimonials
Auricular (ear staple)		
Acupressure		
Yoga		

phase, during which the smoking rate is low, or zero, but the urge is still quite high—this is intensive and lasts several weeks; (5) *extended* period, lasting up to several months, during which the smoker has to cope with continuing urges; (6) *resolution*—urges have ceased; if nonsmoking is to continue, nonsmoking attitudes must develop.[10]

Motivation is crucial—but how does one affect it? Incentives and family and peer pressure can all be used but cannot always be manipulated. Figure 8.5 illustrates the steps in motivating a smoker to quit.

Implementation

Once the smoking-cessation program is planned, implementation of the education and service components can begin. We will assume that participants will not be referred to outside agencies. Typically, inhouse programs use educational materials from relevant resources and personnel from community agencies. The health/fitness specialist usually serves as a coordinator and facilitator.

Education Component

The purpose of the education component is to help participants become more knowledgeable about smoking and about cessation methods. Self-care methods, education programs, and group and individual counseling are all useful.

The *Bibliography on Smoking and Health* provides many references to useful books.[11] Some manuals are more effective used alone, and others are more effective when used with guidance.

Individual and group counseling methods are used by many programs. The 5-Day Plan, American Cancer Society, and American Lung Association program representatives are willing to conduct, or to instruct someone else to conduct, their agencies' programs onsite with minimal obligations, responsibilities, and costs to the sponsoring facility. National office addresses of useful agencies are listed in Appendix B. If your health/fitness facility cannot support its own counseling program, arrange for your participants to attend offsite.

Service Component

The remainder of cessation techniques are service-related. Aversive behavior modification involves action-related strategies; specific environments are required. Hypnosis requires a skilled therapist. Medication-centered methods require a prescribing physician; if over-the-counter medication is used, you may still wish to have a medical consultant.

There are no clear-cut boundaries between the education and service components, because essentially any smoking cessation technique will have a service aspect, even though it may be an education approach.

Some businesses offer incentives to help employees quit smoking. A variety of such programs are described in an *Employers Kit* compiled by Action for Smoking and Health (ASH). Most offer monetary rewards for quitting, avoiding verification of self-report or penalties for relapse. The Texas Division of Dow Chemical distributed to quitters tickets for an end-of-year raffle of a motor boat. Intermatic opened an "I Quit Smoking" window that covered bets up to $100 from employees who bet they could quit—the company doubled the bets if the employee succeeded, and added additional bonuses. Speedcall and Leslie Manufacture and Supply offer exsmokers a weekly bonus equivalent to the estimated weekly cost of a 2-pack-a-day habit. Few controlled studies have investigated the effectiveness of monetary incentives but, even if they do not increase quit rates, they certainly raise motivation and rally social support. Programs that combine incentives with training in nonsmoking skills should produce the best results.

The general problem with all smoking-cessation techniques is not to obtain an initial change in behavior, but to sustain that change. Almost any intervention can be effective in eliminating or drastically reducing smoking behavior, but the changes tend to be relatively short-lived. Because the severity of withdrawal symptoms causes most relapses to smoking, teach behavior therapy either before cessation or at the very beginning.

Because there is no one best method of cessation, consider the relative costs when you choose a method. Obviously, group programs are more cost-effective than are individual sessions. Behavior-modification programs show

▌ **Figure 8.5** How to motivate a smoker to quit. (From Burton, D. Motivating   ▌
smokers to assume personal responsibility for quitting. In *Progress in smoking
cessation.* New York: American Cancer Society, 1978.)

1. Reason
   a. Make sure he or she has a personal reason sufficient to lead to his or
      her becoming motivated.
   b. Present to him or her all alternative reasons for consideration.
2. Fringe benefits
   Bring to her or his awareness all of the fringe benefits she or he stands to
   gain from stopping. Some examples are: saving money, smelling better,
   not offending other people, and feeling proud of being successful.
3. Irrational components
   a. Loneliness: smoking comforts a lonely person by representing the
      familiar, always there and always counted on. Calling attention to this
      universality may be enough for some smokers to overcome this
      obstacle.
   b. Laziness: most people are resistant to making changes of any kind
      because it takes effort, whereas maintaining status quo takes no
      effort. Confront the smoker with this so he or she cannot mask with
      rationalizations; give detailed behavioral instructions required to quit
      during program.
   c. Euphoria: the expansive state of mind some people enter when
      things are going well for them. Everything is great, I am not vulner-
      able, so I can smoke. Encourage development of key sentences—an
      own personal reason for stopping that is often repeated and becomes
      a part of the unconscious.
   d. Overriding interpersonal conflicts: two individuals support one
      another's smoking, or a smoker is motivated to smoke to spite some-
      one who nags him or her to quit. Call attention to this dependent,
      destructive interaction; smoking is a totally independent and per-
      sonal habit.
   e. Fear of going crazy: fear of anxiety and being overwhelmed. Assure
      individual there is no recorded case of anyone going crazy as a result
      of stopping smoking.
   f. Fear of decreased function: might have decreased concentration and
      be very tense. Teach relaxation exercises.
   g. Incomplete identity: if smoking is an integral part of a person, coun-
      sel on finding other positive inner personality traits, and teach to
      look outside self, pursue hobby.
   h. Fear of failure resulting in loss of self-esteem: anyone can stop smok-
      ing. Address his or her particular anticipated difficulties.
4. How-to steps
   Tell the smoker just what to do, behaviorally, to get rid of his or her
   smoking habit. This step is accomplished in the cessation program itself.

the most cost-effectiveness per unit of abstinence, with education and group support being next. Aversive conditioning techniques can be quite cost-effective when used in groups. Hypnosis shows the least cost-effectiveness.

We can construct an implementation schedule for Mr. Hacker. At noon on Friday, before the 5-day plan, Mr. and Ms. Hacker attend a 30-minute introductory session, held in the employee lounge by a health educator from Hospital A-OK. She gives an overview of what will happen during the five sessions and reminds participants that their cigarettes will be collected Monday night. She asks them to begin analyzing which cigarettes are the most important to them. Each individual then shares what aspects of quitting are worrying him or her the most. When the Hackers return for the first nightly session, an internist talks about how many people smoke and reviews some health aspects of smoking. The health educator explains that there are three types of addiction: nicotine, psychological, and neuromuscular. On day 2, the health educator discusses how habits are formed and broken and suggests ways of substituting new behaviors, and a cardiologist explains the cardiovascular effects of smoking. For 5 nights, Mr. Hacker hears the health educator and a specialist talk and learns some behavioral tips. He receives group support for his nonsmoking. At the end of the last session, he is encouraged to attend ongoing monthly follow-up sessions.

Because there is a large relapse rate among participants who stop smoking, develop follow-up programs for those who fall off the wagon. Have an ongoing monthly ex-smoker meeting to provide support and motivation, and review the specific techniques used in your cessation method. It may be more effective for the participants themselves to conduct all or part of each session; have them give personal advice on approaches that proved effective for them. Withdrawal symptoms appear within hours of stopping and may persist for several years; they consist of changes in physiological, psychological, and behavioral variables. In the affective domain, cessation commonly causes increases in craving, anxiety, irritability, aggressiveness, and hostility.

Assuming that some people will continue to smoke, you can help them find less dangerous ways to smoke. Cigar and pipe smoking is less dangerous, but probably only because people inhale less smoke: do not recommend that a cigarette smoker switch to pipe or cigars—he or she may continue to inhale, but the tobacco will be stronger and will have no filtering. Variations in smoking rate usually reflect an attempt to regulate nicotine blood levels. Serious smokers smoke to prevent withdrawal. If a new brand contains less nicotine, the smoker probably will just smoke more cigarettes, thus inhaling higher levels of carbon monoxide and other gases.[12] Give special concern to those individuals who are unable to quit or who choose not to quit. Do not pass judgment or use intimidation tactics. They may decide to quit in the future; if you alienate them, they are not likely to come to you for assistance. For those who continue smoking, suggest the following guidelines: (1) try to inhale as little as possible and less deeply; (2) try to take fewer puffs of each cigarette, and make each one short, so there is less time to inhale; (3) never smoke the last third of the cigarette—more tar and toxic materials are concentrated in the end; (4) never relight a half-smoked cigarette; (5) take the cigarette out of your mouth between puffs to lessen the amount inhaled.[13]

Evaluation

The smoking-cessation program should be evaluated on the participant and program levels. The participant evaluation involves retesting and determination of current smoking behavior. If carbon monoxide analysis or pulmonary function testing were a part of the initial assessment, they should be repeated at the end of the program.

Program evaluation must include data on the number and percentage of the population of interest recruited, the proportion who complete the program, and the percentage who abstain at least 6 months (preferably, collect data for 1 year or longer). Self-reports of abstinence can be validated through tests of exhaled carbon monoxide or of plasma thiocyanate.

To evaluate the cost–benefit ratio, calculate the cost per participant and divide by the success percentage rate (define "success" as continued abstinence for a minimum of 6 months).

Long-term program evaluation should include data on any variations in absenteeism, health-care costs, discounted lost earnings, fire and accident insurance, on-the-job time lost, property damage, and maintenance. Statistical evidence that any have changed after implementation of the program can be valuable in deciding whether to continue that specific programming. Keep in mind, however, that some of these cost sources may show minimal, if any, direct short-term change.

▌ Summary

This chapter discussed the importance of substance-abuse control programs. We presented different methods of implementing programs, using smoking-cessation programming as a model. Methods of assessing participants were presented and the effectiveness of each method was found to be related to the nature of dependency. Outside resources can help you implement this program. Illustrations of in-house program implementations were provided, as well as means of evaluating program effectiveness.

▌ References

1. National Chamber Foundation. *A national health care strategy; how business can promote good health for employees and their families.* Excelsio, MN: Interstudy, 1978.

2. Danaher, B. Smoking cessation programs in occupational settings. *Public Health Reports* 95:149, 1980.

3. Orleans, C., and Shipley, R. Worksite smoking cessation initiatives: Review and recommendations. *Addictive Behaviors* 7:1, 1982.

4. Weis, W. *The smoke-free workplace: Cost and health consequences.* Paper presented at the Fifth World Conference on Smoking and Health, Winnipeg, Canada, July, 1981.

5. Kristein, M. Economic issues in prevention. *Preventive Medicine* 6:256, 1977.

6. Parkinson, R., et al. Managing health promotion in the workplace: Guidelines for implementation and evaluation. Palo Alto, CA: Mayfield, 1982.

7. U.S. Dept. of Health and Human Services. *Health consequences of smoking and cancer: A report of the Surgeon General.* 1982.

8. Schwartz, J. (ed). Progress in smoking cessation. *Proceedings of the International Conference on Smoking Cessation.* New York: American Cancer Society, 1978.

9. Benfari, R., and Ockene, J. Control of cigarette smoking from a psychological perspective. *Annual Review of Public Health* 3:101, 1982.

10. Best, J. A. Targeting and self-selection of smoking modification methods. In *Progress in Smoking Cessation*, Schwartz, J. L. (ed). Proceedings of International Society on Smoking Cessation, New York: American Cancer Society, 1978.

11. U.S. Department of Health and Human Services (USDHHS). *Bibliography on smoking and health, 1982.* Washington, DC: USDHHS, Public Health Services, Office on Smoking and Health, 1982.

12. Pechacek, T., and McAlister, A. Strategies for the modification of smoking behavior: Treatment and prevention. In *The comprehensive handbook of behavioral medicine*, Vol. 3, Ferguson, J., and Taylor, C. (eds). New York: Spectrum Publications, 1980.

13. Casewit, C. *Quit smoking.* Glouster, MA: Para Research, 1983.

A p p e n d i x

Smoker's Self-Testing Kit*

These four short tests can help you find out what you *know* about cigarette smoking and how you *feel* about it. They can tell you:

1. Whether you *really* want to quit smoking.
2. What you know about the effects of smoking on health.
3. What kind of smoker you are (*why* you smoke).
4. Whether the world you live in will help or hinder you if you do try to stop.

We believe that if you take a good hard look at the facts and that if you analyze your real feelings you may decide to quit smoking. Tests 1 and 2 are designed to help you take this look at yourself.

Tests 3 and 4 will give you some insight into what kind of smoker you are, and will reveal some of the problems you may run into when you try to quit.

The purpose of the tests is to develop your insight . . . to help you understand your smoking habit and to help you decide what you want to do about it.

After you have taken the four tests, you will go on to an explanation of what your scores mean. Make sure, before reading this explanation, that you have answered each question and totaled your scores on all four tests. *Then* go on to the interpretation of your scores.

---

*Source: Department of Health, Education, and Welfare (DHEW). *Smoker's self-testing kit.* DHEW Publication No. (CDC) 75-8716. Washington, DC: U.S. Government Printing Office, 1975. This kit was developed by Daniel Horn, Ph.D., Director of the National Clearinghouse for Smoking and Health of the Public Health Service, and members of the Clearinghouse staff.

Do You Want to Change Your Smoking Habits?

For each statement, circle the number that most accurately indicates how you feel. For example, if you completely agree with the statement, circle 4, if you agree somewhat, circle 3, etc.
Important: Answer every question.

	completely agree	somewhat agree	somewhat disagree	completely disagree
A. Cigarette smoking might give me a serious illness.	4	3	2	1
B. My cigarette smoking sets a bad example for others.	4	3	2	1
C. I find cigarette smoking to be a messy kind of habit.	4	3	2	1
D. Controlling my cigarette smoking is a challenge to me.	4	3	2	1
E. Smoking causes shortness of breath.	4	3	2	1
F. If I quit smoking cigarettes it might influence others to stop.	4	3	2	1
G. Cigarettes cause damage to clothing and other personal property.	4	3	2	1
H. Quitting smoking would show that I have willpower.	4	3	2	1
I. My cigarette smoking will have a harmful effect on my health.	4	3	2	1
J. My cigarette smoking influences others close to me to take up or continue smoking.	4	3	2	1
K. If I quit smoking, my sense of taste or smell would improve.	4	3	2	1
L. I do not like the idea of feeling dependent on smoking.	4	3	2	1

HOW TO SCORE:

1. Enter the numbers you have circled to the Test 1 questions in the spaces below, putting the number you have circled to Question A over line A, to Question B over line B, etc.
2. Total the 3 scores across on each line to get your totals. For example, the sum of your scores over lines A, E, and I gives you your score on *Health*; lines B, F, and J give the score on *Example*, etc.

Totals

_____ + _____ + _____ = _____
A   E   I   Health

_____ + _____ + _____ = _____
B   F   J   Example

_____ + _____ + _____ = _____
C   G   K   Esthetics

_____ + _____ + _____ = _____
D   H   L   Mastery

Scores can vary from 3 to 12. Any score 9 and above is *high*; any score 6 and below is *low*.

■ T E S T 2 ■
What Do You Think the Effects of Smoking Are?

For each statement, circle the number that shows how you feel about it. Do you strongly agree, mildly agree, mildly disagree, or strongly disagree?
Important: Answer every question.

	strongly agree	mildly agree	mildly disagree	strongly disagree
A. Cigarette smoking is not nearly as dangerous as many other health hazards.	1	2	3	4
B. I don't smoke enough to get any of the diseases that cigarette smoking is supposed to cause.	1	2	3	4
C. If a person has already smoked for many years, it probably won't do him much good to stop.	1	2	3	4
D. It would be hard for me to give up smoking cigarettes.	1	2	3	4
E. Cigarette smoking is enough of a health hazard for something to be done about it.	4	3	2	1
F. The kind of cigarette I smoke is much less likely than other kinds to give me any of the diseases that smoking is supposed to cause.	1	2	3	4
G. As soon as a person quits smoking cigarettes he begins to recover from much of the damage that smoking has caused.	4	3	2	1
H. It would be hard for me to cut down to half the number of cigarettes I now smoke.	1	2	3	4
I. The whole problem of cigarette smoking and health is a very minor one.	1	2	3	4
J. I haven't smoked long enough to worry about the diseases that cigarette smoking is supposed to cause.	1	2	3	4
K. Quitting smoking helps a person to live longer.	4	3	2	1
L. It would be difficult for me to make any substantial change in my smoking habits.	1	2	3	4

(continued)

HOW TO SCORE TEST 2:

1. Enter the numbers you have circled to the Test 2 questions in the spaces below, putting the number you have circled to Question A over line A, to Question B over line B, etc.
2. Total the 3 scores across on each line to get your totals. For example, the sum of your scores over lines A, E, and I gives you your score on *Importance*; lines B, F, and J give the score on *Personal Relevance*, etc.

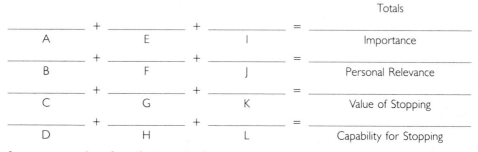

Totals

___ + ___ + ___ = ___			
A	E	I	Importance
___ + ___ + ___ = ___			
B	F	J	Personal Relevance
___ + ___ + ___ = ___			
C	G	K	Value of Stopping
___ + ___ + ___ = ___			
D	H	L	Capability for Stopping

Scores can vary from 3 to 12. Any score 9 and above is *high*; any score 6 and below is *low*.

∎ T E S T 3 ∎
Why Do You Smoke?

Here are some statements made by people to describe what they get out of smoking cigarettes. How *often* do you feel this way when smoking them? Circle one number for each statement.
Important: Answer every question.

		always	frequently	occasionally	seldom	never
A.	I smoke cigarettes in order to keep myself from slowing down.	5	4	3	2	1
B.	Handling a cigarette is part of the enjoyment of smoking it.	5	4	3	2	1
C.	Smoking cigarettes is pleasant and relaxing.	5	4	3	2	1
D.	I light up a cigarette when I feel angry about something.	5	4	3	2	1
E.	When I have run out of cigarettes I find it almost unbearable until I can get them.	5	4	3	2	1
F.	I smoke cigarettes automatically without even being aware of it.	5	4	3	2	1
G.	I smoke cigarettes to stimulate me, to perk myself up.	5	4	3	2	1

▌ T E S T 3 Continued ▌

H. Part of the enjoyment of smoking a cigarette comes from the steps I take to light up.	5	4	3	2	I
I. I find cigarettes pleasurable.	5	4	3	2	I
J. When I feel uncomfortable or upset about something, I light up a cigarette.	5	4	3	2	I
K. I am very much aware of the fact when I am not smoking a cigarette.	5	4	3	2	I
L. I light up a cigarette without realizing I still have one burning in the ashtray.	5	4	3	2	I
M. I smoke cigarettes to give me a "lift."	5	4	3	2	I
N. When I smoke a cigarette, part of the enjoyment is watching the smoke as I exhale it.	5	4	3	2	I
O. I want a cigarette most when I am comfortable and relaxed.	5	4	3	2	I
P. When I feel "blue" or want to take my mind off cares and worries, I smoke cigarettes.	5	4	3	2	I
Q. I get a real gnawing hunger for a cigarette when I haven't smoked for a while.	5	4	3	2	I
R. I've found a cigarette in my mouth and didn't remember putting it there.	5	4	3	2	I

Totals

_____ A	+ _____ G	+ _____ M	=	_____ Stimulation
_____ B	+ _____ H	+ _____ N	=	_____ Handling
_____ C	+ _____ I	+ _____ O	=	_____ Pleasurable Relaxation
_____ D	+ _____ J	+ _____ P	=	_____ Crutch; Tension Reduction
_____ E	+ _____ K	+ _____ Q	=	_____ Craving; Psychological Addiction
_____ F	+ _____ L	+ _____ R	=	_____ Habit

Does the World Around You Make It Easier or Harder to Change Your Smoking Habits?

Indicate by circling the appropriate numbers whether you feel the following statements are true or false. *Important: Answer every question.*

		true or mostly true	false or mostly false
A.	Doctors have decreased or stopped their smoking of cigarettes in the past 10 years.	2	1
B.	In recent years there seem to be more rules about where you are allowed to smoke.	2	1
C.	Cigarette advertising makes smoking appear attractive to me.	1	2
D.	Schools are trying to discourage children from smoking.	2	1
E.	Doctors are trying to get their patients to stop smoking.	2	1
F.	Someone has recently tried to persuade me to cut down or quit smoking cigarettes.	2	1
G.	The constant repetition of cigarette advertising makes it hard for me to quit smoking.	1	2
H.	Both government and private health organizations are actively trying to discourage people from smoking.	2	1
I.	A doctor has, at least once, talked to me about my smoking.	2	1
J.	It seems as though an increasing number of people object to having someone smoke near them.	2	1
K.	Some cigarette commercials on TV make me feel like smoking.	1	2
L.	Congressmen and other legislators are showing concern with smoking and health.	2	1

M. The people around you, particularly those who are close to you (e.g., relatives, friends, office associates), may make it easier or more difficult for you to give up smoking by what they say or do. What about these people? Would you say that they make giving up smoking or staying off cigarettes more difficult for you than it would be otherwise? (Circle the number to the left of the statement that best describes your situation.)

3 They make it much more difficult than it would be otherwise.
4 They make it somewhat more difficult than it would be otherwise.
5 They make it somewhat easier than it would be otherwise.
6 They make it much easier than it would be otherwise.

HOW TO SCORE:
1. Enter the numbers you have circled on the Test 4 questions in the spaces below, putting the number you have circled to Question A over line A, to Question B over line B, etc.
2. Total the 3 scores across on each line to get your totals. For example, the sum of your scores over lines A, E, and I gives you your score on *Doctors*; lines B, F, and J give the score on *General Climate*, etc.

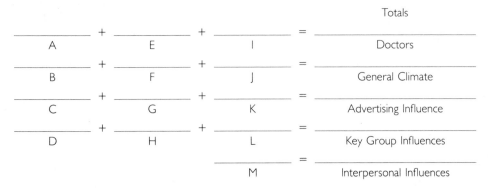

Totals

_____ + _____ + _____ = _____
  A   E   I   Doctors

_____ + _____ + _____ = _____
  B   F   J   General Climate

_____ + _____ + _____ = _____
  C   G   K   Advertising Influence

_____ + _____ + _____ = _____
  D   H   L   Key Group Influences

_____ = _____
  M   Interpersonal Influences

    Scores can vary from 3 to 6: 6 is *high*; 5, high middle; 4, low middle; 3, *low*. Learn from the next section what your scores mean.

You have now taken the four tests and are ready to read the explanation of what your scores mean.

▌ T E S T   1 ▌
Do You Want to Change Your Smoking Habits?

Why do you want to quit smoking? Are your reasons strong enough for you to make the effort to quit? Do you have enough reasons? This is something only you can decide.

Four common reasons for wanting to quit smoking cigarettes are: Concern over the effects on *health*; desire to set an *example* for others; recognition of the unpleasant aspects (the *esthetics*) of smoking; and desire to exercise *self-control*.

Test 1 of the Smoker's Self-Testing Kit was designed to measure the importance of each of these reasons to you. The higher you score on any category, say *health*, the more important that reason is to you. A score of 9 or above in one of these categories indicates that this is one of the most important reasons why you may want to quit.

1. HEALTH

Research during the past 10 or 15 years has shown that cigarette smoking can be harmful to health. Knowing this, many people have recently stopped smoking and many others are considering it. If your score on the *health* factor is 9 or above, the health hazards of smoking may be enough to make you want to quit now.

If your score on this factor is low (6 or less), look at your scores on Test 2. They tell how much you know about the health hazard. You may be lacking important information or may even have incorrect information. If so, health considerations are not playing the important role they should in your decision to keep on smoking or to quit.

2. EXAMPLE

Some people stop smoking because they want to set a good example for others. Parents do it to make it easier for their children to resist starting to smoke; doctors do it to influence their patients; teachers want to help their students; sports stars want to set an example for their young fans; husbands want to influence their wives, and vice versa.

Such examples are an important influence on our behavior. Research shows that almost twice as many high school students smoke if both parents are smokers compared to those whose parents are nonsmokers or former smokers.

If your score is low (6 or less), it may mean that you are not interested in giving up smoking in order to set an example for others. Perhaps you do not appreciate how important your example could be.

3. ESTHETICS (the unpleasant aspects)

People who score high, that is, 9 or above, in this category recognize and are disturbed by some of the unpleasant aspects of smoking. The smell of stale smoke on their clothing, bad breath, and stains on their fingers and teeth might be reason enough to consider breaking the habit.

4. MASTERY (self-control)

If you score 9 or above on this factor, you are bothered by the knowledge that you cannot control your desire to smoke. You are not your own master. Awareness of this challenge to your self-control may make you want to quit.

Summary of Test 1

Test 1 has measured your attitude toward four of the most common reasons why people want to quit smoking. Consider those that are important to you. Even if none are important, you still may have a highly personal reason for wanting to change your habit. All in all, you may now see that you have reasons enough to want to quit smoking.

If you are still not sure, study the interpretation of your scores on Test 2 (the next test) to determine what you know about the effects of smoking on your health and what part that knowledge may play in your decision.

▌T E S T 2▐
What Do You Think the Effects of Smoking Are?

To attempt to give up smoking you must do more than simply acknowledge that "cigarette smoking may be harmful to your health." You must be aware that smoking is an *important* problem, that it has *personal* meaning for you, that there is *value* to be gained from stopping, and that people are *capable* of stopping. Test 2 measures the strength of your recognition of each of these factors.

If your score is 9 or above on any factor, that factor supports your desire to try to stop smoking. If your score is 6 or below, that factor will not help you, but note that you may have scored low because you lack correct information. For every factor for which you *do* have a low score, read the accompanying explanatory material with special care.

1. IMPORTANCE

Cancer, heart disease, respiratory diseases—all related to smoking—are among the most serious to which man is exposed. You should not shrug off the growing evidence that they cause death and severe disability. Yet you may be doing this if your score is 6 or lower on the first part of Test 2.

Research has shown that one death in every three is an "extra" death among men who die between the ages of 35 and 60, because cigarette smokers have higher death rates than nonsmokers. One day of every five lost from work because of illness, 1 day in every 10 spent in bed because of illness, 1 day of every 8 days of restricted activity—all are "extra," because cigarette smokers suffer more disability than nonsmokers.

2. PERSONAL RELEVANCE

Some smokers kid themselves into thinking: "It can't happen to me—only to the other guy." If you score 6 or below, you may be one of these people.

Your reasoning may go something like this: "I don't really smoke enough to be hurt by it. It takes two packs a day over a period of many years before harmful effects show up."

Unfortunately, this is not true. Even people who smoke less than half a pack a day show significantly higher death rates than nonsmokers. Breathing capacity can diminish after only a very few years of regular smoking. Even what used to be considered light smoking, such as half a pack a day, can be harmful.

3. VALUE OF STOPPING

Evidence shows that there are benefits to health when you give up smoking—even if you have smoked for many years. A score of 6 or lower indicates that you do not realize this.

There are real advantages in giving up smoking even for long-term smokers; people who quit before any symptoms of illness or impairment occur suffer lower death rates than those who continue to smoke, and reduce the likelihood of serious illness.

People who have had heart attacks and those with stomach ulcers and chronic respiratory diseases should definitely give up smoking. It is difficult if not impossible to control such illnesses if they do not.

4. CAPABILITY FOR STOPPING

If your score is 6 or lower on this part of the test, you believe that it will be hard for you to quit. But you may find encouragement in the fact that over 20 million adults are now successful ex-smokers. Of these, over 100,000 doctors, well over half of those who were ever cigarette smokers, have successfully quit.

In the following Test, No. 3, you will gain some insight into the reasons why you smoke. With this new knowledge, it may be easier for you to give up smoking than you thought it would be. At any rate, you must develop confidence that it is possible for you to control your smoking; if you do not, you are less likely to succeed in your attempt to quit.

Summary of Test 2

Review your scores on the four factors that this test measures. For those on which you scored in the *middle* or *low* brackets, study the explanatory material. If the explanation does not answer all your questions, you may get additional material from the Public Health Service, your local health department, and such agencies as the National Tuberculosis and Respiratory Disease Association, American Cancer Society, American Heart Association, or your public library.

Now, you should be ready to decide whether or not you are going to try to give up smoking. If you have strong enough reasons to do so, if you know enough about the real effects of smoking, if you have not been led astray by misinformation, and if you will not try to fool yourself, you are ready.

▌ T E S T 3 ▌
Why Do You Smoke?

What kind of smoker are you? What do you get out of smoking? What does it do for you? This test is designed to provide you with a score on each of 6 factors which describe many people's smoking. Your smoking may be well characterized by only one of these factors, or by a combination of factors. In any event, this test will help you identify what you use smoking for and what kind of satisfaction you think you get from smoking.

The six factors measured by this test describe one or another way of experiencing or managing certain kinds of feelings. Three of these feeling-states represent the *positive* feelings people get from smoking: (1) a sense of increased energy or *stimulation*, (2) the satisfaction of *handling* or manipulating things,

and (3) the enhancing of *pleasurable feelings* accompanying a state of well being. The fourth is the *decreasing of negative feelings* by reducing a state of tension or feelings of anxiety, anger, shame, etc. The fifth is a complex pattern of increasing and decreasing "craving" for a cigarette representing a psychological *addiction* to cigarettes. The sixth is *habit* smoking which takes place in an absence of feeling—purely automatic smoking.

A score of 11 or above on any factor indicates that this factor is an important source of satisfaction for you. The higher your score (15 is the highest), the more important a particular factor is in your smoking and the more useful the discussion of that factor can be in your attempt to quit.

A few words of warning: If you give up smoking, you may have to learn to get along without the satisfactions that smoking gives you. Either that, or you will have to find some more acceptable way of getting this satisfaction. In either case, you need to know just what it is you get out of smoking before you can decide whether to forego the satisfactions it gives you or to find another way to achieve them.

1. STIMULATION

If you score high or fairly high on this factor, it means that you are one of those smokers who is stimulated by the cigarette—you feel that it helps wake you up, organize your energies, and keep you going. If you try to give up smoking, you may want a safe substitute—a *brisk walk* or moderate exercise, for example—whenever you feel the urge to smoke.

2. HANDLING

Handling things can be satisfying, but there are many ways to keep your hands busy without lighting up or playing with a cigarette. Why not toy with a pen or pencil? Or try doodling. Or play with a coin, a piece of jewelry, or some other harmless object.

There are plastic cigaettes to play with, or you might even use a real cigarette if you can trust yourself not to light it.

3. ACCENTUATION OF PLEASURE—PLEASURABLE RELAXATION

It is not always easy to find out whether you use the cigarette to feel *good*, that is, get real, honest pleasure out of smoking (Factor 3) or to keep from feeling so *bad* (Factor 4). About two-thirds of smokers score high or fairly high on *accentuation of pleasure*, and about half of those also score as high or higher on *reduction of negative feelings*.

Those who do get real pleasure out of smoking often find that an honest consideration of the harmful effects of their habit is enough to help them quit. They substitute eating, drinking, social activities, and physical activities—within reasonable bounds—and find they do not seriously miss their cigarettes.

4. REDUCTION OF NEGATIVE FEELINGS, OR "CRUTCH"

Many smokers use the cigarette as a kind of crutch in moments of stress or discomfort, and on occasion it may work; the cigarette is sometimes used as a tranquilizer. But the heavy smoker, the person who tries to handle severe personal problems by smoking many times a day, is apt to discover that cigarettes do not help him deal with his problems effectively.

When it comes to quitting, this kind of smoker may find it easy to stop when everything is going well, but may be tempted to start again in a time of crisis. Again, physical exertion, eating, drinking, or social activity—in moderation—may serve as useful substitutes for cigarettes, even in times of tension. The choice of a substitute depends on what will achieve the same effect without having any appreciable risk.

5. "CRAVING" OR PSYCHOLOGICAL ADDICTION

Quitting smoking is difficult for the person who scores high on this factor, that of *psychological addiction*. For him, the craving for the next cigarette begins to build up the moment he puts one out, so tapering off is not likely to work. He must go "cold turkey."

It may be helpful for him to smoke more than usual for a day or two, so that the taste for cigarettes is spoiled, and then isolate himself completely from cigarettes until the craving is gone. Giving up cigarettes may be so difficult and cause so much discomfort that once he does quit, he will find it easy to resist the temptation to go back to smoking because he knows that some day he will have to go through the same agony again.

6. HABIT

This kind of smoker is no longer getting much satisfaction from his cigarettes. He just lights them frequently without even realizing he is doing so. He may find it easy to quit and stay off if he can break the habit patterns he has built up. Cutting down gradually may be quite effective if there is a change in the way the cigarettes are smoked and the conditions under which they are smoked. The key to success is becoming *aware* of each cigarette you smoke. This can be done by asking yourself, "Do I really want this cigarette?" You may be surprised at how many you do not want.

Summary of Test 3

If you do not score high on any of the six factors, chances are that you do not smoke very much or have not been smoking for very many years. If so, giving up smoking—and staying off—should be easy.

If you score high on several categories you apparently get several kinds of satisfaction from smoking and will have to find several solutions. Certain combinations of scores may indicate that giving up smoking will be especially difficult. Those who score high on both Factor 4 and Factor 5, *reduction of negative feelings* and *craving*, may have a particularly hard time in going off smoking and in staying off. However, there are ways to do it; many smokers represented by this combination have been able to quit.

Others who score high on Factors 4 and 5 may find it useful to change their patterns of smoking and cut down at the same time. They can try to smoke fewer cigarettes, smoke them only half-way down, use low-tar-and-nicotine cigarettes, and inhale less often and less deeply. After several months of this temporary solution, they may find it easier to stop completely.

You must make two important decisions: (1) whether to try to do without the satisfactions you get from smoking or find an appropriate, less hazardous substitute, and (2) whether to try to cut out cigarettes all at once or taper off.

Your scores should guide you in making both of these decisions.

∎ T E S T 4 ∎
Does the World Around You Make It Easier or Harder to Change Your Smoking Habit?

What will happen when you try to quit smoking? Aside from the problems that may arise within yourself because of the strength of the smoking habit and what you get out of it, to what extent will you get help from what is happening around you?

This test will help you identify which of 5 factors may be of particular importance to you in providing support to your efforts to quit smoking. A factor on which your score is 5 or 6 represents a part of your environment that can be a help to you. A factor on which your score is 3 or 4 indicates a situation that may hurt your chances of staying off cigarettes.

1. DOCTORS

Many people are influenced by what their physicians do and say about the smoking problem. We know that the overwhelming majority of doctors accept cigarette smoking as a serious health hazard and that well over half of the doctors who used to smoke have given it up. If you score 5 or 6 on this factor, talk to your doctor about smoking and get his support.

2. GENERAL CLIMATE

A score of 3 or 4 on this factor indicates that the environment in which you live and work will not be very helpful in your effort to quit smoking. You may need to seek a more congenial environment. If so, make a point of talking to or associating with people who are trying to stop smoking or who have succeeded in doing so. Also, avoid places where smoking is permitted in favor of places where smoking is prohibited.

3. ADVERTISING INFLUENCE

A score of 3 or 4 on this factor indicates that you are strongly influenced by cigarette advertising. You may have to avoid exposing yourself to these influences until you can withstand them. Reducing your television viewing or watching educational television may help.

4. KEY GROUP INFLUENCES

Knowing the position taken by certain "key groups" can be very important for some people, and a score of 5 or 6 on this factor indicates that you are aware of the influence of such groups. Some people are strongly influenced by the actions of the federal government, some by public and private health agencies, others by schools. All these are on public record that smoking is harmful and all are engaged in programs to reduce cigarette smoking.

5. INTERPERSONAL INFLUENCES

For most of us there are certain people who are particularly important to us. What these people think, do, and say can make a big difference in the way we behave. For some it is a husband or a wife. For others it is their children or their parents. For still others it is the people at work. Because there are so many possible influences, it is difficult to determine which ones are important to you through a simple set of questions. Your answer to Question M should serve as a guide in this area. If your score is 5 or 6, the people who are important to you are likely to be helpful in your effort to quit smoking. If, however, your score is 3 or 4, these important people may not be helpful unless you actively seek their support.

Summary of Test 4

Your chances of staying off cigarettes permanently depend to a large extent on the support you get from the world around you. Your scores on this test identify the "helps" and "hindrances" in your own environment. With this knowledge, you may be able to find ways to improve your chances.

◼ Conclusions

You have completed both parts of the Smoker's Self-Testing Kit. As noted earlier, it was designed (1) to help you decide whether you want to give up smoking, (2) to give you some understanding of the problems you might run into, and (3) to provide some guidelines on how to meet these problems. If you need further help, talk to your physician. Health agencies, both public and private, can provide you with more information and tell you about programs in your own community that may help you to stop smoking.

By 1973, over 30 million adults in the United States had succeeded in breaking their cigarette smoking habits. It's a good group to join. Do it now.

Organizations and Services

Action on Smoking and Health (ASH), 2013 H. Street N.W., Washington, DC 20006

American Cancer Society (ACS), 777 Third Avenue, New York, NY 10017

American Health Foundation—Smoke Cessation System, 320 East 43rd Street, New York, NY 10017

American Heart Association (AHA), 7320 Greenville Avenue, Dallas, TX 75231

American Journal of Acupuncture, 1400 Lost Acre Drive, P.O. Box N-2, Felton, CA 95018

American Lung Association (ALA), 1740 Broadway, New York, NY 10019

Biofeedback Society of America, 4301 Owens, Wheatridge, CO 80303

British Medical Association, BMA House, Tavistock Square, London, England WCIH 9JP

Center for Health Promotion and Education, Centers for Disease Control, 1600 Clifton Road, Atlanta, GA 30333

Department of Health Education, Porter Memorial Hospital, 2525 South Downing, Denver, CO 80201

Federal Trade Commission, Office of Public Information, Pennsylvania Avenue and 6th Street, N.W., Washington, DC 20508

5-Day Plan to Stop Smoking, Seventh-Day Adventist Church, Narcotics Education Division, 6840 Eastern Avenue N.W., Washington, DC 20012

Group Against Smoking Pollution (GASP), P.O. Box 242, Brookline, MA 02146

Live for Life, Breathe for Life, Johnson & Johnson, New Brunswick, NJ 08903

Narcotics Education, Inc., P.O. Box 4390, Washington, DC 20012

National Center for Health Education, 211 Sutter Street, San Francisco, CA 94108

National Health Information Clearinghouse, P.O. Box 1133, Washington, DC 22013

National Heart, Lung and Blood Institute, Building 31, Room 4A-21, National Institutes of Health, Bethesda, MD 20205

National Interagency Council on Smoking and Health, 419 Park Avenue South, Suite 1301, New York, NY 10016

Office of Cancer Communications, National Cancer Institute, National Institutes of Health, Bethesda, MD 20205

Office on Smoking and Health, 158 Park Building, 5600 Fishers Lane, Rockville, MD 20857

Schick Laboratories, 1901 Avenue of the Stars, Suite 1530, Los Angeles, CA 90067

SmokEnders, 50 Washington Street, Norwalk, CT 06854

Superintendent of Documents, U.S. Government Printing Office, Washington, DC 20402

The Tobacco Institute, 1875 I Street N.W., Washington, DC 20006

Valley of the Sun Company (self-hypnosis cassette tapes), Box 38, Malibu, CA 90264

NUTRITION

Healthy Eating

The health/fitness specialist promoting wellness in the workplace must be concerned with proper nutrition. This is especially true if onsite eating facilities are available to employees, because then some control over food selection can be exercised. Regardless of eating facilities, however, nutrition education and information programming are necessary for the overwhelming number of nutritionally illiterate in our workforce.

Because most staff in a health/fitness program are not highly trained in nutrition, a resource person in food services usually is required to implement a nutrition service. Moreover, the education component requires someone with a solid background. Before we recommend specific procedures for promoting proper nutrition, we will present an overview of nutrition.

Supermarket shelves provide a variety of some 10,000 processed and packaged articles; it is not surprising that Americans are often at a loss when trying to choose nutritious foods. "A single food may appear fresh, canned, frozen concentrated, or dehydrated and instantized. Add to that the many new techniques of preparation—heat-and-eat, brown-and-serve, shake-and-bake, boil-in-bag, brown-in-bag, shake, tote or toast."[1] Brody estimates that more than 50% of the foods we eat are processed and packaged and, of those, 50% did not exist 10 years ago.[2] To compound the confusion is the more than

$2 billion dollars per year of advertising, much of which is misleading. Poor eating habits are an understandable result.

Most Americans do not receive adequate nutrition education, and it is little wonder that their diet is no longer wholesome. Since 1900, there has been a 31% increase in fat consumption in the United States, and a 36% increase in the ingestion of sucrose and other sugars. During the same period, we have reduced our complex carbohydrate intake by 43%; beef consumption has risen 72% since 1910, and flour and cereal products are now eaten 54% less often than in the past. Sugar- and fat-laden ice cream products are now consumed an astounding 1426% more often than in 1910. Fat- and cholesterol-rich animal sources now make up 70% of our national protein intake and 3 of every 5 calories eaten come from fats or added sugars.[2] The U.S. diet is generally deficient in fiber and is much too high in sodium. The rate of caffeine and alcohol consumption also is cause for alarm.

Contemporary eating habits reflect the premium placed on the ease of preparation of our meals. Unfortunately, quality and nutritional value have been sacrificed for convenience and speed. Living life in the fast lane has dramatically changed our nutritional habits, and fast foods may be considered the bastard offspring of our hurried way of life. Fast foods typically are rich in fats, sodium, and sugar, low in vegetables and fiber, and overabundant in calories and protein.

Corporate and institutional cafeterias often are as guilty as the burger chains of serving processed foods with nutritional deficiencies. Fast foods also tend to play a dominant role in our eating behaviors at home, where our nutritional habits are shaped from early childhood. Because healthy eating habits usually are not learned during childhood or maintained during adulthood, nutritional enhancement projects in the health/fitness program should address both the participant and his or her family.

▌ Basic Nutrition

Basic nutrition concepts serve as a foundation for understanding and planning sound nutrition programs. Six classes of nutrients enable the body to function properly: carbohydrates, proteins, fats, vitamins, minerals, and water.

Carbohydrates, which are metabolized into glucose, are the main source of energy for the body. Carbohydrates are necessary for fat metabolism to occur and, when eaten in adequate quantity, they free protein for structural maintenance, repair, and growth.

The distinction between *complex* and *simple* carbohydrates is important. Of total dietary calories, 48% should come from complex carbohydrate sources and only 10% should come from simple carbohydrates. Complex carbohydrates are found in foods that also supply protein, fat, vitamins, and minerals. Their best forms are fresh fruits and vegetables and whole grains and cereals. Simple carbohydrates such as sucrose or honey containing fructose supply empty calories. Foods that contain empty calories have low nutrient values for protein, vitamins, and minerals in relationship to their contributing caloric content. Overabundance of such foods in our diet has been linked to many diseases, including tooth decay, obesity, diabetes, and heart disease. On the other hand, complex carbohydrates contain dietary fiber that may reduce the risk of contracting diseases such as colon cancer, diverticulitis, and hiatus

hernia. Dietary fiber is deficient in most U.S. diets. Fiber is a nondigestable component of fruits, vegetables, and whole grains that supplies bulk to help satisfy appetite and aids in efficient digestion and elimination of food. Table 9.1 gives the amount of fiber found in some common foods.

Protein is a major constituent of the cells of the body. It makes up nearly 2000 enzymes in the body, and it is required for blood clotting, acid–base regulation, muscle contraction, and hormone synthesis. Body proteins are composed of amino acid "building blocks." Those we must ingest are called *essential amino acids*. Proteins that have all the essential amino acids in the correct proportions are *complete*; those that do not are *incomplete*. The U.S. recommended daily allowance (RDA) is 0.8 grams of protein per kilogram of body weight and should provide about 12% to 15% of total daily calories. The need for protein is not substantially increased by increased physical activity, although growth of new tissue does require supplemental protein. Children, pregnant women, and burn victims, for example, require additional protein. In the United States, protein is most often obtained from animal sources, but fruit, vegetable, and grain products are good sources of incomplete proteins—they can be combined correctly to form complementary amino acid balances and thus produce complete proteins. Food combinations that form complete proteins are lentils with wheat or rice; legumes with cereals; soybeans with rice; and leafy vegetables with seeds, whole grains, or yeast.[5]

Fat is important as the body's greatest store of potential energy; whereas carbohydrates and proteins contain 4 calories per gram, lipids contain 9. Fat deposits cushion and protect vital organs, serve as insulation, and transport the fat-soluble vitamins A, D, E, and K. Because it remains in the digestive tract longer than other nutrients, fat helps delay hunger pangs. During prolonged exercise, glucose stores are diminished and fat is metabolized increasingly as a source of energy. Humans can remain healthy on a diet of only 10% of calories as fat, although the RDA is 25% to 30% of the total daily calories.

▌ T A B L E 9 . 1 ▌
Dietary Fiber in Food

Food	Serving Size	Weight (g)	Fiber (g)
Breads and crackers			
Graham crackers	2 squares	15	1.5
Rye bread	1 slice	25	2.0
Rye crackers	3 wafers	20	2.3
Whole-wheat bread	1 slice	25	2.4
Cereals			
All-Bran or 100% Bran	1 cup	70	23.0
Bran Buds	¾ cup	60	18.0
Cracked wheat (bulgur), dry	⅓ cup	50	5.6
Grape-Nuts	⅓ cup	45	5.0
Grits, dry	¼ cup	45	4.8
Rolled oats, dry	½ cup	50	4.5
Shredded wheat	2 biscuits	50	6.1
Fruits			
Apple	1 small	90	3.1
Applesauce	½ cup	120	1.7
Banana	1 medium	100	1.8
Cantaloupe, cubes	¾ cup	120	1.4
Cherries, raw	10	70	0.8
Grapefruit	½	200	2.6
Grapes, raw	16	60	0.4
Orange	1 small	90	1.8
Peach, raw	1 medium	100	1.3
Peaches, canned slices	½ cup	120	1.3
Pear, raw	1 medium	120	2.8
Pears, canned	½ cup	125	1.4
Plum, raw	2 small	90	1.6
Strawberries	½ cup	125	2.6
Tangerine	1 medium	100	2.1
Vegetables			
Beans, green	½ cup	50	1.2
Beets, cooked	⅔ cup	100	2.1
Broccoli, cooked	¾ cup	75	1.6
Cabbage, cooked	¾ cup	100	2.2
Cabbage, raw	1 cup	75	2.1
Carrots, cooked	¾ cup	100	2.1
Carrots, raw	1 medium	100	3.7
Cauliflower, cooked	½ cup	100	1.2
Cauliflower, raw	1 cup	100	1.8
Celery, cooked	⅔ cup	100	2.4
Celery, raw	2½ stalks	100	3.0
Corn kernels	⅔ cup	110	4.2
Cucumber	½ of 7-inch cucumber	100	1.5
Kale, cooked	½ cup	100	2.0
Kidney beans, cooked	1 cup	75	3.6
Lentils, cooked	½ cup	100	4.0
Lettuce	1 cup	50	0.8
Parsnips, cooked	¾ cup	120	5.9

■ T A B L E 9 . 1 ■
CONTINUED

Food	Serving Size	Weight (g)	Fiber (g)
Peas, cooked	½ cup	60	3.8
Potatoes, cooked	⅔ cup	90 (raw)	3.1
Rice, brown, cooked	1 cup	65	1.1
Rice, white, cooked	1 cup	65	0.4
Spinach	2 large leaves	50	1.8
Summer squash, cooked	½ cup	100	2.2
Summer squash, raw	1 5-inch squash	100	3.0
Turnips, raw	1 cup	100	2.2

Source: The fiber analyses were prepared by Dr. James W. Anderson, professor of medicine and clinical nutrition at the University of Kentucky Medical Center in Lexington, Kentucky, and appear in Brody, J., *Jane Brody's nutrition book*, New York: W. W. Norton, 1981, pp. 146–147. Used by permission.

The type of fat one ingests is as important as the amount. A balance of 33% saturated, 33% monounsaturated, and 33% polyunsaturated fat consumption is currently recommended. Cholesterol should be limited to 300 mg per day, because it may increase the risk of developing atherosclerosis, which can lead to myocardial infarction or stroke.

Vitamins are organic substances that serve crucial functions in most body processes, including the regulation of metabolism, facilitation of energy release, and bone and tissue synthesis. Because these substances are needed in such small amounts, they are sometimes called *micronutrients*. Their sources and RDAs are listed in Table 9.2.

Minerals are metallic elements that function in cellular metabolism. They are important in the regulation of cellular chemical reactions, in the synthesis of biologic nutrients, as a component of hormones, and in reactions that release energy during protein, carbohydrate, and fat catabolism. Sources and RDAs are listed in Table 9.3.

Minerals also are needed in only small amounts. Salt, for example, is readily available in many foods and many people consume it in amounts far beyond the recommended 5 grams (1 teaspoon) per day: hypertension appears to be correlated with excessive salt intake.

Water can be classified as a sixth nutrient.

Water makes up nearly 60% of the body's weight and is a medium for transport and for all metabolic reactions. It is essential for heat absorption and joint lubrication, and it helps give structure and form to the body.[3] There is no RDA for water, but 6 to 8 glasses of liquid per day generally are recommended.

The need for all the six classes of nutrients in the proper proportions was highlighted in 1977 by the work of the Senate Select Committee on Nutrition and Human Needs.[4] According to their report, six of the ten leading causes of death in the United States have been linked to diet: ischemic heart disease, diabetes, stroke, and bowel, breast, and colon cancer. The committee suggested improvement of the American diet by reducing fat, cholesterol, sugar, and salt consumption and by increasing complex carbohydrate intake.

RDAs for many essential nutrients have been published since 1943 by the National Research Council Committee on Dietary Allowances (NRC). These are revised about every 5 years. The NRC provides detailed guidelines for food choices. One of the most important recommendations from the NRC for *all* Americans is that the diet should include a *wide variety* of foods to assure that adequate amounts of all necessary nutrients are consumed.

Another guide useful for choosing nutritional foods is the basic four food group system,

■ T A B L E   9 . 2 ■
Vitamins: Sources and Daily Requirements

Vitamin	Sources	RDA
A	Liver; eggs; cheese; butter; fortified margarine and milk; yellow, orange, and dark-green vegetables and fruits (e.g., carrots, broccoli, spinach, cantaloupe). Vitamin A is preformed in animal foods. In plants, the yellow-orange "provitamin," called carotene, is converted to an active vitamin in the body.	Women: 800 μg*; men: 1000 μg*
B6	Whole-grain (but not enriched) cereals and bread; liver; avocados; spinach; green beans; bananas; fish; poultry; meats; nuts; potatoes; green leafy vegetables.	Women: 2 mg; men: 2.2 mg
B12	Only in animal foods: liver; kidneys; meat; fish; eggs; milk; oysters; nutritional yeast.	Women and men: 3 mg
Biotin	Liver; kidneys; dark-green leafy vegetables; wheat germ; dried beans and peas. Stored in the body so that daily consumption is not crucial.	Women and men: 100–200 μg
C	Citrus fruits; tomatoes; strawberries; melon; green peppers; potatoes; dark-green vegetables.	Women and men: 60 mg
D	Fortified milk; egg yolk; liver; tuna; salmon; cod liver oil. Made on skin in sunlight, but required in diet by dark-skinned persons in cold climates, babies, and those confined indoors.	Women and men: 5 μg
E	Vegetable oils; margarine; wheat germ; whole-grain cereals and bread; liver; dried beans; green leafy vegetables.	Women: 8 mg; men: 10 mg
Folacin (folic acid)	In all plants and animals, especially liver; kidneys; whole-grain cereal and bread; nuts; eggs; dark-green vegetables. Also made by intestinal bacteria. Lost in refined and heavily processed foods.	Women and men: 400 μg
K	Green leafy vegetables; cabbage; cauliflower; peas; potatoes; liver; cereals. Except in newborns, made by bacteria in human intestine.	Women and men: 70–140 μg*
Niacin (B3)	Liver; poultry; meat; tuna; eggs; whole-grain and enriched cereals, pasta, and bread; nuts; dried peas and beans. Body can convert tryptophan in protein into niacin.	Women: 13 mg; men: 18 mg
Pantothenic acid	Egg yolk; liver; kidneys; dark-green vegetables; green beans. Made by microorganisms in the intestinal tract.	Women and men: 4–7 mg*
Riboflavin (B2)	Liver; milk; meat; dark-green vegetables; eggs; whole-grain and enriched cereals, pasta, and bread; mushrooms; dried beans and peas.	Women: 1.2 mg; men: 1.6 mg
Thiamin (B1)	Pork (especially ham); liver; oysters; whole-grain and enriched cereals, pasta, and bread; wheat germ; oatmeal; peas; lima beans. May also be made by intestinal microbes.	Women: 1 mg; men: 1.4 mg

Source: Adapted from Brody, J. *Jane Brody's nutrition book.* New York: W. W. Norton, 1981, pp. 159–164.
*Estimated safe and adequate intake.

▌ T A B L E 9 . 3 ▌
Minerals: Sources and Daily Requirements

Mineral	Sources	RDA
Calcium	Milk and milk products; sardines; canned salmon eaten with bones; dark-green leafy vegetables; citrus fruits; dried beans and peas.	Women and men: 800 mg
Chloride	Table salt and other naturally occurring salts.	Women and men: 1700–5100 mg*
Chromium	Meat; cheese; whole-grain breads and cereals; dried beans; peanuts; brewer's yeast.	Women and men: 0.05–0.2 mg*
Copper	Oysters; nuts; cocoa powder; beef and pork liver; kidneys; dried beans; corn-oil margarine.	Women and men: 2–3 mg*
Fluorine	Fish; tea; most animal foods; fluoridated water; foods grown with or cooked in fluoridated water.	Women and men: 1.5–4 mg*
Iron	Liver (especially pork, followed by calf, beef, and chicken); kidneys; red meats; egg yolk; green, leafy vegetables; dried fruits (raisins, apricots, and prunes); dried beans and peas; potatoes; blackstrap molasses; enriched and whole-grain cereals.	Women: 18 mg; men: 10 mg
Magnesium	Leafy, green vegetables (eaten raw); nuts (especially almonds and cashews); soybeans; seeds; whole grains.	Women: 300 mg; men: 350 mg
Manganese	Nuts; whole grains; vegetables and fruits; tea; instant coffee; cocoa powder.	Women and men: 2.5–5 mg*
Molybdenum	Legumes; cereal grains; liver; kidney; some dark-green vegetables.	Women and men: 0.15–0.5 mg*
Phosphorus	Meat; poultry; fish; eggs; dried beans and peas; milk and milk products; phosphates in processed foods, especially soft drinks.	Women and men: 800 mg
Potassium	Orange juice; bananas; dried fruits; meats; bran; peanut butter; dried beans and peas; potatoes; coffee; tea; cocoa.	Women and men: 1800–5600 mg*
Selenium	Seafood; whole-grain cereals; meat; egg yolk; chicken; milk; garlic.	Women and men: 0.05–0.2 mg*
Sulfur	Beef; wheat germ; dried beans and peas; peanuts; clams.	Not established

Source: Adapted from Brody, J. *Jane Brody's nutrition book.* New York: W. W. Norton, 1981, pp. 184–188. Used by permission.
*Estimated safe and adequate intake.

which is simpler to follow than the detailed criteria of the RDAs (Table 9.4).

A common point of confusion is how activity level influences nutritional requirements. In general, a person who increases physical activity does not require a diet any different from that recommended for all Americans, except that increased energy (calorie) expenditure obviously increases the need for energy intake (unless the participant is trying to lose weight). Contrary to popular belief, even protein needs are not significantly raised by exercise and usually are met satisfactorily by the larger amount of food an active person eats. The NRC recommends about 2000 calories per day for adequate energy and nutrient for an inactive 120-pound adult

■ T A B L E 9 . 4 ■
The Basic Four Food Groups

Food	Amount per Serving	Servings per Day
Milk Group		
Milk	8 ounces (1 cup)	Children 0–9 years: 2–3
Yogurt, plain	1 cup	Children 9–12 years: 3
Hard cheese	1¼ ounces	Teens: 4
Cheese spread	2 ounces	Adults: 2
Ice cream	1½ cups	Pregnant women: 3
Cottage cheese	2 cups	Nursing mothers: 4
Meat Group		
Meat, lean	2–3 ounces cooked	2 (can be eaten as mixtures of animal
Poultry	2–3 ounces	and vegetable foods; if only vegetable
Fish	2–3 ounces	protein is consumed, it must be
Hard cheese	2–3 ounces	balanced)
Eggs	2–3	
Cottage cheese	½ cup	
Dry beans and peas	1–1½ cups cooked	
Nuts and seeds	½–¾ cup	
Peanut butter	4 tablespoons	
Vegetable and Fruit Group		
Vegetables, cut up	½ cup	4, including one good vitamin C
Fruits, cut up	½ cup	source like oranges or orange juice
Grapefruit	½ medium	and one deep-yellow or dark-green
Melon	½ medium	vegetable
Orange	1 medium	
Potato	1 medium	
Salad	1 bowl	
Lettuce	1 wedge	
Bread and Cereal Group		
Bread	1 slice	4, whole grain or enriched only,
Cooked cereal	½–¾ cup	including at least 1 serving of
Pasta	½–¾ cup	whole grain
Rice	½–¾ cup	
Dry cereal	1 ounce	

Source: Brody, J. *Jane Brody's nutrition book.* New York: W. W. Norton, 1981, p. 18. Used by permission.

woman. If the same woman is training for a marathon however, and running 70 miles each week, McArdle estimates that she will need an additional 900 calories or more per day to maintain her weight and stamina.[3] Remember that the additional calories should be obtained from a wide variety of foods, with an emphasis on complex carbohydrates and ingestion of adequate fluids, especially in hot or humid weather.

The health/fitness specialist can ameliorate the confusion reflected by the inadequacy of the typical contemporary American's diet through nutrition education and information. The aim of nutrition education is to enhance the participants' knowledge and appreciation of good food selection, preparation, and eating habits, and to teach them about the health problems arising from poor nutrition. The topics you should address include: the basic food groups, how to reduce fat in your diet, how to avoid salt, how to increase fiber, how to eat well while on the run, how to eat well while on the road, how to buy wholesome foods, how to be a healthy vegetarian, what food supplements you need, how to eat properly during pregnancy, how to feed people of different ages, how to read nutrition information labels, how to eat properly for weight control, and how to select low-caloric-density foods.

You can help educate employees by using: newsletters, paycheck stuffers, computer-assisted instruction, reference materials, cafeteria posters, color-coded food selections in the cafeteria, caloric and nutritional values added to menus or posted on vending machines, and demonstrations of nutritious meal preparation. An awareness and promotion program should elicit inquiries about ways to enhance nutrition. Some people will be simply curious; others will be committed to altering their eating behaviors. It is this latter group that forms the nucleus of your nutrition program group. Those participants with serious medical problems, such as diabetes, alcoholism, or extreme obesity, should be referred to medical or community agencies for treatment.

■ Needs Assessment

Nutritional assessment is the first step in program delivery. To advise an individual regarding nutrition, the health/fitness specialist must first determine the participant's current nutritional status. The specialist can put the participant at ease by explaining the various procedures of the assessment process and the significance of each of them.

Any one or a combination of four processes is used for this assessment. The first is clinical observation, which includes a brief physical examination and screening for obvious signs of health and disease. The second is anthropometric measurements, which determine body composition. The third is dietary evaluation, which uses a 24-hour recall, diet history, or food diary to reveal current eating habits. Finally,

biochemical tests are used to ascertain the nutrient constituents of the blood and urine.

Clinical Observation

Clinical assessment should include an abbreviated physical examination, during which the health/fitness specialist takes simple measures such as blood pressure and pulse rate. Table 9.5 lists some important overt indicators of physical health status that should be assessed. If an individual appears to be in very poor physical health, a thorough examination by a physician should be arranged. Healthy people usually look well-nourished and free from illness, but the health/fitness specialist should learn the observable signs of illness that indicate the need for referral to a physician.

Anthropometric Measurements

There are many ways to assess body composition; however, most of the technical approaches are expensive and time-consuming. Body density provides the most accurate indication of the fat-to-lean ratio and in turn provides a means of determining a target body weight of the participant. The methods most often used include skinfold thickness, bone diameter, and girth measurements (see Chapter 7).

Dietary Evaluation

Diet can be evaluated by dietary recall: the health/fitness specialist asks the participant to name all foods eaten in the last 24 hours. More accurate data are obtained from the food intake record, which participants fill out for 3 days (not more than 1 weekend day). The dietary recall can supplement a food intake record by indicating participants' levels of awareness of their eating habits.

Another recent approach to nutritional assessment uses computers. Nutrimed of Richardson, Texas, has developed a computerized nutritional evaluation that is accurate, easy to use,

▌ T A B L E 9 . 5 ▐
Clinical Observation in Nutritional Assessment

Area	Observations	Area	Observations
Body size and stature	Large or small frame; thin, obese, muscle wasting; symmetry in size and shape of body parts	Hair	Distribution, density, luster, grooming, color
		Nails	Length, grooming, thickness, ridging, color of nailbed, spoon shaped
Posture	Erect, rigid, slumping, stretched out	Clothing	Appropriate for age and climate; cleanliness, neat or disheveled
Body movements	Strength, speed, symmetry of movements; tremors, twitching; purposefulness	Speech	Clarity, speed, loud or soft, hoarse, whining, halting, stuttering
Skin	Color, luster (dull, shiny), turgor, sags, wrinkles, lesions, edema, perspiration	Mental status	Alert, responsive, lethargic, listless, apathetic
Tongue, gums, and mucous membranes	Edema, lesions, raw, red or pale color, changes in papillae on tongue	Mood	Smiling, frowning, presence of anxiety indicated by tapping fingers or feet, wringing hands, cold moist palms, furrowed brow
Teeth	Missing, caries, grey or white spots on enamel (mottled enamel)	Presence of discomfort or pain	Moaning, writhing, guarding of a body part

Source: Suitor, C. W., and Hunter, M. F. *Nutrition: Principles and application in health promotion.* Philadelphia: J. B. Lippincott, 1980, p. 228. Used by permission.

and inexpensive. Other providers also offer this service.

Biochemical Evaluation

Another indicator of nutritional status is biochemical assay of particular constituents in the blood and urine. Evaluation usually includes measurement of: (1) serum albumin, hemoglobin, hematocrit; (2) lymphocytes, delayed sensitivity to common antigens; and (3) urinary creatinine and blood urea nitrogen. Measures of serum lipids (total cholesterol, HDL to LDL cholesterol ratio, and triglycerides), uric acid, glucose, electrolytes, and the presence of nutritional anemia are particularly relevant.

Ms. Goldstein is a 35-year-old computer scientist. Her assessment is within normal limits on all measures except her body composition, which is too high in fat, and diet, which has

excesses of protein and deficiencies of iron (Figure 9.1). Essentially, her observable health is normal, yet her sedentary lifestyle and dietary excesses have resulted in excess body fat.

Goal Setting

Unlike assessment, much of which can be performed in a group, goal setting is individual. The counseling provided by the health/fitness specialist is critical. After determining nutritional status, the specialist can help the participant set appropriate and realistic goals. The specialist explains what nutrients constitute a healthy diet and makes recommendations for dietary changes. A graph that shows how the participant's status compares to the average population may be useful.

▌Figure 9.1 Ms. Goldstein's nutritional assessment data. **▌**

Name: Ms. Goldstein
Date: 2-8-85

	Results	Norms
1. Clinical observation		
Height	65 in./165 cm	65 in./165 cm
Weight	150 lb/68.2 Kg	124 lb/56.2 Kg
Pulse	69 bpm	72 bpm
Blood Pressure	115/85 mmHg	120/80 mmHg
Temperature	98.6° F	98.6° F
Other	within normal limits	
2. Anthropometric measurements		
Percent fat	35%	25%
Fat weight	52.5 lb/23.8 Kg	39 lb/13.61 Kg
Lean weight	97.5 lb/44.3 Kg	95 lb/43.11 Kg
3. Dietary evaluation		
Food intake:		
Average calorie intake	1584 Kcal	1600–2400 Kcal
Average energy expenditure	1784 Kcal	1700–2050 Kcal
Average energy balance	+/⊖ 200 Kcal	⊕/– 100 Kcal
Nutrient excesses	Protein	Fat
		Protein
		Sugar
		Sodium
Nutrient deficiencies	Iron	Iron
		Calcium
4. Laboratory test results	within normal limits	

To guide the participant in setting appropriate dietary goals, the specialist needs to explain what is considered to be a healthy diet. The National Dairy Council's *Guide to Good Eating* probably is the most easily understandable and commonly available poster for this purpose. Participants can be given a miniature version to carry until they are familiar with the basic four food groupings.

The health/fitness specialist should explain that if they eat only the recommended number of servings from each group, participants will consume only about 1200 calories; larger servings and/or additional choices from the fruit/vegetable and grain categories will provide the necessary additional calories required for optimal health. Once participants understand the constituents of a nutritious diet, the specialist can make specific, individual recommendations for appropriate changes in eating habits. Figure 9.2 is a sample form for recommendations and guidelines, which the specialist can customize to fit the individual's needs.

Specific goals you may wish to discuss with the participant include: increase consumption of low-caloric-density foods, such as vegetables, cereals, and fruits; decrease consumption of high-caloric-density foods, such as red meats, candy, and desserts; alter poor eating behaviors, such as eating on time cues rather than when hungry, eating too fast, and eating during television viewing; increase consumption of high-fiber foods, such as cereals, tubers, and vegetables.

■ **Figure 9.2** Nutritional recommendations and guidelines. ■

Recommendations:

1. Increase/decrease calorie intake from _____ cal to _____ cal.

2. Increase/decrease fat intake from _____% to _____% of total.

3. Increase/decrease complex carbohydrate intake from _____% to 55% to 60% of total calories.

4. Increase/decrease protein intake from _____% to _____% of total calories.

5. Limit salt intake to 5 grams per day or less.

6. Limit cholesterol intake to 300 mg per day or less.

7. Vary your selections from the basic four food groups as much as possible. Choosing a wide variety of foods is the best way to ensure you will consume all the nutrients you need.

Guidelines:

1. Write down your caloric intake, if necessary, until you have a good idea of your daily intake.

2. Eat more vegetable and less animal fat.

3. Eat as few refined and processed products as you can.

4. Eat more poultry and fish and less red meat.

5. Remove the salt shaker from the table and watch for sodium content on labels.

6. Eat fewer eggs and whole-milk cheeses; use low-fat dairy products.

7. Try new foods you have not eaten before; make each day's menu different.

■ Planning

The planning stage of nutrition counseling is crucial. The specialist must use every possible means to capture participants' interest in improving their diet; she or he must also spark the participant's imagination by teaching creative methods for diet improvement.

Suggestions must be easy to follow to prevent participants from becoming confused or bored. Of course, the strategies the specialist recommends depend on each individual—on how motivated the participant is, how radical the necessary changes in diet are, and how accurate the participant's current nutritional knowledge is.

The basic four food groups and the Senate Select Committee guidelines (Figure 9.3) provide a foundation for healthy eating habits and diet planning. In addition, some participants may need more detailed information about specific aspects of good nutrition planning.

There are two keys for obtaining the required nutrients—variety and moderation. The specialist should advise participants to try new foods as well as to prepare old foods in new ways, and to eat as many different kinds of foods as possible (sampling them all in modest amounts, of course). In general, recommend that participants eat prudently: cut down on fat, sodium, and sugar; increase high-fiber foods; take in only moderate amounts of caffeine and alcohol; and maintain ideal weight. Introduce the concept of caloric density, and explain how foods of high caloric density contain excess calories and usually fewer nutrients than do those of low caloric density (see Chapter 7).

Encouragement is important during the counseling session. The specialist should strive to capture participants' interest in better health through improved diet. Take heed, however, that the more changes that are required, the more difficult it will be to bring about those changes: old eating habits are not easily broken. The novelty of a new way of eating often intrigues the participant at first but, as the newness wears off, additional help may be needed. It is helpful to discuss the difficulty of sticking

■ **Figure 9.3** U.S. Senate Select Committee guidelines. (From Suitor, C. W., ■ and Hunter, M. F. *Nutrition: Principles and application in health promotion.* Philadelphia: J. B. Lippincott, 1980, p. 48.)

U.S. Dietary Goals

1. To avoid overweight, consume only as much energy (calories) as is expended; if overweight, decrease energy intake and increase energy expenditure.

2. Increase the consumption of complex carbohydrates and "naturally occurring" sugars from about 28 percent of energy intake to about 48 percent of energy intake.

3. Reduce the consumption of refined and processed sugars by about 45 percent to account for about 10 percent of total energy intake.

4. Reduce overall fat consumption from approximately 40 percent to about 30 percent of energy intake.

5. Reduce saturated fat consumption to account for about 10 percent of total energy intake; and balance that with polyunsaturated and monounsaturated fats, which should account for about 10 percent of energy intake each.

6. Reduce cholesterol consumption to about 300 mg. a day.

7. Limit the intake of sodium by reducing the intake of salt to about 5 grams a day.

Dietary goals are not meant to be rigid rules but are meant to indicate a healthful direction which people might take when deciding how they want to eat.

The goals suggest the following changes in food selection and preparation:

1. Increase consumption of fruits and vegetables and whole grains.

2. Decrease consumption of refined and other processed sugars and foods high in such sugars.

3. Decrease consumption of foods high in total fat, and partially replace saturated fats, whether obtained from animal or vegetable sources, with polyunsaturated fats.

4. Decrease consumption of animal fat, and choose meats, poultry and fish which will reduce saturated fat intake.

5. Except for young children, substitute low-fat and non-fat milk for whole milk, and low-fat dairy products for high fat dairy products.

6. Decrease consumption of butterfat, eggs and other high cholesterol sources. Some consideration should be given to easing the cholesterol goal for premenopausal women, young children and the elderly in order to obtain the nutritional benefits of eggs in the diet.

7. Decrease consumption of salt and foods high in salt content.

---

to the new regime day after day, week after week, and to suggest ways to deal with problems when they arise. The specialist should also discuss the likelihood of occasional relapse, reassuring clients that this should not discourage them from sticking to their long-term goals. The specialist's own zeal for healthy eating can be a great source of infectious enthusiasm and motivation.

The specialist also should plan group

education. Decide: class size (10 to 12 is recommended); class time and location; lesson content; speakers and outside resources; course evaluation; and synergistic effects of other programming such as exercise and stress management.

You also must plan how participants will monitor their progress. The following are useful techniques: computerized data entry of dietary intakes; periodic reassessment of body weight and composition; support group meetings to discuss progress, share new recipes, and so on; behavior modification progress reports; and incentives for program compliance.

Implementation

The first step in nutrition program implementation might be to suggest that each participant keep a food diary. One simple approach is to check off portions from the basic four food groups as they are eaten. Participants can score their compliance by giving themselves points for eating portions up to the recommended number—and by subtracting points for excesses.

Where appropriate, a health/fitness specialist can also help the implementation of nutrition counseling by encouraging the company food service to follow sound nutritional policies, such as stocking vending machines with fresh fruit, fruit and vegetable juices, and low-fat yogurt instead of candy. Decaffeinated coffee and fresh fruit or rolls should be available for coffee breaks; low-fat milk should be sold in the cafeteria. A well-stocked salad bar complete with low-calorie dressings is another health-conscious cafeteria option. If many participants travel frequently, you can provide guides to assist them in the selection of nutritious foods while eating out.

Participants almost surely will have some difficulty implementing dietary changes, particularly if major alterations are involved. Suggest that the changes progress a little at a time. Instead of switching from whole to nonfat milk, for instance, use low-fat milk at first. If removing the salt shaker from the dinner table is too drastic, gradually reduce its use and do not add salt when cooking—taste for sodium will decline slowly. Most recipes taste just as good when the salt content is halved. Another approach is to follow only one recommendation for the first week, two during the second week, and so on. The group approach is a good way to affect a large number of participants. General Mills, for example, lists the calories for all menu entries served in its dining facilities. Direct ways

to implement nutrition enhancement include (1) classes and demonstrations on healthy food preparation, (2) consumer-education classes on intelligent purchase and selection of food, (3) healthy meal planning in busy lifestyles, and (4) exchange systems for nutrition-conscious consumers.

Evaluation

After the participant has been on a new diet regimen for some time, you should evaluate progress. Recommend that participants return periodically during the first 3 months, bringing along whatever implementation tools they are using, such as food diaries. Evaluate and discuss participants' new eating habits. If participants are following a healthy regimen 80% of the time, they are on the road to nutritional success. It also might be appropriate to reassess body composition at 3 months, especially if a restricted-calorie diet has been used.

If the evaluation shows that the participant has succeeded in altering eating behaviors, offer congratulations and encouragement to continue the good work. If the participant now knows the food groups and recommended guidelines and is meeting his or her goals, the food diary no longer is needed.

If the evaluation pinpoints problems or areas of particular weakness, then try to find out why certain parts of the program are difficult for the participant to follow. It may be necessary to discuss specific goals again, perhaps giving more detailed guidelines.

As in the goal setting and planning session, enthusiasm and motivation are key ingredients of the evaluation process. The specialist must be positive and sympathetic, offering encouragement and assurance that success will come—if gradually—as long as the participants follow their individualized guidelines and adjust to a new way of eating.

The specialist's most important job is to convince participants to try the new program for a reasonable time. If they can be convinced it is worthwhile to stick to the new diet through a transition period, participants probably will become converts simply because they will develop new tastes and will enjoy better health and fitness. Request that participants return for another evaluation after 3 more months, and tell them they can consult you in the meantime if problems arise. Incentive techniques are useful during this period as well.

▌ Summary

There are three types of macronutrients in our foods—carbohydrates, fats, and proteins—and two micronutrients—vitamins, minerals. Water is our remaining essential nutrient. We need adequate amounts of both in our diets to maintain high-level wellness. Changing lifestyles and the demands of work and family frequently influence our good intentions regarding proper nutrition.

We have presented some concepts in this chapter to help the health/fitness professional implement a nutrition program. We discussed assessment techniques to determine the nutritional needs of participants, as well as goal setting and planning. Guidelines to implement and evaluate a nutrition program were discussed.

References ▌

1. Stare, F. J., et al. What everyone should know. In *The complete diet guide for runners and other athletes*, Higdon, H. (ed). Mountain View, CA: World Publications, 1978.

2. Brody, J. E. *Jane Brody's nutrition book.* New York: W. W. Norton and Company, 1981.

3. McArdle, W. D., Katch, F. I., and Katch, V. L. *Exercise physiology: Energy, nutrition, and human performance.* Philadelphia: Lea & Febiger, 1981.

4. Senate Select Committee on Nutrition and Human Needs. *Eating in America.* Cambridge, MA: MIT Press, 1977.

5. Hamilton, E. M., et al. *Nutrition: Concepts and controversies*, 3rd ed. St. Paul, MN: West Publishing Company, 1985.

STRESS MANAGEMENT

Stress Awareness (handwritten)

Several years ago, the executive medical director of a well-known silicon valley organization was contacted with the purpose of marketing a "Managing Stress to Increase Productivity" workshop. After polite formalities were out of the way, he indicated that their corporation had no stress. "In fact if anyone is under stress here we would just as soon get rid of them because they must be <u>neurotic</u>." Three years after this interesting interview, this same corporation had an inhouse program that was widely touted as a state-of-the-art stress-management course.

Had this corporation developed massive amounts of stress in the intervening years? No, it seems more likely that, at the time of the initial interview, this corporation was unaware of the true state of affairs. Subsequently, the corporation had had its attention turned to stress because a highly placed executive had had a heart attack. His private physician had communicated, in no uncertain terms, that stress had been at least a significant causal factor.

This is not an unusual occurrence in the corporate setting. Stress-related illness or death among senior management frequently focuses sufficient attention on the problem to warrant wholesale programming in stress management.

This chapter will present a model and informational basis on which to structure an inhouse stress-management program. The use

of external resources either exclusively or in combination with inhouse personnel also will be discussed.

Stress and Distress

Generally speaking, stress is the reaction that each individual has to all of life's stimuli. Stress is not inherently "good" or "bad," although stress has a villainous reputation. This reputation is based on simple misunderstanding of the nature of stress.

Actually, *stress* is simply the body's ability to respond to life. *Distress* is an accumulation of normal stress beyond personal limits.

It is interesting that when audiences are asked to describe stress, they most often choose words like *anxiety, overwhelm, danger,* and *illness.* These words are actually descriptive of *distress,* which *Webster's New Collegiate Dictionary* defines as "a state of danger." Distress is very much in evidence in the corporate setting. Distress has four basic manifestations:

1. *Physical symptoms.* Recent research by Pelletier et al. has demonstrated positive correlations between stress and illness.[1] The American Medical Association has stated that 80% of all illnesses are stress related,

and high turnover rates, absenteeism, alcoholism, and drug abuse are the most visible examples of corporate symptoms of distress.

Historically, corporations have not wanted to acknowledge the relationship between stress and these symptoms because to do so might implicate the organization's environment or management style.

Although fast-track corporate cultures may contribute to certain types of stress-related disorders, the American way of life need not be hazardous to your health, as this chapter will demonstrate.

2. *Interpersonal symptoms.* Physical distress and chronic stresses often coincide with increased temper and conflict. When people are tired or ill, their problem-solving abilities are severely impaired.

3. *Emotional impact.* According to Dr. Hans Selye, the founder of the stress theory, the first effect of stress on the human system is the *stage of alarm.*[2] During the alarm stage, our bodies go into a *fight or flight* reaction that is instinctual and unreasoning. Another way of saying this is that in a normal state of *normal* baseline stress, the intellect is in control of the emotions. When the alarm state takes over, emotions are in control of the intellect and behavior may become emotion or instinct driven. Unfortunately, this instinctual response need not be triggered by an actual threat to physical survival. All that is needed is a *perceived* threat to the ego or self-esteem for the fight or flight response to be triggered.

Corporate settings spawn a host of these perceived threats to the survival of self-esteem; for example, difficult people and cost-containment measures often threaten our employment status.

4. *Impaired creativity.* The most subtle effect of distress in the workplace is on creativity. When individuals or workgroups are experiencing distress, their abilities to come up with unique solutions to thorny problems are decreased. Although when we are in distress we are motivated to find solutions, we may not develop appropriate or quality solutions and, as management

theorists have noted, we may solve the wrong problem.

The costs of distress to corporations in dollars and cents are enormous. As stated in Chapter 1, there is documented proof of the human medical costs resulting from risk factors and their related distress-producing behaviors.

The subject of stress is not a mere fad. Distress is a deeply rooted symptom of the age we live in, an age that Drucker terms "turbulent times"[3] and Toffler has dubbed the "information age society."[4]

"It is the curse of a person to be born in a great age" (Chinese proverb, 10th century B.C.). Individuals and organizations are attempting to deal with exponential increases in the rate, depth, and types of change with the same coping strategies learned generations ago. If corporations attempt to manage today's workforce with the autocratic or traditional management styles of the fifties, they become vulnerable to criticism and cannot adequately cope with the changing values of today's employees.

In addition, the information technologies of hardware and software have been both a blessing and a curse. Millions of today's employees are struggling to keep up with the electronic communications revolution. The most hard-hit segment of the workforce may be not those at the bottom but those at the middle and the top. The higher an individual goes, the farther there is to fall.

Changes in information types, formats, and delivery compel managers to join the computer age. Resistance to computer literacy due to entrenched styles of adapting may bring a middle-management ice age. Like the mammoth, many managers may become obsolete. Added to these multiple stresses are shifts in the values and age composition of the workforce, and the increasingly prominent role that women play in altering the culture of a corporation. Both men and women must learn to adapt to these multidimensioned stimuli or they experience distress.

All change, regardless of whether it is positive or negative, is stressful. The basic choice is whether to view change as an opportunity or to react to it as a threat. This choice and the capacity to choose are the areas that may be influenced by a stress-management program in the corporate setting.

Benefits of a Stress-Management Program

There are three immediate benefits of hosting a stress-management program.

One, the public relations benefits of stress management are unlimited. Employees believe that the organization has a real interest in their health. Stress management allows the organization to put money and other resources behind their expressed concerns over employees' stress levels.

Two, if a stress management program is well designed, it provides an opportunity for employees to develop healthy habits that have secondary and tangible benefits to the corporation. Examples of such benefits are: reduced absenteeism; a higher degree of personal responsibility for health; greater personal vitality, which in turn leads to less irritability between employees; and an overall reduction in chronic distress levels.

The third benefit of stress management was measured by Pelletier and his colleagues in a study of 172 corporations with health/fitness programs.[1] Their research indicated that there was a measurable decrease in employee turnover rates and in employees' use of health insurance and sick leave over a 5-year period.

The literature dealing with stress management from the viewpoint of cost–benefit analysis is prolific. Chapter 1 presented an examination of this subject.

Preliminary Decisions

The first step is to identify the target audience or program participants. Is the program going to be offered to, and therefore oriented to, individual random program participants or particular employee groups? Cost is the major factor to consider here; it is generally more cost-effective to tailor a program to fit a particular group than to try to gear it to random individuals. A second benefit resulting from a group participation is peer reinforcement and mutual support in practicing new skills (Figure 10.1).

It is a good idea to designate the initial offering as a *pilot program*. This makes the venture sound less risky to the senior management, who can more easily support an experiment that can be changed and modified than a program that makes a long-term commitment.

A top-down executive-staff-supported stress-management program will have maximum leverage. The likelihood of continued funding for long-term intervention is enhanced if senior management participates.

A third decision is whether to create an in-house program or to use resources in the community. According to Pelletier, who has done the most exhaustive study so far on the costs of health/fitness programs in the corporate setting, it is preferable to use resources available in the community, whenever possible, in the design or implementation of a stress-management program.[1] There are excellent packages that come in video, audio cassette, workbook, and textbook format. You must decide whether it is feasible to develop your own materials, or whether you want to buy them and then tailor them to your specific setting; the latter is likely to be more cost-effective.

A crucial fourth step is establishing realistic goals for your stress-management program. Many corporations have unrealistic expectations based on unspoken assumptions or lack of information. Your goals should be geared to the sophistication level of your target population and the information level of senior management.

It is essential to begin with specific, measurable, and observable goals that are agreed to by the participants and management, so that there is a basis for evaluating the success or failure of the program. The following are realistic expectations for an initial course—participants will be able to:

■ **Figure 10.1** Risks and benefits of group versus individual participation in ■ stress-management courses.

INDIVIDUAL MODEL

Risks	Benefits
Lack of feedback from other participants	Goals tailored to each person
No support group to carry on learning after course	Individualized instruction specific to needs
	Individual gets much attention and feedback
Expensive to develop customized program	
Poor use of director's time versus payoff to corporation	

GROUP MODEL

Risks	Benefits
Peer pressure may be reason for individuals to drop out	Larger population practices health habits
Lack of individualized instruction	Greater payoff in use of director's time
Reduced feedback from instructor to each individual	Use of materials and resources can be spread out among many participants
	Support group for individuals to carry on learning from class

■ Know the difference between stress and distress, and positive and negative stress

■ Identify their own symptoms of distress

■ Develop an action plan for identified symptoms of distress

■ Increase their practice of healthy habits

■ Understand the benefits of exercise, diet, and relaxation training

■ Practice a relaxation exercise

■ Decrease the frequency of distressing habits

■ Understand the role of perception in the formation of negative attitudes

The fifth step is to market the program to both management and the target participants. Stress management is often the most popular and least expensive intervention in the health/ fitness package. The most frequently expressed needs of corporations are exercise and stress-management programs. Generally, stress management is less expensive than an exercise program for employees, and many corporations

are becoming more sensitive to expressions of high distress levels within the organization.

One good way to market a stress-management program to decision makers is to invite the senior management to participate in a full day, offsite seminar given by a highly skilled stress-management consultant. The consultant should have an in-depth understanding of your particular corporate culture. Many programs fail at the outset simply because the pilot program was presented to senior management by inhouse personnel. Generally speaking, a senior manager feels politically unable or unwilling to confide in a more junior person in the organization, and this confidentiality issue can compromise the program's success. In addition, it is difficult to be perceived as an expert by your own company, even though you may have a wealth of knowledge and experience. In short, if you want to get off on the right foot with management, bring in an outside consultant who speaks the same language as the executive group, has a firm grasp of the stress-management field, and is an active practitioner of stress management. A vendor that has previously had success with the organization in a different area and has also demonstrated competence and knowledge in stress management can provide a consultant.

Once you have sold senior management on the benefits of a stress-management program through demonstrating a good cost–benefit ratio and by their direct experience in a pilot program, you have the ability to offer the program throughout the organization. At this point, there are several models available for structuring an organizationwide stress-management program.

Targeting Stress-Management Segments

Top-Down Approach

Within the top-down model, after presentation to the executive group, the next course is given to the upper-middle management or senior staff, depending on the structure of your organization. Subsequent offerings are to middle, lower-middle, or second-line supervisors, then to supervisors, and finally to all staff employees (often called nonexempt personnel).

Bottom-Up Approach

Due to the popularity of stress-management courses and the fact that they generate employee goodwill toward the corporation, there is significant benefit to offering the course to those at the bottom of the corporate ladder. The immediate benefits to selecting this group are smiles and positive attitudes and appeasement of the common employee dissatisfaction with lack of training opportunities.

Self-Selection Approach

Many corporations open the course to all employees regardless of classification on a volunteer basis. The benefit of this approach is also a liability. There is a positive consequence to having managers and their employees in the same course—it communicates, "We know you all have stress and we're going to work on it together." The risk is that many managers will not sign up for a class when their employees also are enrolled. Managers often are hesitant or unwilling to expose their problems, or even to acknowledge that they may have stress, to someone less senior in the organization. One way to alleviate this potential problem is to offer the course at two different times, one for exempt and one for nonexempt employees.

Needs Assessment

It is crucial for the stress-management component to incorporate the information collected in the other areas of the overall health/fitness program. For example, data pertaining to medical screening, cardiovascular endurance, muscular strength, flexibility, endurance, diet, and body composition are all indicators of levels of stress.

In the education assessment, the health/fitness director uses all this information and adds specific measurements collected via the Stress-Pertise test (Figure 10.2) and questionnaires on current methods of coping with stress (Figure 10.3), daily stress and tension (Figures 10.4 and 10.5), *Type A* personality (Figure 10.6), positive stressors (Figure 10.7), and life events (Figure 10.10).

The purpose of the Stress-Pertise test is to develop a baseline measurement of factors influencing successful management of stress. The 20 questions are either taken directly or extrapolated from Selye's research. The correct answer to all questions is *yes*. The questionnaire can be a catalyst for participants to develop interest in the subject because many of the questions (notably 1, 2, 3, 4, 10, 11) often are directly contradictory to participants' beliefs.

The health/fitness specialists should introduce the information in Figure 10.3 with the caveat that they are only gathering information, and that answers are confidential. The data should be used to evaluate current levels of

■ **Figure 10.2** Stress-pertise test. ■

This test is designed to help you assess your knowledge concerning our nation's number one health issue. Please mark either *yes* or *no* for each question, according to whether or not you agree with the statement.

Yes No

1. Stress is unavoidable.
2. A lover's kiss involves the same stress reaction as an interview with a prospective employer.
3. Stress can be good for you.
4. Breathing is stressful.
5. A happy, healthy staff produces more than a staff motivated by fear.
6. The definition of *distress* is *a state of danger*.
7. Stress is cumulative.
8. You can overload the body with stress, causing it to break down.
9. All employees, regardless of position, experience stress. It is a matter of type more than degree.
10. Your attitude about stress can make a difference between health and disease.
11. The right kind of stress can save your life.
12. With the right kind of assistance, employees in a company can get along considerably better.
13. Mental and physical health are interlocking.
14. You can prevent absentee days by promoting healthy habits.
15. Disease is stress related.
16. Producing excellent quality work need not be distressing.
17. Working at any job, however satisfying, is stressful.
18. Humor on the job is appropriate.
19. All those around me, including my clients, suffer if I am *distressed*.
20. I can do something about stress on the job.

Scoring: The correct answer to all 20 items is *yes*. If you answered 15 or more *yes*, you already know the value of a course or materials directly designed to help you manage stress. If you answered *no* to 3 or more, an education on stress and how to approach it positively is essential.

knowledge, experience, and practices, not to criticize or negatively evaluate. The questionnaire in Figure 10.4 can be used over 1 month or less to contrast levels of stress and tension from day to day and to encourage participants to gain awareness of their body–mind on a daily basis. The questionnaire in Figure 10.5 is a nice adjunct. Generally the two will correlate, so that in a period of high distress the daily tension rating also will be elevated.

The concept of *Type A* personalities has become popular. More has been written about the questionnaire in Figure 10.6 than about any single measurement of stress and its correlation with personality. Although the test is an inconclusive measurement of a cause-and-effect relationship of cardiovascular heart disease to behavior, Freidman and Rosenman have sampled many thousands of people and the questionnaire has been a reliable indicator of a

■ **Figure 10.3** Current methods of coping with stress questionnaire. "Stress resides ■ neither in the person nor in the situation alone, but depends on how the person appraises particular events" (D. Lazarus, University of California, Berkeley).

Please mark either *yes* or *no* for each question.

Yes   *No*

____ ____   1. Is my energy level lower than it used to be?

____ ____   2. Do I spend more time worrying than I used to?

____ ____   3. Is my usage of liquor, cigarettes, or tranquilizers increasing?

____ ____   4. Is my sense of satisfaction or pleasure in life not as high as I wish it was?

____ ____   5. Do minor problems and small disappointments throw me into a dither?

____ ____   6. Am I finding it difficult to get along with people, or are people having trouble getting along with me?

____ ____   7. Do I fear people or situations that never used to bother me?

____ ____   8. Do I suffer from self-doubt?

____ ____   9. Do I worry constantly about the future?

____ ____ 10. Do I accomplish more, but feel less satisfied?

____ ____ 11. Am I physically exhausted even when I have not done any physical activities?

Scoring: Give yourself 1 point per *yes* answer and add your total of points. If you had a low score (less than 3 points), you are moving in the direction of wellness. The lower the score, the better.

Total score: _____

Level of effective coping: 0–3 = high; 4–7 = medium; 8–1 = low.

---

correlation between certain personality traits (free-floating hostility, a sense of time urgency, and excessively competitive relationships) and heart attacks. Participants should be encouraged to read the complete book[5] if they get a high score on the test. One further disclaimer: for women, the Type A personality appears to be less of a risk than the *superwoman complex* so often seen in women with dual careers of family and job. Women appear to be motivated more by a desire to please everyone and do a perfect job with family and work than by the competitive, aggressive characteristics of the Type A personality.

A questionnaire that measures the healthy behaviors the participant already has is presented in Figure 10.7. *Positive stress* is defined in

a result-oriented manner. Positive stresses increase immunity by adding to your reserves in the bank account of health.

The scales of satisfaction (Figure 10.8) and frustration (Figure 10.9) and the life events questionnaire (Figure 10.10) are perhaps the most helpful measurements of stress. A high score on the life events questionnaire indicates an increased risk of stress-related illnesses. However, this questionnaire has been administered to over 5000 participants and we have observed that, on the contrary, the participants with high scores often are quite healthy human beings. In general, participants who have high scores on the satisfactions scale and low scores on the frustrations scale are very healthy people.

■ **Figure 10.4** Daily stress and tension rating. ■

Below are four pairs of adjectives that describe relative stressfulness or lack of stress. For each pair, there is a scale that goes from 5 to 0. The numbers have the following meanings:

5 = *Very* relaxed, congenial
4 = *Moderately* relaxed, congenial
3 = *Slightly* relaxed, congenial
2 = *Slightly* tense, irritable
1 = *Moderately* tense, irritable
0 = *Very* tense, irritable

Note that there is no neutral rating, because the absence of any feeling of relaxation or tenseness does not seem a likely mental state. Please check under the number that most closely reflects how you have generally felt today for each pair of adjectives. Your ratings may vary from one pair of adjectives to another. That is, you may feel "very tense" and mark "0" on that scale, but feel only "slightly irritable" and mark "2" on that scale.

	5	4	3	2	1	0	
Relaxed	___	___	___	___	___	___	Tense
Unhurried	___	___	___	___	___	___	Hurried, sense of time urgency
Congenial	___	___	___	___	___	___	Irritable
Serene	___	___	___	___	___	___	Apprehensive, worried

Scoring: Add up your total number of points by giving yourself 5 points for every check you made in the "5" column and so on.

Total score: ___

Current level of tension: 0–6 = high; 7–13 = medium; 14–20 = low.

The instructor can give feedback about the information gathered on all these forms in one-to-one meetings. Out of this database will come the second phase: goal setting. Goal setting must be holistic. Participants should take into account their current health practices, diet, exercise, and any other factors that affect stress tolerance, rather than setting goals solely on levels of tension, attitudinal characteristics, or positive–negative stress practices.

friends, and job satisfaction. These three areas must be dealt with both internally and externally. Internally, participants must alter their attitudes so that they can cope effectively with their lifestyle and can form a congruence between their values and their daily expression of these values. External intervention by participants in the management of their own lives could include changing of friends and support groups or learning to problem solve in areas in which they have been avoiding personal accountability.

■ Goal Setting

Education Component

The three spheres that participants will want to set goals in to improve their stress-management capabilities are self-development, family and

Service Component

In the area of self-development, participants examine physical health, educational needs, interest in hobbies, and skills or mental developmental needs (attitudes, beliefs, and values),

▌ Figure 10.5 Tension-level test. ▌

Please make a check in the space to the left of each statement.

Often	*A few times a week*	*Rarely*	
———	———	———	1. Once I find the time, it is hard for me to relax.
———	———	———	2. I have a difficult time finding enough time to relax.
———	———	———	3. I take tranquilizers (or other drugs) to relax.
———	———	———	4. I find it difficult to concentrate on what I'm doing because of worrying about other things.
———	———	———	5. I can't turn off my thoughts away from work enough to feel relaxed and refreshed the next day.
———	———	———	6. I have tension/migraine headaches, or neck/shoulder pain, or insomnia.
———	———	———	7. I eat/drink/smoke in response to tension.
———	———	———	8. People at work/home arouse my tension.
———	———	———	9. I feel tense, anxious, or have nervous indigestion.

Scoring: Give yourself 2 points for each *often* answer, 1 for each *a few*, and 0 for each *rarely*. Total your points.

Total Score	Tension Level
14–18	Dangerous
10–13	Some risk
6–9	Average
3–5	Below average
0–2	Clear sailing—keep it up!

Total score: ——— 0–5 = low; 6–12 = medium; 13–18 = high.

---

and identify an appropriate method for addressing their top priorities through self-education using books, courses, or tapes or through one-to-one assistance from a teacher.

To set goals regarding their support system, participants examine the strengths and weaknesses of their familial and interpersonal network, looking specifically for significant individuals who are positive stresses (they feel better after being with them) and for people who are negative stresses.

In professional development, participants examine present skill levels for their current functions and responsibilities and determine if there are skills that need to be upgraded to alleviate distress or produce positive stress.

Some case studies will illustrate the process. Each individual performs a distinctly different function and exhibits different needs and goals.

Case Studies ▌
Ms. Green

Ms. Green is a 25-year-old, healthy, motivated woman. Her family has no history of degenerative illness. Her last physical examination was done less than 1 year ago. Ms. Green has a history of vigorous physical activity through various competitive sports. She has just been promoted from a nonexempt employee to a first-line supervisor and has recently developed infrequent problems with disruptive sleep patterns and occasional headaches. She has targeted the increased stress of her new job as the primary factor in her motivation to attend a stress-management program.

Ms. Green scored very low on the informational assessment and high on the Type A questionnaire, and her physical assessment is in the

Figure 10.6 Type A personality assessment form. (Revised from the structured interview from the Forum on Type A behavior, National Heart/Lung/Blood Institute. Ray M. Rosenman, MD, 1981.)

Two San Francisco scientist/internists, Meyer Friedman, M.D., and Ray H. Rosenman, M.D., have identified a pattern of attitudes and behavior that they have linked to an elevated risk of heart disease. They have named this pattern Type A behavior and have written a book, *Type A Behavior and Your Heart* (Alfred A. Knopf, 1974), to describe it and its effects. Here is how they define Type A behavior: "It is a particular complex of personality traits including excessive competitive drive, aggressiveness, impatience, and a harrying sense of time urgency. Individuals displaying this pattern seem to be engaged in a chronic, ceaseless race and struggle—with themselves, with others, with circumstances, with time, sometimes with life itself." The opposite of Type A behavior is called Type B, and studies have shown that Type B personalities get just as much (if not more) work done in an allotted amount of time, without the upsets, distress, and health hazards.

Please answer *yes* or *no* for each item.

Yes *No*

____ ____ 1. Do you feel your job carries heavy responsibility?

____ ____ 2. Would you describe yourself as a hard-driving, ambitious type of person?

____ ____ 3. Do you usually try to get things done as quickly as possible?

____ ____ 4. Would family members and close friends describe you as hard-driving and ambitious?

____ ____ 5. Have people close to you ever asked you to slow down in your work?

____ ____ 6. Do you think you drive harder to accomplish things than most of your associates?

____ ____ 7. When you play games with people your own age, do you play just for the fun of it?

____ ____ 8. If there's competition in your job, do you enjoy this?

____ ____ 9. When you are driving and there is a car in your lane going far too slowly for you, do you mutter and complain? Would anyone riding with you know that you are annoyed?

____ ____ 10. If you make an appointment with someone, would you be there on time in almost all cases?

____ ____ 11. If you were kept waiting, would you resent it?

____ ____ 12. If you see someone doing a job rather slowly and you know you could do it faster and better yourself, does it make you restless to watch him or her?

____ ____ 13. Would you be tempted to step in and do it yourself?

____ ____ 14. Do you eat rapidly? Walk rapidly?

____ ____ 15. After you've finished eating, do you like to sit around the table and chat?

____ ____ 16. When you go out to a restaurant and find eight or ten people waiting ahead of you for a table, will you wait?

____ ____ 17. Do you really resent having to wait in line at the bank or post office?

____ ____ 18. Do you always feel anxious to get going and finish whatever you have to do?

____ ____ 19. Do you have the feeling that time is passing too rapidly for you to accomplish all the things you'd like to get done in one day?

____ ____ 20. Do you often feel a sense of time urgency or time pressure?

____ ____ 21. Do you hurry in doing most things?

Scoring: Questions 7, 15, and 16: give yourself 1 point for each *yes* answer.
On the rest of the questions, give yourself 1 point for each *no* answer.

Total score: _____

Add up your points for all questions. The higher your score, the less Type A behavior or attitudes you exhibit.

Level of Type A (unhealthy) behavior: 0–7 = High; 8–13 = Medium; 14–21 = Low.

(*continued*)

■ **Figure 10.6** Continued ■

Tips to Reduce Type A Behavior

- Don't rush your life unnecessarily (hurry sickness). Slow down your pace of eating, drinking, driving, and working when appropriate.
- Prioritize the things to be done; do one thing at a time and delegate whenever possible.
- Give yourself plenty of time for each task or event. Don't schedule appointments too close together.
- Learn to say "no." You can't do everything. This will help reduce the number of deadlines in your life, self-imposed or otherwise.
- Avoid hurried sandwiches at your desk, and reduce working lunches. Get away, give yourself a break.
- Avoid taking your work home. It will be there tomorrow; finish it then.
- Keep fresh and spontaneous. Don't do things the same way all the time.
- Become more flexible and less a perfectionist.
- Increase listening time and decrease talking time. Type A people have a tendency to verbalize too much.
- Spend more time cultivating relationships with Type B people.
- Get up 30 minutes early to give yourself more quality time to visit with your family and dress without rushing.
- Set aside an hour a day for you to be alone, to relax, read, walk, or just reflect.
- Insist on having a time and place at home in which you can be alone without interruptions.
- Remember that no one else can do for you what you can do for yourself.

above-average range. The health/fitness director contracts with Ms. Green to set the following goals.

Behavioral goals: (1) to develop a scheduled break of 15 minutes each day to reflect and practice relaxation; (2) to increase by 20% the evenings devoted to doing something that is frivolous and fun. *Learning goals:* (1) to understand the differences between positive and negative stress by the third week of class; (2) to identify three triggers in her life that cause a state of alarm and either devise ways to eliminate them or change her reaction to them by the end of the class. *Physical goals:* (1) to spend 20 minutes per day, three times per week, doing some form of relaxation training; (2) to take a yoga class that will teach her stretching techniques and to incorporate 10 minutes of stretching in her aerobics program.

During the course, Ms. Green's progress with each objective will be discussed in small groups and with the instructor. An ongoing check-in with the director could be established to maintain her focus on the successful completion of each objective.

Mr. Nolan

Mr. Nolan is a 55-year-old man who has been a middle manager for the company for 15 years. He is on the job in the manufacturing division 60 to 70 hours per week. Mr. Nolan has had numerous warnings from physicians about his weight, which is 30 pounds over the average for his height and age. He is moderately healthy as a result of playing golf three times each week for the last 12 years. He walks 6 miles each day that he plays golf and walks with his wife on weeknights for 15 to 20 minutes at a brisk pace. Mr. Nolan has been advised by his doctor to take some precautions to ensure that he does not become a victim of cardiovascular disease. He has a two-generation family history of death resulting from myocardial infarction. He is thus highly motivated to attend the stress course.

Mr. Nolan scored high on the Type A

Figure 10.7 Positive stressors questionnaire. *Positive stressor*: a person, group, organization, event, or situation that makes you feel better about yourself and more alive and vital.

Please put a check by those you practice regularly:

_____ 1. Deep relaxation techniques

_____ 2. Meditation

_____ 3. Aerobic exercise

_____ 4. Engaging in a sport you enjoy

_____ 5. Taking a fun class

_____ 6. Spending at least 1 hour per day for yourself and by yourself

_____ 7. Writing in a diary or journal

_____ 8. Learning a new skill

_____ 9. Developing a new interest

_____ 10. Relaxing with a hobby

_____ 11. Taking a walk

_____ 12. Communicating with a safe (accepting) person

_____ 13. Taking action on an unresolved situation or relationship

_____ 14. Using your own unique way to relax (for example, reading, cooking)

_____ 15. Practicing time management

_____ 16. Clarifying your life goals and values

_____ 17. Practicing deep breathing, especially in distressing situations

Scoring: Give yourself 1 point for each check you made, and add up your points.

Total score: _____

The more of these you include in your life, the better, and the more negative stress in your life, the more positive stressors you need to stay healthy. It is important to achieve a balance. Those people who feel they cannot afford the time for positive stressors are exactly the people who need them the most! Any score below 4 deserves increasing, and scores of 6 and above most likely mean you have already learned how to be good to yourself—congratulations!

0–3 = low; 4–5 = medium; 6 or more = high.

questionnaire. He acknowledges that he is a workaholic but says that he "loves it." He also scored high on the Stress-Pertise questionnaire. He knows a great deal about stress because his son has given him books and articles on the subject. His physical assessment discloses an immediate need for weight loss and for relaxation training that might counterbalance his high level of activity. A contract with Mr. Nolan might include the following.

Physical goal: (1) to lose 40 pounds—2 pounds per week over the next 20 weeks—by eating 1000 calories less per day of foods that are nutritionally sane, safe, and balanced and by exercising aerobically at his exercise heart rate three times per week for 13 to 20 minutes. *Behavioral goals:* (1) to develop an effective system of goal setting and assigning priorities that allows him to work no more than 50 hours per week; (2) to delegate work to his subordinates, so that he decreases by 25% the work he takes home each week. *Learning goals:* (1) to read and discuss in the stress-management class *Type A Behavior and Your Heart* by Freidman and Rosenman[5] by the end of the class sessions; (2) to develop a scheduled relaxation break 4 times

▌ **Figure 10.8** The scale of satisfaction. ▌

Please mark the statement that most closely describes your response to the questions, and give yourself the appropriate number of points according to which column you have marked (column 4 = 4 points, and so on).

Column 4 = yes, definitely
Column 3 = yes, somewhat
Column 2 = I feel neutral
Column 1 = no, somewhat
Column 0 = no, definitely

  4   3   2   1   0

Work

____ ____ ____ ____ ____ 1. Is the work you do challenging?
____ ____ ____ ____ ____ 2. Do you feel you are given adequate responsibility?
____ ____ ____ ____ ____ 3. Do your employers give you the authority to carry out your responsibilities?
____ ____ ____ ____ ____ 4. Is the work you are in right for you?
____ ____ ____ ____ ____ 5. Do you have the right amount of supervision to assist you in carrying out your functions?
____ ____ ____ ____ ____ 6. Are the people you work with for the most part supportive?

Finances

____ ____ ____ ____ ____ 7. Is your career path satisfying your financial needs?
____ ____ ____ ____ ____ 8. Is your lifestyle better than it was 3 years ago?
____ ____ ____ ____ ____ 9. Are you able to save money?
____ ____ ____ ____ ____ 10. Do you feel prepared (or can you prepare when you want to) for retirement?
____ ____ ____ ____ ____ 11. Is spending money not associated with anxiety for you?
____ ____ ____ ____ ____ 12. Is your spouse or partner supportive of your income level?*

Friends

____ ____ ____ ____ ____ 13. Do you have a safe person with whom you can talk about almost anything?
____ ____ ____ ____ ____ 14. Outside your immediate family, do you have a support system—that is, people who accept you and give you positive strokes?
____ ____ ____ ____ ____ 15. Do you have fun socializing?
____ ____ ____ ____ ____ 16. Do you like listening to other people's problems?
____ ____ ____ ____ ____ 17. Are your friendships marked by mutual respect?
____ ____ ____ ____ ____ 18. Do you have a close friend of the opposite sex?

Home life

____ ____ ____ ____ ____ 19. Do you have an enjoyable hobby?
____ ____ ____ ____ ____ 20. Can you relax at home?
____ ____ ____ ____ ____ 21. Do you enjoy spending a quiet evening at home?
____ ____ ____ ____ ____ 22. Is your home supportive of your self-nurturing as well as the nurturing of your friends?
____ ____ ____ ____ ____ 23. Do you have a sense of pride about where you reside?

■ Figure 10.8 Continued **■**

Sexuality

___ ___ ___ ___ ___ 24. Do you enjoy your own sensuality?

___ ___ ___ ___ ___ 25. Do you get pleasure from sex?

___ ___ ___ ___ ___ 26. During sex with your partner do you never fantasize about new or different sexual partners?*

Spouse or partner

___ ___ ___ ___ ___ 27. Are you satisfied with your marital or single state?

___ ___ ___ ___ ___ 28. Given a chance to change your present marital or single state, would you choose to keep it the same?

___ ___ ___ ___ ___ 29. Does your partner let you know he or she cares about you?*

___ ___ ___ ___ ___ 30. Do you feel free to discuss openly matters that cause conflict with your partner?*

___ ___ ___ ___ ___ 31. Do you and your partner laugh and have fun together?*

Humor

___ ___ ___ ___ ___ 32. Do you laugh often?

___ ___ ___ ___ ___ 33. Do you attend humorous movies, plays, and so on?

___ ___ ___ ___ ___ 34. Can you laugh at yourself?

___ ___ ___ ___ ___ 35. Can your sense of humor get you through difficult times?

___ ___ ___ ___ ___ 36. Is laughter your best medicine?

Meaning

___ ___ ___ ___ ___ 37. Do you feel you are making a valuable contribution to the world?

___ ___ ___ ___ ___ 38. Do you feel needed, appreciated, and special to people important to you?

___ ___ ___ ___ ___ 39. Can you see a clear direction toward which your life is heading?

___ ___ ___ ___ ___ 40. Do your past, present, and future fit into a reasonably coherent whole? (Can you see beyond the negative parts of your life to a larger and more important meaning?)

___ ___ ___ ___ ___ If you were terminally ill and the doctor gave you 1 year to live, would the way you chose to live that last year be essentially similar to your present way of living?

*Do not answer unless involved in a partnership. Instead, add 15 points to your total score.

Total score: ___

Scoring scale:

0–90 =	*Low* satisfaction. Grounds for danger. Start goal setting to convert the lack of satisfaction to a positive feeling.
90–135 =	*Medium* satisfaction. There may be areas of your life that need work that the questionnaire will have helped you see more clearly. Where did you indicate dissatisfaction (low scores)? Look carefully for patterns of dissatisfaction.
135 or more =	*High* level of satisfaction. Correlates with wellness.

■ Figure 10.9 The scale of frustration. ■

Please mark the statement that most closely describes your response to the questions, and give yourself the appropriate number of points according to which column you have marked (column 4 = 4 points, and so on).

Column 4 = yes, definitely
Column 3 = yes, somewhat
Column 2 = I feel neutral
Column 1 = no, somewhat
Column 0 = no, definitely

  4   3   2   1   0

Energy level

____ ____ ____ ____ ____ 1. Does life seem "too much" often?

____ ____ ____ ____ ____ 2. Does your job leave you exhausted?

____ ____ ____ ____ ____ 3. Do you feel overextended?

____ ____ ____ ____ ____ 4. Is it impossible to do things properly because you have too much to do?

____ ____ ____ ____ ____ 5. Are your weekends taken up with recuperating from the weekdays?

Health

____ ____ ____ ____ ____ 6. Do you often have headaches?

____ ____ ____ ____ ____ 7. Do you suffer from aches and pains?

____ ____ ____ ____ ____ 8. Do you often feel depressed?

____ ____ ____ ____ ____ 9. Do you have trouble getting to sleep?

____ ____ ____ ____ ____ 10. Is sex an unwelcome activity in your life?

Trust and control

____ ____ ____ ____ ____ 11. Do you feel as if others control your time/environment?

____ ____ ____ ____ ____ 12. Do you have no people you trust with your innermost feelings?

____ ____ ____ ____ ____ 13. Are people hurtful to you often?

____ ____ ____ ____ ____ 14. Do you feel that you are unable to make a contribution to your job and/or family and friends?

____ ____ ____ ____ ____ 15. Is "powerless" a way you would describe yourself?

Habits

____ ____ ____ ____ ____ 16. Do you use alcohol or drugs to relieve anxiety?

____ ____ ____ ____ ____ 17. Do you find you cannot relax without a pharmacological aid?

____ ____ ____ ____ ____ 18. Do you overeat, binge, or starve yourself?

____ ____ ____ ____ ____ 19. Do you smoke cigarettes?

____ ____ ____ ____ ____ 20. Do you not exercise often (3–4 times per week)?

Total score: ____

Scoring scale:

0–16 = *Low* frustration. This score probably coincides with a high satisfaction score. If you have a low satisfaction score as well as a low frustration score, look for signs of boredom and apathy.

16–32 = *Medium* level of frustration. It is time to discover if there are specific frustrations you can do something about immediately, as well as to make long-range plans for eliminating frustrations.

32 or more = *High* frustration. This is a sign of either acute and chronic distress or a very perfectionistic individual. It is essential to change your attitudes or to do something about the frustrations, one at a time. Make sure you do something!

per week through napping, relaxation exercise, autogenics, or taking a hot bath.

Mr. Nicholson

Mr. Nicholson is a 62-year-old long-term employee who works in the finance division. He smokes 2 packs of cigarettes per day, drinks at least 4 ounces of whiskey per day, and has not exercised regularly for 18 years. Mr. Nicholson is in the company's preretirement counseling program and has been identified as being at high risk of life-threatening illness when he retires. The corporate physician has been consulted about Mr. Nicholson's condition and has talked with him about participating in some aspect of the organization's fitness program. Mr. Nicholson has chosen the stress-management class, although he states, "It's not going to change my habits."

Mr. Nicholson scored low on the Type A behavior questionnaire and on the knowledge assessment. He is described as unhealthy and unmotivated on his physical assessments.

Physical goals: (1) to explore the range of possible aerobic activities by participating at least once in a swimming class, walking program, or other exercise of his choice; (2) to develop a minimum commitment to aerobic conditioning, such as walking for 30 minutes three times per week. *Behavioral goals:* (1) to interview three retirees who have an interesting hobby or activity and to gather ideas for his own retirement by the end of the stress course; (2) to plan at least one activity per week that includes another person and is fun. *Learning goals:* (1) to explore the subject of positive stresses and incorporate a positive stress into his life 30 minutes per day, 5 days per week, for the next 6 months; (2) to read one book on longevity or aging that includes information on the positive aspects of aging (for example, a popular book by George Burns, Norman Cousins, or Ruth Gordon).

Case Review

In each of the three case examples, the process is similar: (1) assess the three areas for current habits, knowledge, and actions; (2) contract with the participant individually, in writing, for at least one goal in each of the three areas; (3) monitor progress both during and after the class through individual, informal interviews or group discussions; (4) celebrate any successes and devise ways to turn failures into ongoing projects and recommitments to "small wins."

Planning

A successful stress-management program can be delivered in a variety of ways at a range of costs and in various formats. We will examine each option and discuss its pros and cons.

Inhouse Programs

It is generally more cost-effective to give an inhouse stress program using internal resources, and training personnel or bringing in an external consultant when no inhouse personnel are available. The benefits of offering an inhouse course are low cost, more efficient coordination, minimal travel expenses, and ease in monitoring and maintaining the quality of the course.

If you hire an external consultant, the costs in most cases range from $25 to $150 per participant per day. The price is dependent on the experience of the consultant, class materials to be used, and travel and hotel expenses of the consultant.

In selecting a consultant, *caveat emptor*. A sizeable amount of external consultants' pricing depends solely on what the traffic will bear. Get more than one bid and take the time to negotiate the price with your chosen consultant.

Materials The cost of stress-management materials depends largely on the format and medium involved. A simple photocopied handout, with no additional materials, can cost less than $5 per participant. Commercially available workbooks cost between $7 and $15 per person.

It is a good idea to give each participant a cassette tape that reviews the relaxation response. These tapes may have music in the

■ **Figure 10.10** The social readjustment rating scale. "We have the two essential strategies for ■
coping: the way of avoidance or the way of attention. . . . We have the biological capacity to deny
our stress—or transform it by paying attention to it" (Marilyn Ferguson, *The Aquarian Conspiracy*).
(From Holmes, T. H., and Rahe, R. H. The social readjustment rating scale. *Journal of Psychosomatic
Research* 11:213–218, 1967. Copyright 1967 Pergamon Press, Ltd. Used by permission.)

The following is a list of events that may have occurred in your life within the last year. If an event did
occur, give yourself the mean value number of points in the space provided to the left, marked *past*. If
you can reasonably anticipate that an event will occur in the year to come, give yourself the mean value
number of points in the *future* space.

Mean value	Past	Future	Life event
100	_____	_____	1. Death of spouse
73	_____	_____	2. Divorce
65	_____	_____	3. Marital separation
63	_____	_____	4. Detention in jail or other institution
63	_____	_____	5. Death of a close family member
53	_____	_____	6. Major personal injury or illness
50	_____	_____	7. Marriage
47	_____	_____	8. Being fired from work
45	_____	_____	9. Marital reconciliation
45	_____	_____	10. Retirement from work
44	_____	_____	11. Major change in the health or behavior of family member
40	_____	_____	12. Pregnancy
39	_____	_____	13. Sexual difficulties
39	_____	_____	14. Gaining a new family member (through birth, adoption, oldster moving in)
39	_____	_____	15. Major business readjustment (merger, reorganization, bankruptcy)
38	_____	_____	16. Major change in financial state (a lot worse off or a lot better off than usual)
37	_____	_____	17. Death of a close friend
36	_____	_____	18. Changing to a different line of work
35	_____	_____	19. Major change in the number of arguments with spouse (either a lot more or a lot less than usual, regarding child-rearing, personal habits)
31	_____	_____	20. Taking on a mortgage greater than $10,000 (to purchase a home, business)
30	_____	_____	21. Foreclosure on a mortgage or loan
29	_____	_____	22. Major change in responsibilities at work (promotion, demotion, lateral transfer)
29	_____	_____	23. Son or daughter leaving home (marriage, college)
29	_____	_____	24. In-law troubles
28	_____	_____	25. Outstanding personal achievement
26	_____	_____	26. Beginning or ceasing formal schooling
26	_____	_____	27. Spouse beginning or ceasing work outside the home
25	_____	_____	28. Major change in living conditions (building a new home, remodeling, deterioration of home or neighborhood)

▌ Figure 10.10 Continued ▌

24	___	___	29. Revision of personal habits (dress, manners, associations)
23	___	___	30. Troubles with the boss
20	___	___	31. Major change in working hours or conditions
20	___	___	32. Change in residence
20	___	___	33. Change to a new school
19	___	___	34. Major change in usual type or amount of recreation
19	___	___	35. Major change in church activities (a lot more or a lot less than usual)
18	___	___	36. Major change in social activities (clubs, dancing, movies, visiting)
17	___	___	37. Taking out a mortgage or loan of less than $10,000 (to purchase a car, television, freezer)
16	___	___	38. Major change in sleeping habits (a lot more or a lot less sleep, or change in part of day when asleep)
15	___	___	39. Major change in number of family get-togethers
15	___	___	40. Major change in eating habits (a lot more or a lot less food intake, or very different meal hours or surroundings)
13	___	___	41. Vacation
12	___	___	42. Christmas or major holiday
11	___	___	43. Citation for minor violations of the law (traffic tickets, jaywalking, disturbing the peace)

Scoring: Add your total number of points, keeping both columns separate. Of those people with over 300 life change units for the past year, almost 80% become ill in the near future; of those with 150 to 299, about 50% become ill; of those with less than 150, only about 30% become ill. The higher your life change score, the harder you should work (and relax!) to stay well.

0–150 = low; 150–299 = medium; 300 or more = high.

Preventive measures:

The following are suggestions for using the social readjustment rating scale to help you maintain your health and prevent illness:

1. Become familiar with the life events and the amount of change they require.
2. Put the scale where you and the family can see it easily several times a day.
3. With practice, you can recognize when a life event happens.
4. Think about the meaning of the event for you and try to identify some of the feelings you experience.
5. Think about the different ways you might best adjust to the event.
6. Take your time in arriving at decisions.
7. If possible, anticipate life changes and plan for them well in advance.
8. Pace yourself, even if you are in a hurry.
9. Look at the accomplishment of a task as a part of daily living and avoid looking at such an achievement as a "stopping point" or a time for letting down.

background, although it is not essential. Such tapes cost about $10 each.

If you intend to offer the class to a significant percentage of the organization's workforce, the purchase of a film or video may be justified. Examples of quality productions available are "Managing Stress to Increase Productivity" from Productivity Specialists in Palo Alto, California, which costs $1200 for eight 25-minute modules, and McGraw-Hill's "Stress Management" film from CRM Productions, which costs about $800. Addresses and additional resources can be found in the Appendix.

Course location   The course location depends on whether there is adequate classroom space available—of course, it is always more expensive to rent space. The criteria for selecting a room are: good air circulation; a carpeted floor if possible; sufficient floor space for participants to do the deep-relaxation training exercises lying down; controls for dimming lights or a low watt lamp to turn on during relaxation. Most important, the chairs must support the participants' spines and be conducive to a full day of sitting—and to deep relaxation should students decide to sit in a chair while practicing the relaxation exercise.

As mentioned, we recommend that you first offer a pilot program to senior managers. Hold the class offsite—for example, in a hotel meeting room or a lodge—so that participants are not distracted by telephone messages or day-to-day operations. For all subsequent classes, if there are no onsite facilities, explore the options of social-service agencies, hotels, colleges, schools, or churches, which may rent space. Depending on where you are, costs for rented space range from $35 per day in social-service settings to $150 per day for hotel rooms.

Course scheduling   Stress-management programs either are an integral and required part of the core health/fitness program or are considered ancillary and nonessential programs that employees are "encouraged" to attend outside of work hours. When you schedule your course, you must decide which type of program you are going to offer. Does senior management want the program to be a core part of the health/fitness program? If yes, offer it during a full workday to senior and middle-management staff, and offer either 1 day or 2 half days to middle managers and staff. Are senior managers in favor of offering the stress course but not convinced that it is as important as the exercise component of the fitness program? If yes, offer the course in the evening, at lunchtime, or in the late afternoon in 1- to 3-hour segments totaling 8 hours.

Does the business operate on a 24-hour schedule—for example, three shifts per day? In this case, the course may be offered at three separate times for each shift, for 1 hour per week for 8 classes or as a 1-day workshop. You must decide whether people on the night and graveyard shifts are interested in attending and whether it is worth the effort to schedule early-morning and late-afternoon sessions for them. Often the simplest solution is to offer a 1-day class and assume that those who are motivated will find ways to attend.

One additional method for ensuring that all who wish to learn about stress management have the opportunity to do so is to purchase a video or film and have it available for viewing on a regular basis in different locations close to individuals' worksites.

Offsite Programs

Providers of stress-management programs fall within three general types: health promoters, management developers, and quick fixes. We will explore each type and discuss some of their benefits and risks.

Health promotion   Many cities have social service agencies like YMCAs, hospitals, or private health-promotion programs that offer stress management. Typically, the instructor is a health-care professional, such as a nurse or physician, who is interested in the topic. Such providers may have done research in the field and may have acquired "canned" materials or developed their own program. The obvious advantage of such providers is that they are readily available and often inexpensive. An additional advantage may be that they eliminate the confidentiality problem that onsite programs may pose. Many employees believe there is a stigma attached to having stress, and they may not want others to know they are attending a class.

To assess course quality, we recommend that you read the course objectives, review any handouts or books for the course, preview films or videos, and interview the instructors to decide whether what they are covering and how they are covering it fit with your needs.

In one case of a poor fit, a provider in a local community chose an instructor from a religious group that represented itself as being composed of "stress-management instructors." The employees found that the instructor taught a type of meditation and emphasized a spiritual perspective without giving information about the physiology of stress or exploring work-related stress issues. The health/fitness director could have avoided an embarrassing situation by interviewing the prospective instructor.

Management development Often, stress management is an integral part of a management-development course. Community colleges, universities, private consulting firms, and packaged management-development courses generally can supply materials and instructors.

There are sound reasons to offer stress management as a part of either an ancillary or a core management-development program:

1. Managers experience stress because they are responsible for motivating others. Often managers want to know how to recognize stress in their employees so that they will know how to approach and help an employee under pressure.

2. Middle management has the unique position of receiving constant pressure from above to produce results and of having to get work done through others.

3. Management-development courses often focus on interpersonal skills, which are important to the survival of a manager. Effective interpersonal relations can be improved when each individual is aware of and responsible for his or her own stress/distress.

4. Burnout, which is endemic to many management positions, can be decreased through stress-management practices, such as relaxation training, exercise, goal setting, and positive problem solving.

A management-development course in the area of stress should focus on topical areas that are distinct from those of a health-promotion or general stress course offered to all employees. Managers have special needs. Our experience is that physicians, health educators, and fitness consultants often are not appropriate instructors because managers do not find them credible. If the consultant has not had management experience recently, his or her validity as an expert will be doubted before the course begins. We recommend using management consultants who are proficient in stress theory and techniques and who can tailor their remarks to a management group.

The content is different from the general interest stress-management course in the following ways:

1. Course content should reflect the managers' need to view themselves as a special population with specific concerns. Sufficient time should be allotted to discussions on the unique stresses of managers.

2. Class discussion and small group exercises with an emphasis on increased participation are a key to success. Managers find the lecture format condescending, and they generally will reject the course if they cannot communicate their own reactions, ideas, and questions throughout the day.

3. The format of a management course must either be a 1-day class or 2 half-day classes. Giving the class in the evening or in 1 or 2 hour segments will not work. Managers want the information *now*, and will not allocate more than 1 day to the subject.

4. Managers like to go offsite, to a hotel, lodge, or other pleasant location. There is good reason to get them away from the office—onsite courses allow them to go back to their offices at breaks and lunch,

and it is not uncommon never to see them again. If they are away from the office, there is less likelihood of their not completing the class.

Quick fixes The dozens of management and general interest courses available through the American Management Association, community colleges, and other agencies are excellent resources if you are not planning the stress-management component as an integral, ongoing part of your health/fitness program. Selected employees who have been targeted as needing stress-management instruction can be sent relatively inexpensively to quick-fix courses. The disadvantages of quick fixes are that they are generally "canned" and not tailored to your corporate setting, and the instructors' credentials and knowledge base often are scanty—they may have read two books on stress and become self-proclaimed experts. To get the best bang for the corporate buck, we suggest an inhouse course tied to the training and development catalog, approved and possibly previewed by senior management, and designed to be content-specific to each segment of the attending population.

▊ Implementing an Inhouse Program

If you have planned ongoing courses and if the target population is over 1000 employees, you should consider training your own instructors and developing your own materials.

The most likely choices for instructors are the health/fitness director and the members of the training and development staff. We have found knowledgeable and interested persons in the human resources department that were ideal candidates.

Training the Trainer

To get an instructor up to speed in the stress-management field, three areas can be studied. (1) The instructor should be an active practitioner of some kind of relaxation-training technique and be able to speak from her or his own experience concerning its efficacy. (2) A regular aerobic exercise program must be a part of his or her weekly routine. (3) The instructor can study the program by John Adams of University Associates of San Diego on how to start a stress-management program internally,[6] or your corporation may choose to purchase a video-based program like ours, which is entitled "Managing Stress to Increase Productivity" and provides eight video modules to initiate a discussion for group learning.

The stress-management instructor can lose more credibility by not being a physically fit and balanced individual than by not knowing the intellectual concepts of the stress theory. It is far easier to pick up theory than it is to counterfeit wellness. Participants want to be motivated to manage their stress when they attend a course, and the best motivator is one whose inspiration is coupled with personal commitment to behavioral objectives.

Sample Program

"Positive Stress for Promoting Health" is a general-interest course offered to all employees regardless of job classification. This 8-week course is conducted both at the lunch hour and at 5:30 P.M. (or whenever the shifts change/employees go home) for 1 hour per week.

Participants must be interested in improving their abilities to manage stress in a positive, healthy way. They need not have a stress-related problem or concern to attend. The course focuses on the positive aspects of stress and on how to eliminate or decrease negative stresses in their lives.

The instructor is the company's health/fitness director, Susan Jones. Ms. Jones is a regular jogger, has been practicing relaxation techniques for the past 8 months and is avidly interested in how stress can be dealt with in positive ways.

Participants are asked to pay one-half of the fee and the company pays the other half. (If participants pay some percentage of the fee,

▮ Figure 10.11 Sample course outline for an inhouse program. **▮**

Hour One. Needs assessment questionnaires will measure prior knowledge and current behaviors that produce or help manage stress; these will be correlated with a physical assessment from the exercise component of the corporate fitness program; participants will discuss results with instructor; individual course objectives will be written by participants with the instructor's assistance.

Hour Two. Hans Selye's research findings on stress theory will be outlined; participants will be introduced to relaxation training, autogenic training, or alternate tensing and relaxing exercises; group will discuss the relaxation training in terms of results, benefits, and problems.

Hour Three. The definition of distress and causes of negative stress will be outlined; participants will identify sources of distress in their lives and discuss in small groups the alternative strategies for coping successfully with their current distressors.

Hour Four. Participants will be given handouts from Benson's book *The Relaxation Response*[7]; the class will examine what happens physically and mentally during relaxation; instructors will lead participants through a relaxation exercise from Dr. Benson's book, and the class will compare it to the previous week's relaxation techniques.

Hour Five. The instructor will review with participants their progress toward fulfilling the be-

havioral objectives identified in session one of the course; the class will identify any obstacles to successful completion of defined objectives and will renegotiate timelines or quantify their commitment with the instructor. The life events, frustrations, and satisfactions questionnaires will be completed in class; the class will discuss the correlation between change and stress.

Hour Six. The class will discuss the effect of deep relaxation exercises on stress; participants will review the frustrations and satisfactions questionnaires and identify a frustration in their lives; they will develop written solutions to areas of frustration and discuss them in small groups.

Hour Seven. The concept of positive stress will be defined; the participants will discuss positive stresses in their lives; the class will examine the positive benefits of exercise, humor, diet/nutrition, and effective communication.

Hour Eight. Individuals' objectives will be monitored; participants will increase commitments to following through by enrolling group support or making individual agreements with the instructor.

A pre- and posttest questionnaire may be used for the course. The Stress-Pertise test is appropriate for this purpose and can be used as is or in a slightly modified form.

---

even less than 50%, they have a greater commitment to attending all sessions.) Figure 10.11 gives a sample course outline.

▮ Evaluation

An essential component of the evaluation phase of a stress-management course is to determine what the administration of the organization views as success. The contract for defining the content and objectives of a course should be derived from the expectations of management. When initially developing an evaluation methodology, the health/fitness specialist should request a written list of the expectations that management has of the course. The specialist can

negotiate with the management group those expectations that he or she thinks are clearly unrealistic, and suggest other goals that are more in line with the content and direction of the course. For example, it is not uncommon for management to expect instant stress relief, radical improvement in labor relations, cessation of turnover, and an immediate reduction in absenteeism and use of sick leave. Realistic results from any course are more likely to be a noticeable "smile effect" due to employees' gratitude, an increase in productivity for specific individuals, and a better understanding of symptoms of stress.

The organizations that have the best overall success in their stress-management program link the program to other training and development core courses or make it an integral part of the health/fitness program. In addition, they view it as a long-term commitment—results are expected to appear gradually over years rather than months or weeks. The benefits of reduced sick leave, absenteeism, or insurance liabilities rarely are seen in the short run.

Finally, it is important to develop an evaluation tool based on the original course objectives.

Stress-management courses sometimes are in danger of being viewed by results-oriented managers and executives as nonessential. Although many health/fitness specialists have the good fortune of strong organizational support, it is prudent to document thoroughly all visible signs of success.

A summary report of participants' questionnaires or a more formal evaluation based on both subjective data and an evaluation by the participants' managers may be used to sell the idea of continuing stress management for all employees to the decision makers in management.

▌ Summary

We have provided the background information necessary to market stress management to decision makers as well as concrete suggestions for structuring a stress-management program in your organization. An inhouse program that makes use of an already-developed workbook and relaxation tape in the long run may be the best and easiest strategy for implementation. If inhouse resources are not available, make use of community resources and external consultants.

Stress management is one of the most popular courses in American corporations. In all likelihood, the health/fitness specialist will become the corporate hero or heroine for helping employees with their palpable and often overwhelming stress.

References ▌

1. Pelletier, K. *Mind as healer, mind as slayer.* New York: Delta, 1977.

2. Selye, H. Health care monster blamed for firm's costs. *The Washington Post*, April 12, 1984.

3. Drucker, P. *Drucker on management.* Audio cassette series. New York: AMACOM, 1974.

4. Toffler, A. *The third wave.* New York: William Morrow & Co., 1980.

5. Freidman, M., and Rosenman, R. H. *Type A behavior and your heart.* New York: Alfred A. Knopf, 1974.

6. Adams, J. D. *Understanding and managing stress.* San Diego, CA: University Associates, 1980.

7. Benson, H. *The relaxation response.* New York: William Morrow & Co., 1975.

A p p e n d i x ■

Stress Management Resources and Materials

General Resource

- Pelletier, K., et al. *A summary of corporate study on health programs.* California Nexus Foundation, 2152 Union Street, San Francisco, CA 94123. $20.00.

Audio Tapes and Study Guide

- Emmett Miller, M.D., Source Cassettes, P.O. Box W, Stanford, CA 94305.
- Levinson, E. "The Distress Destroyer," 1160 California Avenue, Palo Alto, CA 94306.

Workbooks

- Adams, J. D. (ed). *A workbook in changing life styles.* University Associates, P.O. Box 26240, 8517 Production Avenue, San Diego, CA 92126.
- Levinson, E. *Managing stress to increase productivity.* Wadsworth Publishing Company, 10 Davis Drive, Belmont, CA 94002.

Videos/Films

- "Stress Management," CRM, McGraw-Hill, P.O. Box 641, DelMar, CA 92014.
- "Managing Stress to Increase Productivity," Productivity Specialists, 1160 California Avenue, Palo Alto, CA 94306.

C H A P T E R **11**

LOW-BACK–PAIN MANAGEMENT

Low-back pain (LBP) is frequently a problem for adult Americans. Nachemson comments that, during their active lives, 80% of the people in industrialized countries suffer back pain of various duration, intensity, and disability.[1] The pain and discomfort associated with LBP frequently are so acute that daily routines are completely disrupted. LBP presently is the largest single cause of lost work hours in business and industry. Bonica estimates that the cost of all complications of LBP, including outpatient fees, loss of work productivity, and compensation payments, could be as high as $50 billion annually.[2] LBP remains one of the few widespread, serious health problems that modern medicine has yet to conquer. In fact, there is considerable controversy among the medical specialties regarding the cause, treatment, and management of LBP; any LBP-prevention program should adopt a prudent approach.

Health/fitness professionals should not be diagnosticians, but should implement physician-prescribed exercise regimens for the acutely impaired. Mildly impaired and asymptomatic individuals may seek LBP-prevention classes offered by health/fitness programs. It is important to distinguish between *primary prevention* (involving individuals with no prior history of significant LBP) and *secondary prevention* (directed toward those who have evident clinical back disease or injury). Clinical screening performed by the corporate medical specialist identifies participants who should be referred to

physicians for evaluation and secondary prevention. Figure 11.1 illustrates the triage for the two groups within the health/fitness program.

Health/fitness specialists should assess and educate participants regarding possible predisposing factors that may precipitate LBP. Through proper education and appropriate exercise programs, health/fitness practitioners may significantly decrease the severity, if not the incidence, of LBP.

Thus, one step in the primary prevention program is to identify individuals at risk for LBP. A few common symptoms may be clues. Kraus describes the "classical back patient" as exhibiting one or more of the following characteristics: (1) excess weight, (2) extremely lordotic posture (abnormal curvature of the spine forward), (3) absence of a regular exercise program, (4) weak abdominal muscles, (5) tight hamstrings or hip flexors, (6) weak or tight back muscles, and (7) general tension.[3]

Other factors also seem to predispose to LBP. A recent study found a significant positive correlation between individual strength (in relation to the physical demands of work) and lower frequency of LBP.[4] It also found that factors such as smoking, chronic cough, anxiety, depression, and aging seem to be associated with increased incidence of LBP.

Posture also plays a role in the prevention or causation of LBP. Active or dynamic posture is extremely important when transporting objects. Magora reports that in many instances the

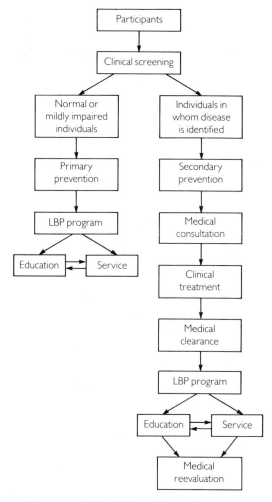

Figure 11.1 Triage of participants to the primary- and secondary-prevention components of the LBP program.

persons who either sat for prolonged periods of time or were unable to sit at all during the working day.[5] The need to avoid a prolonged posture and the importance of good body mechanics while standing or sitting can be taught in the health/fitness environment.

Secondary prevention, for individuals with demonstrable back disease, begins following clinical evaluation and treatment and subsequent medical clearance to institute appropriate exercise programs. In addition to orthopedic physicians, the specialists who assess secondary LBP and treat it include osteopaths, physiatrists, physical therapists, internists, gynecologists, urologists, psychologists, psychiatrists, chiropractors, and acupuncturists. Needless to say, each specialist has a different professional perspective on and bias toward the assessment, diagnosis, and treatment.

This diversity of opinion arises consequent to the multiple origins of LBP. A variety of causative factors may be involved, including trauma, congenital abnormalities, postural defects, tumors, arthritis, tension, referred pain from other tissues, miscellaneous nerve or blood-vessel disease, and psychosomatic illness. A well-designed LBP program must be appropriate for individuals with LBP of diverse origins.

Corporate communities are beginning to realize the need for and advantages of LBP-rehabilitation and *healthy back* programs. Commercial *back schools* have proved successful, expanding from only three facilities operating in 1973 to over 100 in 1983. The corporate setting is an ideal site to promote healthy backs through preventive education and service programs. Although numerous health/fitness specialists in business and industry choose to use programs at community or commercial agencies, such as the YMCA or a "back school," a comprehensive health/fitness program can provide the education and services necessary to promote healthy backs and manage LBP. Well-developed LBP-management programs can offer substantial benefits to business and industry in increased productivity and lower compensatory payments.

Health/fitness practitioners can use a variety of strategies when implementing a preventive

incidence of LBP may be lowered after employees are trained to use proper lifting techniques.[5] Static posture, exemplified when sitting or standing, also may contribute to LBP; Anderson notes that sitting in bent-over work postures increases the risk of LBP.[6] Also, it is important to change posture while working. Magora found a higher incidence of LBP in back-care program. Naturally, the specialist's budget often determines the extent of the intervention. Educational materials in a variety of forms, including written pamphlets, group presentations, posters, or films, can address topics such as basic anatomy, the role of exercise, and the importance of posture. Individualized written modules that require active participation and personalized goal setting often are useful. Community-based or inhouse exercise classes can be held; attendance can be mandatory or optional. Inhouse courses can be developed for various topics, such as relaxation training or lifting techniques. Secondary prevention often involves clinical treatment by appropriate specialists.

▌ Needs Assessment

The seemingly ubiquitous nature of LBP requires a thorough assessment of lifestyle. By evaluating participants' knowledge and fitness level, you can obtain an individualized, comprehensive view of direct needs. The initial baseline values determined during the educational and service evaluations permit periodic reassessment and comparison.

The role of the health/fitness professional includes implementing a primary-prevention plan for participants and supervising the prescribed exercise programs of individuals referred by medical specialists. You can provide education in both the primary and secondary programs.

Before you plan your education program, assess participants' knowledge. Determine what patients know about LBP (1) types, (2) causes, (3) treatments, (4) prevention techniques, (5) suitable exercises, and (6) proper body mechanics. If you wish, use the result to create homogeneous groups for your LBP-management programs.

The practitioner influences attitudes to achieve positive behavior modification. Attitudinal adjustment toward prudent LBP management can be encouraged through many avenues, including education, counseling, and improved physical conditioning. The needs

assessment should be tailored to the health status and educational level of each individual. Figures 11.2 through 11.5 are assessment instruments that may be used or adapted to gather data for the educational assessment.

Assess needs for the separate primary and secondary prevention service components. Secondary prevention usually begins with implementation of physician-prescribed exercises. As individuals demonstrate improved health status and receive medical clearance, they may progress to the primary prevention program. The primary program includes evaluation of posture and lifting techniques, assessment of flexibility and strength, and appraisal of relaxation skills.

Proper body mechanics (that is, good posture and movement) play a critical role in preventing LBP not only when lifting objects but in all the activities of daily living. Poor body mechanics place the muscles and vertebrae at a distinct disadvantage. Eventually, the muscles cannot support this added stress and pain occurs. This is especially true in the lumbar region (the lower area of the back), where poor posture and muscle weakness exaggerate the normal curvature (lordosis). Thus, static posture while standing or sitting is surprisingly important in the prevention of LBP.

Begin the evaluation of body mechanics with an appraisal of standing posture. In correct posture, a line dropped from the ear will go through the tip of the shoulder, middle of the hip, back of the kneecap and front of the anklebone. Encourage the participant to have the chin tucked in, head up, back flattened, and pelvis held straight.

Dynamic posture—posture when transporting objects—also is important. Critique and evaluate the participant's ability to: (1) bend the knees (not the back) when lifting objects, (2) use the leg muscles to provide force, (3) hold the object close to the body, keeping the trunk erect, (4) lift objects only chest high, (5) pivot the body rather than twist, and (6) get help if the object is too heavy. Figure 11.6 can be used to record the results.

The health/fitness specialist can evaluate an individual's risk of LBP through a variety of

A. Demographic data

    1. Name _____   4. Height _____   7. Address _____
    2. Age _____   5. Weight _____   _____
    3. Sex _____   6. Physician _____   8. Phone (work) _____
                                                                    (home) _____

B. Occupation

    1. Occupation _____
    2. Exercise requirements of occupation (check one)
        a. Light _____   c. Heavy _____
        b. Moderate _____
    3. Have you ever been absent from work as a result of low-back pain? Yes _____ No _____
       If yes, how often? Rarely _____ Annually _____ Monthly _____
    4. If your absence from work due to low-back pain is rare, how often do you have low-back pain but
       continue to go to work? _____

C. Medical history

    1. Do you presently have recurring low-back pain? Yes _____ No _____
       If so, how often? _____
    2. Please check each of the areas where you have had pain during the past 2 months.
       Neck _____   Abdomen _____
       Upper back and shoulders _____   Legs _____
       Lower back _____
    3. Have you had previous treatment for your back pain? Yes _____ No _____
       If yes, which of the following provided treatment?
        a. Physician _____   d. Physical therapist _____
        b. Surgeon _____   e. Chiropractor _____
        c. Osteopath _____   e. Other _____ (Please describe) _____
        _____
    4. If surgery was performed, please describe.
        a. Nature _____
        b. Date _____
        c. Surgeon (name, address) _____
    5. If you have had previous treatments, how would you rate their success?
       Complete _____ Moderate _____ Slight _____ None _____
    6. Do you have any other handicaps that need to be considered in providing you with an education
       and/or exercise program to prevent low-back pain? Yes _____ No _____. If yes, please
       describe. _____
       _____
    7. If you were referred by a doctor, what were the reasons?
        a. Rehabilitation after injury _____   d. Alternative to surgery _____
        b. Rehabilitation after surgery _____   e. Other _____
        c. Prevention _____
    8. What do *you* think is the cause of your low-back pain?
        a. Congenital anomaly _____   f. Related disease _____
        b. Injury _____   g. Overweight _____
        c. Disc problems _____   h. Excessive exercise _____
        d. Tension_____   i. Other _____
        e. Arthritis _____

▌ Figure 11.3   LBP knowledge test.   ▌

Select the *one* best answer.

A.   Causes

___ 1. Low-back pain sometimes is caused by:
   a. Excessive stress and anxiety
   b. Poor lifting habits
   c. Typing
   d. "a" and "b"
   e. "a," "b," and "c"

___ 2. Low-back pain sometimes is caused by:
   a. Obesity
   b. Racially determined factors
   c. Trauma or injury to the lower back
   d. "a" and "c" only
   e. "a," "b," and "c"

___ 3. Low-back pain can be caused by:
   a. Laughing
   b. Crying
   c. Joking
   d. Poor posture when sitting or standing

___ 4. Low-back pain often can be prevented by:
   a. Drinking coffee
   b. Learning proper stress management
   c. Swearing
   d. Eating the right foods
   e. None of the above

___ 5. Low-back pain sometimes can be caused by:
   a. Overuse of the back, e.g., in doing the same exact task with no variations
   b. Congenital defects and growths in the lower back
   c. Unknown causes, possibly vitamin or mineral deficiency
   d. None of the above
   e. "a," "b," and "c"

B.   Treatments

___ 6. Low-back pain frequently is diagnosed and treated by:
   a. Osteopaths
   b. Physicians
   c. Surgeons
   d. Chiropractors
   e. All of the above

___ 7. Low-back pain should be treated by:
   a. Going for a massage
   b. Seeking medical attention
   c. Going to a sauna
   d. Drinking alcohol
   e. Ignoring the problem

___ 8. What is the best way to lift an object off the floor?
   a. Bend and drag object along the floor
   b. Lift with a straight back
   c. Bend and lift with the legs, keeping a straight back
   d. Squat, then bend and lift
   e. Push object along the floor with your foot

___ 9. What exercise is useful in relieving a sore back?
   a. Basketball
   b. Relaxation techniques
   c. While sitting, gently bending over, drawing knees and chest together
   d. "b" and "c" only
   e. "a," "b," and "c"

___ 10. Low-back pain can be prevented by which types of exercises?
   a. Gentle static stretching of back muscles
   b. Relaxation techniques
   c. Abdominal exercises
   d. All of the above
   e. None of the above

C.   General Knowledge

___ 11. What percentage of adult Americans experiences low-back pain?
   a.   20%
   b.   40%
   c.   60%
   d.   80%
   e.   100%

___ 12. Of the Americans who once experienced low-back pain, what percentage becomes chronic sufferers?
   a.   10%
   b.   25%
   c.   50%
   d.   75%
   e.   90%

___ 13. What age group seems to be most prone to have low-back pain?
   a.   10–20 years
   b.   20–30 years
   c.   25–50 years
   d.   50–70 years

___ 14. How long does it take to recover fully from an *untreated* backache that is not due to an organic problem?
   a.   1–2 days
   b.   1–2 weeks
   c.   1–2 months
   d.   1–2 years
   e.   None of the above

___ 15. The best way to avoid low-back pain is to:
   a.   Manage stress
   b.   Use proper body mechanics
   c.   Avoid obesity
   d.   Exercise regularly
   e.   None of the above
   f.   All of the above

Answers: 1. e   4. b   7. b   10. d   13. c
                  2. d   5. e   8. c   11. d   14. c
                  3. d   6. e   9. d   12. c   15. f

Scoring: 13–15 correct is good; 10–12 correct is average; below 10 correct is poor.

■ Figure 11.4 LBP participant learning style questionnaire. ■

Rank the following ways of learning by giving your preferred method a ranking of 1, the next best method a 2, and so on, until you have ranked all the methods indicated.

I prefer to learn by:

Ranking

_____   1. Reading about it in a book.
_____   2. Seeing and hearing it in a film.
_____   3. Doing an activity and applying my learning from other methods.
_____   4. Discussing the material in groups.
_____   5. Teaching a lesson on the material to be learned.
_____   6. Working problems.
_____   7. Using programmed learning texts.
_____   8. Listening to lectures.
_____   9. Listening to tapes.
_____ 10. Looking at pictures or posters.
_____ 11. Listening to rhymes and songs about the material.
_____ 12. Other (please list) _____

Evaluation: Evaluate preferred learning styles by comparing responses in the following categories:

Looking/listening styles: 2, 4, 8, 9, 10, 11; reading styles: 1, 6, 7; combination styles: 3, 4, 5, 6.

■ Figure 11.5 LBP behavioral inventory. ■

Number the behaviors as follows: do very frequently (1); do usually (2); unsure (3); do seldom (4); do rarely (5).

 1. Practice relaxation _____
 2. Lift with a straight back _____
 3. Sit with a straight back _____
 4. Deal with problems as they arise rather than accumulating them _____
 5. Listen to advice from my physician _____
 6. Warm up before exercises _____
 7. Maintain a proper body weight _____
 8. Stand erect rather than slumping _____
 9. Use a seat belt and shoulder harness when driving _____
10. Exercise my whole body so as to prevent one part from becoming overdeveloped _____
11. Play games, sports, and so on according to the limitations of my fitness level (don't overdo on weekends) _____

The H/F practitioner should discuss this inventory question-by-question with the participant to reinforce proper behavior and teach new positive behaviors.

■ Figure 11.6 Lift and push/pull mechanics test. **■**

Give the participant a large plastic beach ball and have him or her demonstrate lifting.
Place an X beside each of the following that is properly executed. The participant:

1. Got as close to the ball as possible   _____
2. Adopted a staggered stance prior to lifting   _____
3. Squatted to grasp the ball (rather than bent at the waist)   _____
4. Tucked in the chin when lifting   _____
5. Exhaled when actually lifting   _____
6. Kept the load close to the body during the lift   _____
7. Lifted with the legs rather than the back   _____
8. Came to an upright position without hunched shoulders   _____

Have the participant alternately push against the wall and pull on a door knob.
Place an X beside each of the following that is properly executed. The client:

9. Adopted a staggered stance   _____
10. Transferred weight to proper foot when pushing (rear) and pulling (front)   _____
11. Kept the elbows bent during execution   _____
12. Kept the chin tucked during execution   _____
13. Noticeably contracted the abdomen during execution   _____
14. Noticeably exhaled during execution   _____
15. Performed the action without "jerky" movements   _____

---

fitness measures. Range of motion (flexibility) and muscular fitness tests should include measurements of all the affected joints and muscle groups of the lower back and lower extremities. These include muscle testing of the pelvis, low back extensors, hip extensors, hip aductors, hip flexors, hip rotators, hamstring group, abdominal group, and the tensor fasciae latae. Range-of-motion measurements should evaluate hip flexor and hamstring tightness as well as low back and hip mobility.

You do not need an elaborate array of equipment to evaluate strength and flexibility. Manual muscle testing and observation of participants' ability to perform exercise procedures provide an adequate assessment of minimal fitness levels.

Manual muscle testing involves placing the muscle group that is to be tested in a position whereby contraction of that muscle group will move the limb against gravity. Instruct the participant to perform the maneuver and to *hold* the extremity when near the limit of available

motion at this point; then apply smooth constant pressure against the limb in the direction just traveled for approximately 3 seconds. When normal muscular strength is present, the limb should not give way or return to the beginning position. In fact, following release of the applied resistance, the muscle should rebound to the fully flexed attitude. The participant must understand that maximum resistance or effort should be applied during all strength testing. This method of testing is appropriate for hip, thigh, and leg musculature.

Abdominal and back extensor strength evaluations simply require observation. The classic test of abdominal strength is the bent-knee sit-up. The participant should be instructed to keep the arms across the chest, holding on to the shoulders, as he or she attempts to sit up while keeping the feet in contact with the floor. Care should be taken to keep the knees bent to emphasize a curling up and then uncurling, and to avoid having the feet held or placed under an object. Adequate strength is demonstrated if the participant can perform 3 to 5 sit-ups, although this is a minimal fitness measurement.

To assess muscular strength of the back extensors, the subject lies prone, with a pillow under the abdomen and places hands behind the head and lifts the trunk backward, avoiding holding the breath. The examiner should secure the feet and lower back while this maneuver is performed; participants demonstrate satisfactory strength if they can hold the position for 10 seconds.

The sit-and-reach test evaluates flexibility of the back extensors and hamstrings. The individual sits on the floor with the legs straight, 6 inches apart. Place a yardstick between the legs, extending beyond the feet. The measurement at the heel level should be at the 15 inch level of the yardstick. Tell the participant to keep the knees straight and slide the arms forward as far as possible without bouncing. A reach to within 1 inch of the heels (14 inches on the yardstick) or beyond is adequate.

Hip flexor motion can be assessed easily: place the participant on a table or plinth in the supine position. He or she then brings both knees to the chest, and then holds one leg while letting the other leg down until it is flat on the table. The back should not arch. If the participant cannot flatten the leg on the table, hip flexor tightness is present. Figure 11.7 shows the Kraus–Weber tests for the hip flexors, abdominal muscles, and back muscles.

Another area that must be assessed is the individual's ability to deal with stress. Stress often is a precipitating factor in LBP. In fact, stress may be the missing link in many cases in which medical experts cannot explain LBP. This relationship is based on the premise that emotional stress creates additional muscular tension. Weak and fatigued muscles are particularly susceptible to pain, because increased tension compromises blood flow and results in painful spasms. Anxiety resulting from pain propagates additional tension and thus more anxiety, creating a vicious cycle. Figure 11.8 illustrates some tests of an individual's ability to relax.

Assessment measures are determined by both availability of resources (equipment and personnel) and the accuracy that the specialist desires. The need for equipment, the ability to compare results to normative measures, the scale of measurement (nominal or interval), and the amount of supervision or assistance necessary to perform the assessment all require consideration. For example, a low-budget program could use a photocopy of the self-test in Figure 11.9, which requires only a partner for assistance and provides an assessment of minimal fitness levels in muscular strength and joint flexibility. The Kraus–Weber tests (see Figure 11.7) allow more extensive evaluation of minimal levels of fitness but require personal evaluation by a skilled test administrator. The sit-and-reach measurement allows a comparison to normative values and permits progress to be monitored but also involves the use of minimal equipment and an evaluator. Relaxation evaluation usually involves participant demonstration of appropriate behaviors and a subjective assessment by the health/fitness specialist.

Goal Setting

The needs assessment is a prerequisite for setting individual goals for LBP management. Many individuals exhibit behaviors conducive to a healthy back; others display the opposite. The health/fitness professional identifies these behaviors and provides positive reinforcement or instructive counseling. Educational objectives help the participant recognize and change potentially harmful lifestyles. Homogeneous groups can be developed: behavior modification and reinforcement often are enhanced by groups with similar goals. Individual consultations also are important in setting measurable, obtainable goals for each participant.

Participants in the primary stage of prevention (those without severe or chronic LBP) could set these goals: ability to identify high-risk conditions or behaviors related to LBP; ability to perform mechanically correct lifting, pulling, and pushing; ability to perform preventive exercises properly, using correct technique and

Figure 11.7 The Kraus–Weber tests are used to assess the strength and flexibility of key posture muscles. These tests check minimum muscular fitness of individuals to see if they are strong enough to manage body weight and flexible enough to deal with body size. They are done as slowly and smoothly as possible. Avoid jerky movements. Do not strain. Stop and rest briefly after each test. The tests are done without shoes. (Adapted from Kraus, H., Nagler, W., and Melleby, M. Evaluation of exercise programs for back pain. *American Family Physician* 28:3, 1983. Used by permission.)

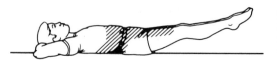

TEST 1. Lie on your back, hands behind your neck, legs straight. Keeping your legs straight, raise both feet 10 inches off the floor and hold for 10 seconds. This is a test of your hip-flexing muscles.

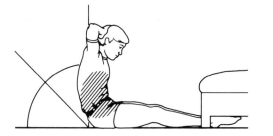

TEST 2. Lie on your back, hands behind your neck, feet under a heavy object which will not topple over. Try to "roll" up to a sitting position. This tests your hip-flexing and abdominal muscles.

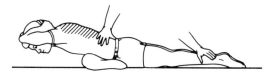

TEST 3. Lie on your back, hands behind your neck, knees flexed, feet under a heavy object which will not topple over. Again try to "roll" up to a sitting position. This is a test of your abdominal muscles.

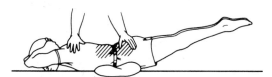

TEST 4. Lie on your stomach with a pillow under your abdomen, hands behind your neck. With someone holding your feet and hips down, raise your trunk and hold for 10 seconds. This tests the upper back muscles.

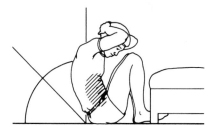

TEST 5. Taking the same position as that used for Test 4, but this time having someone holding your shoulders and hips down, try to raise your legs and hold for 10 seconds. This tests the muscles of the lower back.

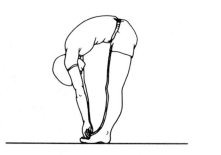

TEST 6. Stand erect with shoes off, feet together, knees stiff, hands at sides. Try to touch the floor with your fingertips. If you can not, try it again. Relax, drop your head forward, and try to let your torso "hang" from your hips. Let gravity help you. Do not jerk or strain. This is a test of muscle tension or flexibility.

■ **Figure 11.7** (Continued.)   Scoring the Kraus-Weber tests. ■

■ *TEST 1 Hip-flexing muscles*   Score 10 if held for 10 seconds. Score 6 if held for 6 seconds, and so on.

■ *TEST 2 Hip flexors and abdominal muscles* Score 10 if subject can come up to a full sit-up position (90°). Score 5 points if subject can raise to 45°; 7 or 8 points if subject can raise her- or himself halfway between 45° and 90°.

■ *TEST 3 Abdominal muscles*   Score the same way as Test 2.

■ *TEST 4 Upper back muscles*   Score 10 if held for 10 seconds, 7 if held for 7 seconds, and so on. Use two pillows to avoid hyperextension of back. Upper body should be held parallel to the floor.

■ *TEST 5 Lower back muscles*   Score 10 if held for 10 seconds, 4 if held for 4 seconds, and so on. Use two pillows to avoid hyperextension of backs. Legs should be held parallel to floor.

■ *TEST 6 Flexibility or muscle tension*   Score in inches, measuring distance from tip of middle finger to floor. For example, − 6″. If fingers just about touch floor, score "touch minus" (T −). If knuckles or finger joints can touch floor, score "touch plus" (T +). Caution that no jerky movements or bounces are to be done to gain inches— these can lead to muscle strain resulting in soreness. Emphasize reaching down toward the floor as far as you comfortably can without forcing. Hang loose.

---

speed of movement; ability to demonstrate stress-management techniques (relaxation skills); acceptable muscular strength and flexibility in the appropriate musculature.

We will use the fictitious Mr. Murry to demonstrate the goal setting for participants in the primary-prevention program. The education assessment indicated that Mr. Murry had a great deal to learn. He exhibited a limited knowledge of the causes of LBP, an improper understanding of its treatment, poor appreciation of stress-management techniques, and mistaken beliefs about the role of exercise in preventing and treating LBP. Not surprisingly, his service assessment revealed complementary results: poor body mechanics, limited strength and flexibility, and improper exercise technique.

The health/fitness specialist establishes the following goals with Mr. Murry for his LBP-management program: knowledge of the various etiologies of LBP pain; recognition of the various treatments for LBP; mastery of relaxation techniques; appreciation of the role of exercise in managing LBP; use of proper body mechanics when lifting, pulling, or pushing; progressive improvements in strength and flexibility; and use of proper technique in the performance of appropriate exercises.

The secondary prevention individuals have demonstrable disease processes and are under medical supervision. The health/fitness specialist can assist referred individuals in many ways, including implementing the prescribed exercise program and, perhaps more important, providing educational services. In secondary prevention, the health/fitness professional works in conjunction with the medical community, reporting progress and discussing projected goals. The program must be sufficiently flexible to allow for the daily fluctuations in an individual's condition. Goals for an individual recovering from LBP include: demonstration of improved knowledge regarding the nature, cause, treatment, prevention, and chronicity of LBP; correct implementation of the prescribed progressive exercise program; performance of correct lifting, sitting, standing, and related biomechanical techniques; and development of a lifestyle that prevents or mitigates recurrence of discomfort.

Progressive improvement may allow an individual, following reevaluation by a medical specialist, to graduate from the secondary- to the primary-prevention program. However, an individual may remain in the secondary stage under medical supervision—for these

■ **Figure 11.8**   Relaxation test. ■

Have the participant lie down on a mat or rug and assume a restful supine position. Shoes should be removed or loosened. Once the participant is comfortable, instruct him or her to demonstrate the methods he or she feels are best to become as relaxed as possible. During the next 2 to 3 minutes, observe the participant and place an X beside each behavior observed. The participant:

1. Begins to breathe more deeply   ____
2. Tends to tense and then release tension from a given body part   ____
3. Tends to have less tension in facial musculation (eyes may even be closed)   ____
4. Assumes a limp position with the arms   ____
5. Has the fingers open and not closed in a fist   ____
6. Has the feet naturally splayed (toes pointed outward) because of gravity's
   influence   ____
7. Has a general appearance of reduced tension in the muscle   ____
8. Tends to let the head drop to one side   ____
9. Has little visible movement after the initial moments of adjustment to
   position   ____
10. Has the appearance of being able to fall asleep   ____

Scoring: 8 or more, good; 5–7, average; less than 4, poor.

participants, the LBP-management program is essential.

■ Planning

The health/fitness professional can use numerous planning strategies in LBP-management programs. The starting point is a careful evaluation of the needs assessment and an examination of the established goals. These data provide an overview of the participants' status that is useful in developing appropriate educational and service methodologies. Determine whether you can develop an *internal presentation*, implemented within the health/fitness program, or wish to use an *external* program, implemented by community or medical agencies. If available resources are limited and there is a clear need for LBP management, offsite programs may be the best strategy.

If available resources are sufficient to provide at least some of the prevention strategies, such as correct lifting procedures, then you can plan a combination of onsite and offsite pro-

grams. For example, exercise classes could be offered through the local YMCA's "Y's Way to a Healthy Back" program, with supplementary educational programs provided inhouse. The self-test could be used with inhouse formal exercise and relaxation classes. Commercial back schools, such as the American Back School, provide extensive training and medical supervision, but at a high price. A hospital contract also provides comprehensive benefits and professional expertise for a corresponding fee. Within the corporation, work with the safety, employee assistance, or personnel department to coordinate a healthy-back program. Decide whether to offer self-instructional packets or formal, structured classes. If the latter, create homogeneous groups and encourage participants to discuss feelings and attitudes about LBP.

Class sessions should be of progressive length as participants reach improved performance levels. Classes should be convenient for participants in time, location, and length of course.

Appropriate planning is essential for secondary-prevention education programs in

Figure 11.9 Four tests for healthy muscles that can be done with a partner. These tests measure minimal levels of muscular strength and joint flexibility for key muscle groups related to your back. Failing any one of these tests indicates that your muscles are underexercised or too tense. This lack of muscular conditioning increases your chances of developing back pain in the future. Before you begin, please note: If you have any back pain or other health problems, consult your physician before taking these tests. Take off your shoes and get comfortable. Don't hurry through the tests. Do not push or strain through the movements. (From Pfeiffer, George J. *Self-Starter: A self-help guide to back care.* Xerox Corporation, 1983, p. 6. Used by permission.)

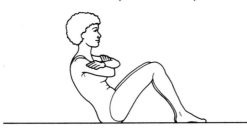

Test 1: Sit-Up/muscular strength in your abdominals

Lie on the floor with your arms across your chest, knees bent, heels flat to the floor. Attempt to sit up, keeping your feet in contact with the floor.

A passing grade: 3 to 5 sit-ups.

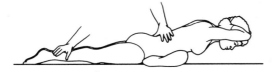

Test 2: Trunk rise/muscular strength in your back extensors

On your abdomen, place a pillow under your abdomen, keep your hands behind your head, with feet and lower back held by your partner. Lift your trunk and hold that position. Do not hold your breath!

A passing grade: holding position for 10 seconds.

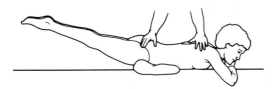

Test 3: Hip extensors/muscular strength in your hip extensors

On your abdomen, with pillow under your abdomen, place your arms under your chin. Have your partner secure your back. Keeping your legs straight, lift them up and hold position.

A passing grade: holding position for 10 seconds.

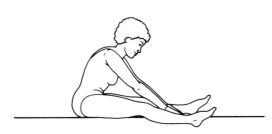

Test 4: Sit and reach/flexibility in your back extensors and hamstrings

Sit on the floor with your legs straight and feet 6" apart. Place a yardstick on the floor between your legs with the 16" mark in line with your heels. Slowly reach forward as far as you can comfortably go. Do not bounce or force the movement. Repeat three times; record your best score.

A passing grade: a reach of 15" or greater.

view of the extended recovery phase and the lifelong risk of reinjury. Knowledge of LBP-management procedures allows participants to adjust, redirect, or adapt prior lifestyles. Consider creating a long-term program with a series of lectures based on degree of recovery, compliance, and knowledge level. You might develop a resource center for self-paced learning for chronic pain individuals. Post illustrations of proper lifting techniques. Finally, schedule periodic conferences in which the participant, health/fitness specialist, and medical director can assess the participant's progress in compliance, understanding, and overall health status.

The service component for secondary-prevention participants should reflect both the recommendations of the referring medical specialist and the individual's own goals and objectives. Knowledge of LBP diagnosis, pharmacological treatment, medical history, prognosis, and exercise prescription are all essential for proper planning. Although participants can benefit from an exercise program in a group setting, sometimes it is helpful for them to undertake personal exercise programs at home, in familiar conditions and surroundings. This reinforces incorporating the exercises into a permanent lifestyle. Group support, on the other hand, often helps people stick to exercise programs, especially in the early stages. Any home program should be less strenuous than that scheduled in a supervised environment where proper instruction in technique and intensity is given. Periodic assessments of those who exercise alone allows the specialist to prescribe an appropriate, progressive program.

Back rehabilitation is individual; exercise therapy programs must leave room for fluctuation while providing an orderly progression of low back load and muscular stress. Each participant can progress or regress through a sequence of exercise depending on his or her current condition.

Plan what you will do if a participant has a severe relapse and is unable to continue in the mainstream of the group program. If participants pay all or part of the fees, definite policies concerning refund procedures are imperative,

and participants must be made aware of (and must acknowledge) these guidelines.

Implementation ▮

Education Component

The participants in an LBP-management education program should become familiar with the terms used for describing the LBP problem and how it is to be managed.

The basic anatomy of the lower back, including the muscular vertebral regions and support structures such as the discs, should be explained to the participants. Figure 11.10 illustrates the essential structure of the back. We recommend the *Back owner's manual*[7] as a teaching aid. Included in this booklet are the mechanics of proper and efficient spinal movement and the concept of leverage, the consequences of improper leverage and incorrect body mechanics such as poor posture, and the do's and don'ts for maintaining a healthy, pain-free back. Use the booklet to teach proper body mechanics, both active (manual handling and lifting) and static (sitting, standing, sleeping). Designate a specific location within the workplace to teach LBP management. When you teach proper lifting and carrying techniques, use objects the participants handle during work, such as drums, sacks, or boxes. Encourage people who must stand for long periods to use a footrest and change their posture frequently to avoid fatigue. Walking, bending and stretching can be used to avoid the prolonged standing posture. If breaks are not possible, then recommend they stand erect, with chin in, head up, back flattened, pelvis held straight, and knees slightly bent. People who work at a cabinet or table should not lean into the structure.

A firm, straight-backed chair usually is best—or a rocking chair may be more restful for relaxed sitting. The chair's seat height should allow the feet to rest on the floor. The seat should be deep enough that the hips are not against the back of the chair. If the chair has armrests, they should be the right height to support the shoulders comfortably. Tell the participant to "sit tall," with hips pushed back in the

❙ Figure 11.10 Anatomy of a normal, healthy back. ❙

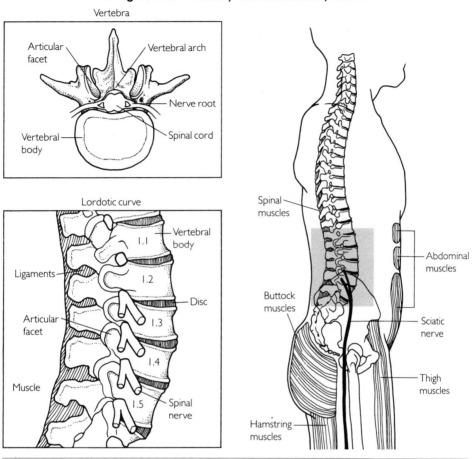

Vertebra

Articular facet

Vertebral arch

Nerve root

Vertebral body

Spinal cord

Lordotic curve

Vertebral body

Ligaments

1.1

1.2

Disc

Articular facet

1.3

1.4

Muscle

1.5

Spinal nerve

Spinal muscles

Abdominal muscles

Buttock muscles

Sciatic nerve

Thigh muscles

Hamstring muscles

chair, thighs parallel to floor, and weight distributed on both thighs and feet. If people must sit for extended periods, they can place one foot on a footrest that raises their knee higher than the corresponding hip; this results in tilting of the pelvis and relieves swayback.

Sleeping posture also is surprisingly important. If participants do not have a firm mattress, they can place a plywood board between the box spring and mattress. Teach participants to sleep on their sides with knees bent and a pillow between their knees (fetal position) or on their back with a pillow underneath their knees. Discourage sleeping face down, as this position increases swaying of the back and strains neck

and shoulder muscles. When driving, move the seat forward to keep the knees bent and higher than the hips. On long trips, stop frequently and get out, stretch, and walk around.

Classes of eight to ten are most effective. The optimal class length is 45 minutes to 1 hour. The program's effectiveness is enhanced by enrollment of all personnel, including top management. Supervisors should receive additional training in the prevention of work-related back injuries.

Many people have misconceptions about LBP that you will need to correct. Some common ones are: (1) LBP always is caused by weak abdominal muscles or a muscle imbalance; (2)

all LBP is the result of a "slipped disc"; (3) the whole disc is displaced when it "slips"; (4) LBP always is recurrent; (5) an x-ray film will reveal any lower back injury; and (6) pain-killing and muscle-relaxing medications are the only approaches to relief of LBP.

Service Component

Implementation of the service component requires close communication and considerable cooperation within the corporate setting. Some minor adaptations can decrease the incidence of LBP among employees dramatically. Unfavorable physical work situations should be altered. In Great Britain, the upper limits of loads lifted have been recommended to be 50 kilograms (110 pounds) for men and 30 kilograms (66 pounds) for women.[8] Although few work environments have adopted such rigid rules, designing work situations to eliminate or lower mechanical stress can reduce the incidence of LBP. Individuals whose work requires lifting should be reassigned to different tasks if they are recovering from LBP, to prevent recurrence of the problem.

The service component can be implemented with relative ease and at low cost. A systematic, progressive preventive exercise program, designed to promote the maintenance of a healthy back, should include individual instruction. After the participants have demonstrated competency, they can be enrolled in a class. Classes should start and end with relaxation exercises.

Tell participants to allow enough time to perform the exercises at home in a relaxed atmosphere. They should exercise on a carpeted floor (not a soft bed), using the same sequence that they perform in class. Warn participants to stop exercising if they experience pain.

Implementing a secondary LBP-management program requires close communication among the clinician, participant, and health/fitness specialist. Unless he or she is a doctor, the health/fitness professional is not legally permitted to practice medicine. Make it

clear that the exercise program is not a therapeutic prescription, and that the specialist's role is only to implement what a physician has recommended.

The participant will already have been seen and evaluated by a clinician before coming to the program. Appropriate therapeutic measures will have been performed and subsequent medical clearance given. Prescribed exercise regimens should be continued or implemented, but remember that exercise is not a panacea and is not appropriate for certain disease states. Exercise usually is effective for treating trauma- or postural-induced LBP.

Relaxation is important in LBP rehabilitation and always should be included in the exercise sessions. Alternating contractions of muscle groups with periods of relaxation is a simple and effective technique. Start with the facial muscles, move down to the upper extremities, and so on down to the toes.

Next perform stretching and strengthening exercises, such as the YMCA routine or the Williams-type flexion series (Figure 11.11).

Participants usually have been given prescribed exercises. The health/fitness specialist should demonstrate each exercise and ensure that the participant uses proper technique.

Faulty posture frequently either causes or intensifies and prolongs LBP. An exercise that helps remedy poor posture is the pelvic tilt. Ensure that the maneuver is performed correctly—incorrect execution may exacerbate LBP. The participant lies on his or her back on a firm surface and flattens the lower back by tucking in the pelvis, which reduces swayback or lordosis. The movement is performed by the combined contraction of the abdominal and gluteal muscles. Placing the participants' hand at the small of the back and having them press down on the hand helps them to understand the intended movement. They must not "bridge" (that is, raise the lower back from the floor), as this will cause hyperextension (an increase in the original curve) rather than flattening. After clients have mastered pelvic tilting in the supine position, they can incorporate it in their lifelong posture. To exercise 1 hour a day while continuing to stand or sit in a faulty manner for the

Treatment of Lumbar Strain

Acute	Chronic and prophylactic
Absolute bed rest	Reduction of weight
Warm tub baths, heat pad, hydrocollator	Correction of posture
Sedation	Firm mattress, bed board
Firm mattress, bed board	Daily low back exercises
Diathermy, massage	Regular sports activity compatible
Local anesthetic infiltration to trigger zones	with age and physique
Occasionally corset, brace or strapping	

Exercises for chronic lumbar strain (starting positions in outline)

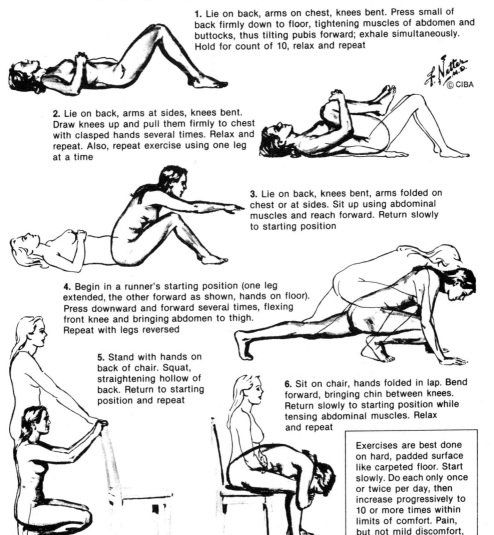

1. Lie on back, arms on chest, knees bent. Press small of back firmly down to floor, tightening muscles of abdomen and buttocks, thus tilting pubis forward; exhale simultaneously. Hold for count of 10, relax and repeat

2. Lie on back, arms at sides, knees bent. Draw knees up and pull them firmly to chest with clasped hands several times. Relax and repeat. Also, repeat exercise using one leg at a time

3. Lie on back, knees bent, arms folded on chest or at sides. Sit up using abdominal muscles and reach forward. Return slowly to starting position

4. Begin in a runner's starting position (one leg extended, the other forward as shown, hands on floor). Press downward and forward several times, flexing front knee and bringing abdomen to thigh. Repeat with legs reversed

5. Stand with hands on back of chair. Squat, straightening hollow of back. Return to starting position and repeat

6. Sit on chair, hands folded in lap. Bend forward, bringing chin between knees. Return slowly to starting position while tensing abdominal muscles. Relax and repeat

Exercises are best done on hard, padded surface like carpeted floor. Start slowly. Do each only once or twice per day, then increase progressively to 10 or more times within limits of comfort. Pain, but not mild discomfort, is indication to stop remainder of the day will lead to no improvement of posture and no decrease in pain.

Another exercise strategy is abdominal strengthening. Bent-knee sit-ups are recommended. Again, form is paramount. The participant is encouraged to curl up, gradually peeling the head and shoulders from the floor and emphasizing tucking the chin to the chest. If abdominal weakness prohibits correct technique, the exercise can be done in reverse—an uncurl instead of a curl up is performed. The participant is instructed to lean back from the fully curled-up position, with nose to knees. After a few degrees of uncurling, the participant returns to the full-curled position. Progressive uncurling with return to the full-flexed position continues until the participant can return from the totally flat (supine) position.

Low-back stretching is best done curled up, in a ball position. The participant gradually draws up both knees to the chest without raising the head from the floor; it is not necessary for the knees to touch the nose. This also may be performed with one leg at a time.

Exercises are often misperformed, and their effects negated, by haste, improper instruction, poor adherence, or the addition of inappropriate drills by the participant. Instruction about the nature of the exercise, proper technique of performance, and anatomical structures involved should be included when the exercise is introduced.

Teach participants to move through a full range of motion when possible and to stop exercising if they experience pain or discomfort. Encourage total relaxation between exercises. Teach the speed at which an exercise should be performed—too slow or too fast a movement rate can cause injury. Instruct participants always to bend their knees when they lie on their back. Encourage them to cease other physical activities, such as games or jogging, during the rehabilitative period.

▮ Evaluation

As we have discussed, evaluation provides information demonstrating the benefits of a pro-

gram or signifying the need for adjustment of the curriculum. Evaluate the participants' success in reaching planned goals. Prepare a cost–benefit analysis of the program, and record any unplanned effects (positive or negative).

The education component can be evaluated by having participants retake the tests used during the needs assessment. Also, include questions regarding job absenteeism related to LBP, usage of back-care techniques, and adherence to appropriate exercise regimens.

To evaluate the service component, retest participants on measures such as the Kraus–Weber, relaxation, and sit-and-reach tests. In addition, have them fill out the program evaluation questionnaire in Figure 11.12.

The health/fitness specialist usually does not test participants involved in the secondary prevention strategy: the clinician who originally diagnosed the difficulty and referred the participant to the program conducts the reevaluation.

Summary ▮

LBP affects a large percentage of our adult population. The greatest incidence occurs during middle age, the period of peak earning potential. The loss of critical work hours in business and industry due to LBP provides ample justification for an LBP-management program.

This chapter presented guidelines for implementing LBP-prevention programs. Corporations can offer inhouse educational programs that provide training in correct lifting and handling techniques, or preventive/therapeutic exercise classes. You might also elect to use community programs or a consultant. Inhouse programs provide a fringe benefit, improve *esprit de corps*, and probably reduce absenteeism and increase productivity.

References ▮

1. Nachemson, A., The lumbar spine: An orthopaedic challenge. *Spine* 1, 1976.

▮ Figure 11.12 Evaluation questionnaire for progress in an LBP program. (Adapted ▮
from Kraus, H., Nagler, W., and Melleby, M. Evaluation of exercise programs for back
pain. *American Family Physician* 28:3, 1983. Used by permission.)

Date _____

We hope you have enjoyed participating in the Y's Way To A Healthy Back. So that we may evaluate the effectiveness of the program, please answer the questions below. Thank you.

1. At this moment I would describe my back discomfort as:
   None at all   Slight   Moderate   Severe   Agony

2. Yesterday, I would have described my back discomfort as:
   None at all   Slight   Moderate   Severe   Agony

3. During the past week, I would have described my back discomfort as:
   None at all   Slight   Moderate   Severe   Agony

4. During the past 6 weeks, I would have described my back discomfort as:
   None at all   Slight   Moderate   Severe   Agony

5. At this moment my back discomfort interferes with my normal routine:
   Strongly disagree   Disagree   Not Sure   Agree   Strongly agree

6. Yesterday, my back discomfort interfered with my normal routine:
   Strongly disagree   Disagree   Not Sure   Agree   Strongly agree

7. During the past week, my back discomfort interfered with my normal routine:
   Strongly disagree   Disagree   Not Sure   Agree   Strongly agree

8. During the past 6 weeks, my back discomfort interfered with my normal routine:
   Strongly disagree   Disagree   Not Sure   Agree   Strongly agree

9. Yesterday, I was uncomfortable:
   Not at all   Once   More than once   Frequently   Constantly

10. During the past week, I was uncomfortable:
    Not at all   Once   More than once   Frequently   Constantly

11. During the past 6 weeks, I was uncomfortable:
    Not at all   Once   More than once   Frequently   Constantly

12. How many times a week do you exercise at home?
    0-2   3-5   6-9   10-15   more than 15

13. How long is your average home exercise session?
    Less than 15 minutes   15-30 minutes   31-45 minutes   over 45 minutes

14. After a home exercise session, I am tired:
    Strongly disagree   Disagree   Not Sure   Agree   Strongly agree

15. After a home exercise session, I am relaxed:
    Strongly disagree   Disagree   Not Sure   Agree   Strongly agree

16. After class, I am tired:
    Strongly disagree   Disagree   Not Sure   Agree   Strongly agree

17. After class, I am relaxed:
    Strongly disagree   Disagree   Not Sure   Agree   Strongly agree

18. I have experienced relief from back discomfort as a result of this course:
    Strongly disagree   Disagree   Not Sure   Agree   Strongly agree

19. Have you participated in any form of exercise while taking this course?   Yes or No
    If yes please describe _____

20. Do you have any suggestions that you feel would improve this program? _____
    _____

2. Bonica, J. Basic principles of managing chronic pain. *Archives of Surgery* 112:783, 1977.

3. Kraus, H. Evaluation of muscular and cardiovascular fitness. *Preventive Medicine* 1:178, 1972.

4. Troup, J. D., Martin, J. W., and Lloyd, D. C. Back pain in industry: A prospective survey. *Spine* 6:6, 1981.

5. Magora, A. Investigation of the relation between low back pain and occupation. *Industrial Medicine*, 39, 1970.

6. Anderson, G. Epidemiologic aspects on low-back pain in industry. *Spine* 6:53, 1981.

7. Krames, L. A., et al. *Back owner's manual.* Daly City, CA: PAS Patient Information Library, 1977.

8. Jayson, M. (ed). *The lumbar spine and back pain.* New York: Grune and Stratton, 1976.

PART 3
MANAGEMENT
OF HEALTH/FITNESS PROGRAMS

CHAPTER 12

PARTICIPANT ADHERENCE

Now that health/fitness programs have become a part of the corporate environment, corporations are finding that participant adherence is a key problem as they attempt to measure the success of company involvement in preventing illness through these programs. The problem of adherence is especially critical in settings that serve a small population. Dropouts in a corporate program with a limited target population are more critical than dropouts in a commercial or community-based program where large target populations are being served. Thus, in programs where limited target populations exist, the health/fitness professional has even more reason to maximize adherence as well as to enroll new participants through a variety of strategies.

Corporations' health-care costs continue to grow. The American Heart Association estimates that recruiting replacements for unhealthy workers sets U.S. industry back more than $700 million each year.[1] This is causing companies to examine other alternatives to reduce absenteeism, improve productivity, improve morale, and decrease workers' compensation related to poor health. Corporations are looking for a solution to extreme health-care costs and are encouraging changes in employee lifestyles to improve the health/fitness of their workforce.

Health/fitness professionals have been dealing with adherence problems for many years. Most experts find that 50% of the individuals who begin an exercise program discontinue it within 6 months: research indicates that this 6-month period is critical to a continuing program that encourages an active lifestyle and health-improving behavior.[2]

Almost everyone would agree that the practice of good health habits and regular physical activity is good for the mind, body, and spirit. The benefits range from improved health, better appearance, and reduced stress to an abundance of energy. Why then is it so difficult to *commit* to a program of improved health/fitness and even more difficult to *stay committed*?

The participants' reasons for dropping out of programs are many, and most are legitimate. The time is not right. The place is inconvenient. Family and work responsibilities interfere. The exercise program is too hard or too easy. The exercise activity or educational program is boring and no fun. However varied such excuses may be, they all boil down to the same fact: the individual has chosen not to participate. Health/fitness professionals must examine all the factors of individual differences to plan programming for adherence.

In this chapter, we will focus on exercise programming techniques that can be used to enhance the program and improve adherence. We will consider leadership, environmental factors, management support, creative programming, family and peer support, and education about health-improving behaviors.

Appropriate communication techniques allow the health/fitness professional to promote participation and assure continued program adherence. Health/fitness counseling on an individual basis gives continued reinforcement to participants. We will suggest communication guidelines to follow when instructing individuals to improve their health/fitness through lifestyle behavioral changes. Finally, continued participant adherence to a healthy lifestyle requires reinforcement and followup on the part of the health/fitness professional.

Individual Factors

Adherence to any health/fitness program component is important, and each area requires unique approaches to promoting adherence. However, we will focus primarily on exercise adherence. Exercise program adherence clearly illustrates participants' continued commitment to a change in lifestyle. Moreover, the spillover effect of enhanced wellness behaviors resulting from the initiation of an exercise program provides a good starting point in affecting other health behaviors, such as nutrition, weight control, substance-abuse cessation, and stress management.

Biological Factors

An individual's biological makeup may influence exercise program adherence. Those individuals who adhere best to exercise prescription often are leaner, lighter, less fit, and more symptomatic with regard to coronary disease at the time of program entry.[3] Thus, exercise screening may predict participant adherence in exercise programs.

The fact that lean, lighter individuals have a better adherence rate suggests that adherence is higher in individuals who have already established some good balanced diet and exercise activity habits. Also, for these individuals the long-term, uphill battle of weight control may not be a factor in their measurement of fitness improvement. These lean and light individuals find it less difficult to move their bodies while participating in exercise routines. A poor self-image or lack of confidence, which often are factors for overweight and out-of-shape persons, probably are not problems for lean and light individuals. Lean, light, unfit participants see benefits of improved fitness much faster than do overweight, unfit participants, and this directly influences their self-motivation to adhere to the program. The plain facts of life versus death provide coronary heart patients a potent natural motivation.

The health/fitness professional should give more personal attention to overweight and unfit individuals, who are more likely to drop out.

Psychological Factors

Psychological differences are another factor that affects adherence to exercise. Individuals who are goal-oriented are likely to carry out their commitment to physical exercise.[4] Self-motivation—or its absence—may be the single most important predictor, capable of identifying reliably those who need help and encouragement to persevere. Individuals who have both low self-motivation and high body fat may have great difficulty adhering to an exercise program. The exercise motivation quiz in Figure 12.1 can help you assess your participants' motivation level. Dishman found a high degree of accuracy for those taking the quiz, when the individual's overall body weight plus an accurate skinfold assessment of percentage of body fat were also taken into account. He points out that a low score on this questionnaire should not provide an excuse not to exercise, but it is an indication that this individual has tendencies that make adherence more difficult. Also, be aware that individuals who adhere to a program for 6 months usually overcome their obstacles to achieving improved physical fitness and wellness.[4]

■ **Figure 12.1**   Motivation assessment scale to determine likelihood of compliance. (From ■ Dishman, R. K., et al. Self-motivation and adherence to habitual physical activity. *Journal of Applied Social Psychology* 10:129, 1980; also from Falls, H. B., et al. *Essentials of fitness.* Copyright © 1980 by Saunders College/Holt, Rinehart and Winston. Assessment scale copyright 1978 by R. K. Dishman; codeveloper W. J. Ickes. Reprinted by permission of CBS College Publishing and R. K. Dishman.)

Directions: Circle the number beneath the letter corresponding to the alternative that best describes how characteristic the statement is when applied to you. The alternatives are

A. *Extremely* uncharacteristic of me
B. *Somewhat* uncharacteristic of me
C. Neither characteristic nor uncharacteristic of me
D. *Somewhat* characteristic of me
E. *Extremely* characteristic of me

A	B	C	D	E	
5	4	3	2	1	1. I get discouraged easily.
5	4	3	2	1	2. I don't work any harder than I have to.
1	2	3	4	5	3. I seldom if ever let myself down.
5	4	3	2	1	4. I'm just not the goal-setting type.
1	2	3	4	5	5. I'm good at keeping promises, especially the ones I make to myself.
5	4	3	2	1	6. I don't impose much structure on my activities.
1	2	3	4	5	7. I have a very hard-driving, aggressive personality.

Scoring: Add together the seven numbers you circled. A summated score equal to or less than *24* suggests drop-out prone behavior. The lower the score, the greater the likelihood toward exercise noncompliance. However, if the score suggests dropout proneness, it should be viewed as an incentive to remain active, rather than a self-fulfilling prophecy to quit exercising.

Social Factors

A third factor in adherence to exercise programs is social influence. Group exercise and health-improving classes are extremely successful; they generate an active interest and awareness that help the individual make positive lifestyle changes.

Most individuals enjoy a social experience with others involved in similar goals and objectives. A class activity provides participants with the opportunity to meet new friends and to belong to a group while engaging in self-improvement. The Danielsons reviewed studies conducted by Abraham Maslow on the hierarchy of needs and their relationship to human health.[5] Referring to Maslow's chart, Figure 12.2, they point out that individuals are en-

gaged in a lifetime of striving to reach the highest strata of the chart; however, they cannot reach the highest level until the basic needs at the bottom—food, shelter, and safety—have been satisfied.

As you follow the *needs type* upward on Maslow's chart it is clear that a basic human need is that of "belonging." Affectionate relationships, strong family bonds, satisfying group memberships, and satisfying team memberships are listed directly above safety. With this in mind, it is easy to see how a successful health/fitness class led by an energetic, caring, and creative instructor can be a strong positive influence on an individual's progress toward self-fulfillment, and can provide continued motivation in group activity. Also note that when an individual reaches the *neutral point* at

Figure 12.2 Maslow's hierarchy of needs. (From Danielson, R. R., and Danielson, K. F. Ongoing motivation in employee fitness programming. In *Employee fitness "the how to ..."*, Proceedings of the Ontario Employee Fitness Workshop. Seneca College, King City, Ontario: Ministry of Tourism and Recreation, March 1979, p. 138. Reprinted by permission.)

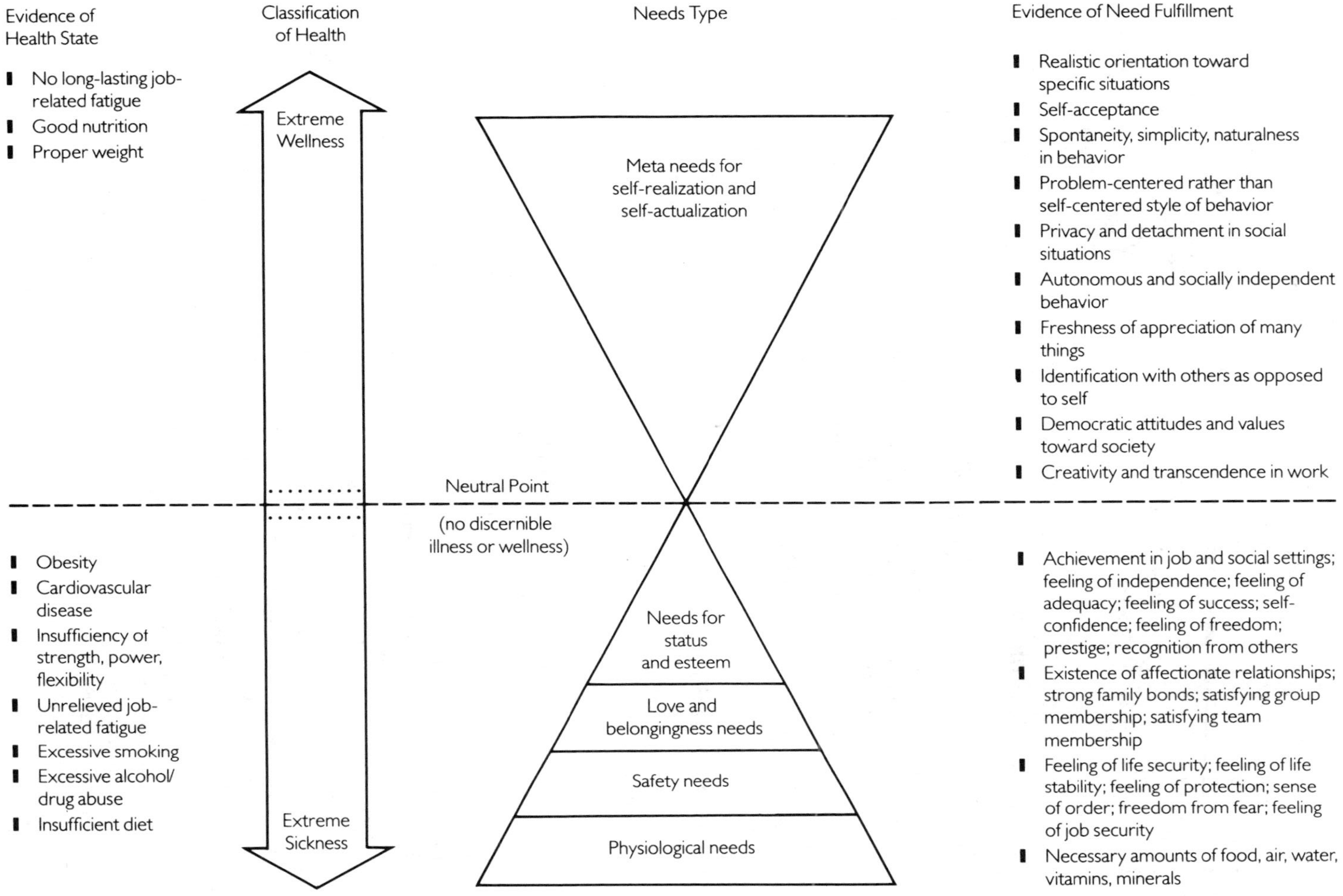

Evidence of Need Fulfillment

- Realistic orientation toward specific situations
- Self-acceptance
- Spontaneity, simplicity, naturalness in behavior
- Problem-centered rather than self-centered style of behavior
- Privacy and detachment in social situations
- Autonomous and socially independent behavior
- Freshness of appreciation of many things
- Identification with others as opposed to self
- Democratic attitudes and values toward society
- Creativity and transcendence in work

- Achievement in job and social settings; feeling of independence; feeling of adequacy; feeling of success; self-confidence; feeling of freedom; prestige; recognition from others
- Existence of affectionate relationships; strong family bonds; satisfying group membership; satisfying team membership
- Feeling of life security; feeling of life stability; feeling of protection; sense of order; freedom from fear; feeling of job security
- Necessary amounts of food, air, water, vitamins, minerals

Needs Type

- Meta needs for self-realization and self-actualization
- Needs for status and esteem
- Love and belongingness needs
- Safety needs
- Physiological needs

Neutral Point
(no discernible illness or wellness)

Classification of Health

Extreme Wellness

Extreme Sickness

Evidence of Health State

- No long-lasting job-related fatigue
- Good nutrition
- Proper weight

- Obesity
- Cardiovascular disease
- Insufficiency of strength, power, flexibility
- Unrelieved job-related fatigue
- Excessive smoking
- Excessive alcohol/drug abuse
- Insufficient diet

the center of the chart—achievement in job and social settings—the continued satisfaction of the belongingness needs and the desire for self-improvement motivate the individual even farther upward. The importance of spouse, family, and peer approval in making health/fitness improvements in lifestyle cannot be overlooked.

■ Adherence Techniques

We have touched upon some of the most important factors that affect an individual's adherence to a program. In designing successful health/fitness programs, the following factors help promote adherence: strong leadership, a pleasant functional environment, strong company support, creative planning, and family and peer support.

Strong Leadership

The most important element in any health/fitness program is the leadership. An enthusiastic leader who is totally committed to the program and its goals can be an excellent role model. He or she can inject vitality into a program, affecting each individual and minimizing creeping boredom. A strong leader encourages fun and play in the exercise activity. The program participant should enjoy the doing, the "getting someplace," as much as the goal or the "arriving."

The importance of strong leadership always has been recognized in the business environment. Effective leaders are elevating, mobilizing, inspiring, exalting, uplifting, exhorting, and evangelizing. [6]The same qualities, with the addition of caring, mark a good health/fitness leader. A health/fitness professional must be a charismatic leader and role model. Leaders who have the ability to involve the participants in dialogues rather than conducting a lecture will make the program more exciting and interesting, encouraging program adherence.

Environment

The program environment is another major factor in program adherence. The appropriateness of the facility and convenience of its location, time of day that the class meets, and the duration of program sessions all affect initial interest as well as the long-term adherence.

The facility, no matter how large or small, must be designed for the best possible delivery of services. It need not necessarily be expensive; however, space and equipment must be safe and the surroundings pleasant. Programs delivered in an environment carefully designed to make the participant feel good about being there have a better chance for success. Exercise rooms must be of adequate size, be well ventilated, have temperature and humidity controls, and be clean and cheerful.

Onsite programs, because they are convenient, will draw more participants and have lower dropout rates than programs held across the street or a few blocks away. There is a strong relationship between program participation and the convenience of the program site.

If the budget allows, other features to be considered are showers, lockers, exercise equipment, juice bars, a pro shop, and enlarged activity facilities such as a running track, racquetball courts, a swimming pool, or a tennis court.

The *times* at which exercise programs are offered is a factor in participants' commitment. Keep in mind that the individuals will be choosing how best to spend their free time. If they must wait around after work or leave the work site and return, they often will decide not to participate. Classes should be held after work unless showers are available. Facilities with showers and other club amenities can enhance program adherence by allowing you to schedule classes throughout the day, particularly if employees have flexible work hours or varied work and travel schedules.

Most people drop out prior to the fifth or sixth week of a program. The program leader should keep participants interested through creative programming while focusing on short-term goals.

The leader should encourage participants to exercise when they are unable to attend classes. People who undertake aerobic exercise outside of class, such as walking, jogging, swimming, or cycling, as well as use music and video tapes designed for exercise at home or on the road, are more likely to make a habit of regular exercise.

Management Support

Program participation or other types of visible support from the company president, chief executive officer, and other senior executives have a positive effect on employees' adherence to health/fitness programs as well as facilitating program operation.

Creative Programming

Creative programming and leadership often are one and the same. A strong, creative leader has that special spark that converts an exercise workout into a "happening," and a boring health-related lecture into a stimulating discussion. Designing the exercise program to "flow" well to music, which sets a happy mood and establishes an appropriate tempo for the warm-up, flexibility, strength, aerobics and cool-down segments of the program, requires skill, strong dedication, planning, and hard work. Some companies sell choreographed exercise routines set to music, and train and certify leaders to deliver the programs. Names and addresses of aerobic dance exercise companies around the world can be obtained by writing Ms. Kathie Davis, Executive Director, International Dance Exercise Association, IDEA, 4501 Mission Bay Drive #2F, San Diego, CA 92109. Another source of information is the national office for the Association for Fitness in Business, 1312 Washington Boulevard, Stamford, CT 06902.

The following professional organizations and agencies can supply names of companies that offer creative programs in your area: The President's Council on Physical Fitness and Sports, 450 5th Street N.W., Room 7103, Washington, DC 20001; Office of Disease Prevention and Health Promotion, 300 7th Street S.W., Room 613, Washington, DC 20201; National Center for Health Education, 211 Suter Street, 4th Floor, San Francisco, CA 94108. You can also call your state department of health, Governor's Commission on Physical Fitness and Sports.

Music The use of music is without a doubt essential to a group exercise class; it is one of the greatest motivational tools available. Music can set a mood, spark energy and excitement, and encourage rhythm and coordination. "Time flies when you are having fun." Vary the music on a regular basis.

Fun Periodically introduce the participants to a fun activity that is not a regular part of the class. This surprise adds spice to the program and gives the participants the feeling they might *miss* the fun if they do not attend each class period. Some ideas for novelty activities are:

▌ Games and relays

▌ Simple inexpensive equipment such as wands, ropes, towels, balls, paper, chairs

▌ Simple dance steps or folk dance formations such as polka, cotton-eyed joe, schottish, disco, square dance

▌ Partner exercises

▌ Circuit and interval training

▌ Low-key contests (high-level competition is not appropriate)

The health/fitness leader who obviously enjoys leading the group will help participants to enjoy their own efforts. Encourage laughter, singing, moaning, and other expressions of involvement from the class members—these give each participant a sense of belonging, a real sense of ownership, which obviously encourages program adherence.

Incentives   Incentives can be rewards given by an individual to him- or herself at the completion of a task well done, or they can be offered by the health/fitness program. Avoid incentives that are counterproductive to the goal. For instance, a calorie-loaded meal or heavy alcohol consumption is not an appropriate reward for reaching a desired weight. Dishman suggests identifying an enjoyable activity and not allowing yourself to do it until your exercise is completed or a goal is reached—think of the activity as dessert.[4] Also, treating yourself to a special day or a purchase you otherwise would not buy is a great way to reward yourself.

Incentives work in business; they work in health/fitness programs as well. Our society encourages us to act by evaluating what we do and rewarding us for "good" behavior. An incentive for an activity can increase the activity's perceived value. A popular weight-training program for the Eugene, Oregon, police department was offered to 20 qualified persons from outside the department. The department's demand for use of this room was great, and if one of the outside 20 people failed to use the room 3 times per week, he or she lost the privilege. The police department believes this increased the paticipants' commitment.[7] Some type of monetary commitment on the part of the participant can act as an incentive to stay with the program. When participants contribute financially to the health/fitness program, they perceive it as having more value and this increases compliance.

Pollock et al. studied an 8-week starter program at the YMCA of Milwaukee using a test to measure the fitness improvement of 892 men and 470 women in the program.[8] They reported that heavier initial body weight of the participant was associated with a greater dropout rate. Furthermore, requiring attendance for reimbursement and having the participant take partial responsibility for payment positively affected program attendance. Four methods of payment were studied, and the results (Table 12.1) clearly show that the most motivating fee-payment designs were b and c, in which participants either were reimbursed dependent on attendance or split the fee with their employer. The group in which the company paid the entire fee with no attendance requirement had the lowest adherence.

Special Events   Provide special events throughout the program. This requires long-term planning, in which participants should be involved. Some ideas are: company-sponsored road races, walks, hikes, bicycle rides, superstar events, and family activities; guest day—bring a friend to class; weight-loss contest; awards and recognition parties; and team activities.

Family and Peer Support

One of the main reasons individuals commit to an exercise program is that friends and family also exercise and encourage their participation. The support of the participant's family is important to all health/fitness programs, be they exercise, nutrition, weight control, or stress management. Group support and the social atmosphere of the class reinforce adherence. When families participate, program growth and participant adherence are greatly enhanced.

Interests developed in the exercise group are naturally extended to home, work, and leisure time. Participants often begin outside exercise activity such as walking, jogging, cycling, or hiking. These out-of-class activities contribute to increased fitness, which allows program goals and benefits to be realized sooner and thus promotes program adherence. In addition, the added social support and comradeship also help to ensure adherence.

Education Component

To promote lifestyle change, the director must plan sound health education. Although participants certainly should be encouraged to exercise regularly, eat nutritional foods, stop smoking, and avoid stress and drug abuse, it is just as important for them to know why they are exercising, what foods are necessary for good health, how they can cope with everyday stress,

▮ T A B L E I 2 . I ▮
Program Attendance in Relation to Method of Payment

Method of Payment	Percent of Total Sessions Attended	Number of Participants
a. Participant paid entire fee	70.7 + 27.2 † ‡	342
b. Participant reimbursed by company if attendance was at least 75% to 90%	80.6 + 23.7* ‡	588
c. Participant and company both paid part	83.7 + 19.2* ‡	140
d. Company·paid entire fee (no attendance requirements)	62.2 + 26.8* ‡	103

Source: Pollock, M. L., et al. Effects of a YMCA starter fitness program. *The Physician and Sportsmedicine* 10:98, 1982. Reprinted by permission.

*p < .01 vs a; † p < .01 vs b or c; ‡ p < .01 vs d.

what causes and how to avoid negative addictions, and what will help them to feel good and have a positive self-image.

The educational component should be part of a support system for promoting adherence. It should not be merely an informational exchange. Good education requires participation in discussion, with the leader actively and voluntarily involving the participants in the learning process.

Brevity is important in delivering class-oriented educational programs. Approximately 50% of the statements made in an educational setting are forgotten by the participants within 5 minutes. Be selective in presenting information and organize data conceptually. Present clear outlines of the class material at the outset of each session. Categorize information when possible; categorizing and labeling improve recall by 50%. Present lessons in order of importance; learners tend to recall and comply with information presented during the first third of a class. Repetitive and multimedia approaches are effective in promoting recall and subsequent behavior: summarizing and repeating are helpful, as is combining visual aids with lectures and discussion. Consider the participants' educational level when presenting written material.

Finally, specificity enhances learning; for example, help participants compute their target body weights rather than simply informing them that they need to lose weight.

Promoting the Program ▮

Communicating information and stimulating awareness of the program are important parts of program promotion. Creating initial interest in participating in health/fitness programs and ensuring continued adherence to those programs are two major obstacles facing health/fitness professionals in any environment. Good promotional techniques successfully combat these problems.

Initial Promotion

After you decide to implement a health/fitness program, identify a group of influential leaders in the organization who support the program and can serve on a wellness committee. This group should plan a timetable of events leading up to the start of the program. Circulate an exciting and nonthreatening description of the program to potential participants. Include a survey that asks questions concerning individual interest in participation, preferred method of program payment, how often to offer the program, and at what times, as well as any other information you need to serve the participants.

If the target population shows sufficient interest, distribute *promotional materials*. Approximately 4 weeks prior to the initiation of the program, use informational posters, brochures, or displays. Ask the wellness committee to help distribute materials. Also announce the program through existing company communications systems, such as paycheck stuffers, newsletters, memoranda, or bulletin boards. Commercial and community health/fitness programs should be advertised in local newspapers, and on television and radio.

One week prior to the start of the program, hold a preview. Ask all interested people to come dressed for exercise to participate in a demonstration of the program and to view slides, videos, or other materials describing the program. The preview provides interested participants an opportunity to meet the instructor, "taste" the program, talk to other participants, and ask questions. The demonstration should be exciting and informative and should include registration for the class. You can hold drawings for free gifts and/or a free program to encourage people to attend. The preview can be followed by refreshments to promote social interaction among the participants, the wellness committee, management, and health/fitness professionals.

Newsletters

Newsletters provide participants with information on just about every aspect of the health/fitness program. They announce special programs and events, recognize individual accomplishments, welcome new participants, disseminate education information and generate greater interest in the program.

If your organization already publishes a company newsletter, design a section of it to relate only to the health/fitness programs.

Record Keeping

Keep careful records to document the effectiveness of the program as evidenced by participants' improvement. Documentation of adherence allows the company to see the overall effectiveness of the program and produce a cost–benefit analysis as it relates to medical insurance cost, absenteeism, productivity, or employee turnover. Accurate program and individual participant records can serve as a continuous promotion within the company. Your records may also interest other companies in health/fitness programs. Finally, participants are motivated to come to class if you keep attendance records, and their achievements can be measured by good record keeping.

Personal Evaluation Questionnaires

Questionnaires can be used effectively to determine attitudinal and behavioral changes in participants. The questions assess relevant present behaviors, such as eating habits, exercise activity, addictions, or handling of stress. These *assessment appraisals* can be developed by the health/fitness professional or can be purchased from an outside company that administers the tests and evaluates the information gathered. You can then give participants personal confidential feedback about problems, goals, and lifestyle by feeding the questionnaire data into a computer program. Participants can receive tailormade dietary, nutritional, exercise, and lifestyle recommendations from the computer.

Fitness Testing

Submaximal fitness tests conducted at regular intervals allow you to track progress, provide participant incentive and motivation, and measure program progress. Fitness testing results can be logged into a computer for continued assessment of improvement. Previous chapters have described appropriate tests for each program.

Health/Fitness Counseling

There is no question that individual counseling in a health/fitness program can promote a higher degree of program adherence. The prime objective of any health/fitness program is to achieve a high level of participation at a reasonable cost. Fitness Systems has prepared a manual with suggestions on how to enhance program participation; they note that level of participation is directly related to the amount of personal attention offered and the convenience for the participants of the program.[9]

The ideal situation is a program conducted at the worksite that includes regular individual counseling for all program participants. Naturally, this individual attention by the health/fitness staff is an additional cost factor; many companies will not find it practical. Some provide employee assistance programs, which offer counseling for participants; others restrict this service to high-level executives or participants at a high risk; still others charge additional fees for individual exercise prescription and continued assessments.

The health/fitness leader always should be available before and after the class to counsel participants informally, exchange ideas, and answer questions. Whether counseling is formal or informal, individual or group, good communications occur when a person understands what the leader intended to convey. The basic attitude of the effective counselor is one of concern and compassion; he or she provides appropriate feedback, if it is solicited.

▌Followup Programs

Individuals who have taken the risk, paid the price, and reaped the benefits of regular participation in a health/fitness program that involves lifestyle change have indeed taken a giant step. They are well on the road to self-responsibility for an active and productive life. Learned behavioral changes produce lifestyle change. The successful participant is "hooked"; he or she usually will continue to practice good habits of health and fitness for life. However, you must provide followup programs for motivated individuals to help them sustain behavioral change and, perhaps more important, to collect data about what you can do to create exciting and stimulating programs to encourage new participants. Can you identify needs for interesting new programs? For example, could you help older employees plan for an active retirement and provide them with health/fitness programs? Are special programs needed for exercise class dropouts, the physically restricted, mothers to be, new mothers, or busy executives who often live in hotel rooms and travel in airplanes? Followup programs keep health/fitness program participants from regressing to old behaviors.

Summary   ▌

Corporations are looking for ways to reduce their health-care costs. Employers have always known that a healthy, well-adjusted employee tends to be a productive worker. The practice of prevention through quality health-promotion programs at the worksite thus is one way to increase employee productivity. However, just providing programs and encouraging participation will not guarantee the program's success.

In this chapter, we examined many factors that affect the participant's initial entry in and continued adherence to the program. In planning, implementing, and delivering health-promotion programs, the employer must consider several factors, including the characteristics of the employees that the program serves; the enthusiasm and professional skills of the program director and staff; the convenience, size, and environment of the program space; the financial and personnel resources that management is willing to provide; and the means the company has available to promote the program.

The biggest problem for health-promotion programs is participant dropout. We have provided some techniques to help you promote program adherence and thus discourage program failure. When participants enjoy the program, learn how to make changes, and achieve improvement, your program will succeed.

■ References

1. Employee fitness: Corporate philosophy for the 1980's. Health and fitness: The corporate view. Madison, WI: *Athletic Business* (formerly *Athletic Purchasing and Facilities*), July 1980, p. 3.

2. Dishman, R. K. Health psychology and exercise adherence. *Quest* 33:168, 1982.

3. Dishman, R. K. Biologic influence and exercise adherence. *Research Quarterly for Exercise and Sport* 52:143, 1981.

4. Dishman, R. K., et al. Self-motivation and adherence to habitual physical activity. *Journal of Applied Social Psychology* 10:129, 1980.

5. Danielson, R. R., and Danielson, K. F. Ongoing motivation in employee fitness programming. In *Employee fitness "the how to . . . ,"* Proceedings of the Ontario Employee Fitness Workshop. Seneca College, King City, Ontario: Ministry of Tourism and Recreation, March 1979, pp. 139–140.

6. Peters, T. J., and Waterman, R. H., Jr. *In search of excellence lessons from America's best-run companies.* New York: Harper & Row, 1982, pp. 83–84.

7. Villeneuve, K., et al. Employee fitness: A bottom line payoff. *Journal of Physical Education, Recreation, and Dance* 54:35, 1983.

8. Pollock, M. L., et al. Effects of a YMCA starter fitness program. *The Physician and Sportsmedicine* 10:98, 1982.

9. Corporate fitness programs: Trends and results. Los Angeles: Fitness Systems, 1980, p. 13.

THE MANAGEMENT ROLE

This chapter outlines a generic model of the organizational structure and management process used in implementing a health/fitness program. Examples of organizational structures are given for the corporate, community, and commercial settings, and then a model of the management process in a corporate setting is presented.

We will look primarily at the management of inhouse health/fitness programs. Externally delivered services designed around solid market surveys, business plans, and management principles also can serve as examples.

▌ Getting Started

Starting an internal health/fitness program in an organization has been described thoroughly by the American Heart Association's *Heart at Work* coordinator's guide[1] and the American Heart Association Texas Affiliate's guidelines for implementing employee fitness programs.[2] These guidelines can help any organization in the corporate, community, or commercial settings plan a wellness program. Getting started requires three major steps: (1) select appropriate leadership to coordinate the program; (2) develop a program to meet the needs and interests of employees and management; and (3) plan facilities or use existing resources to carry out the program.

Select a program coordinator, preferably a person within the organization who has a personal commitment to health and fitness. This person has the responsibility to coordinate all the available resources to implement the program.

An advisory group for the health/fitness program can help to develop the program in the beginning and to promote the program later. This group should consist of the health/fitness director, the project coordinator, and representatives from management, medical, personnel, union, safety, legal, communications, and nonexempt employee groups. Employee involvement fosters the feeling that the employees have some degree of ownership in the program.

If the company has no medical director, arrange medical guidance with local medical resources. Medical guidance lends credibility to the program and increases the chances that safe procedures will be used.

Next, conduct a survey of the specific needs and interests of the company and its employees. The sample needs assessment forms in Appendixes A and B may be modified to suit your organization. The participant survey should not ask questions that might increase employee expectations beyond the capability of the organization; it should ask for preferences on times, days, activities, and programs that the organization can offer. For example, if the organization

■ T A B L E 13.1 ■

Approximate Costs for Exercise Program Resources

$0–$10 Per Month Per Employee	$10–$50 Per Month Per Employee	> $50 Per Month Per Employee
Self-help exercise programs	Public school and college health/fitness programs	Private health/fitness facilities
Walk, jog, cycle routes	YMCA facilities and programs	Dance/exercise studios
Parks and recreation facilities	Hospital facilities and programs	Commercial health clubs
Public school and college facilities	Contract exercise instructors	Inhouse exercise programs
Community agency programs (social service/ health)		

Source: American Heart Association (AHA). *Heart at work:* Exercise program. Austin, TX: AHA. 1984, p. 6. Used by permission.

can offer programs only before or after work hours, do not ask whether people prefer noon meetings.

After you conduct the survey, plan the program relative to the costs involved and the resources needed to carry out the plan. Corporate costs range from nothing to more than $600 per participant per year.[1] Table 13.1 summarizes the available exercise program resources and their approximate monthly cost per employee. Some of the costs may involve only a one-time charge.

For a relatively low cost, you can provide awareness and self-help educational materials to encourage employees to start health/fitness programs on their own. Display posters in entrances and exits, lunchrooms, and break locations. Announce program information in newsletters, on bulletin boards, and in paycheck stuffers.

Self-help educational materials include health-hazard appraisals, which examine medical history, health habits, and lifestyle and recommend actions for reducing disease risk and improving personal health. Health/fitness self-tests, such as the *Canadian Home Fitness Test*,[3] evaluate resting heart rate, walk tests, ideal body weight, flexibility, and strength to

help individuals identify current health/fitness status and areas that need to be improved. Good self-help educational material outlines goals, such as written guidelines on starting an exercise program with regard to type of activity, frequency of participation, and the intensity and duration of effort. Information on monitoring progress and maintaining positive living habits also should be included.

You may want to promote employee participation in external health/fitness programs, such as those offered by your local department of parks and recreation.

Encourage employees to hold small group meetings at lunch and to go for walks or runs together. Recommend that people walk to and from work, around shopping centers, and on jogging paths.

A company wishing to utilize outside resources to deliver its health/fitness program should ask the following questions in judging the quality of the resource. *Staff:* Are staff members professionally trained in physical education, exercise science, health promotion, or medicine? Are staff members certified by a national organization such as the American College of Sports Medicine or any medical certifying body? Do staff members have consulting expertise and experience? Do staff members have experience at administering a health/fitness program? *Program:* What program components are offered? Will the program components offered meet the goals of the contracting organization? Are the program recommendations safe? Are they designed with an individual's safety in mind? What is the insurance coverage of the organization? Is it adequate in relationship to program and facility? *Facilities:* What specific facilities are offered? Will the facilities meet the program requirements? *References:* What present and previous clients has the outside resource serviced? Will the outside resource provide a list of all present and previous clients for a reference check? *Ownership:* Who owns the outside resource? How long has the current ownership been in place? What is the turnover rate in ownership and staff at the outside resource?

If you decide to implement an inhouse program, its ultimate success will depend on the selection of good staff. In any organizational structure, the manager sets the tone for the program's operation—the program takes on a "flavor" of the manager's style. We will examine the organizational structures of health/fitness staff in the corporate, community, and commercial settings.

▌ Organizational Structure

The organizational structures of health/fitness programs differ among the corporate, community, and commercial settings due to the obvious differences in their purposes.

Corporate Setting

Organizational strategies for corporate health/fitness programs were presented in Chapter 4. The health/fitness director usually reports to the personnel or medical department manager. In rare instances, the health/fitness director answers to the chief executive officer of the company.

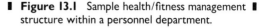

Figure 13.1 Sample health/fitness management structure within a personnel department.

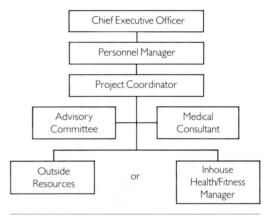

We recommend that you designate a project coordinator to be responsible for hiring the health/fitness director or contracting with outside resources to deliver the health/fitness program. The project coordinator usually is a member of the personnel or medical department. An example of a typical management structure within a corporate setting is illustrated in Figure 13.1.

Community Setting

As reviewed in Chapter 4, organizational structures in community health/fitness programs depend on the type of agency and the purpose of the service provided. For example, in a large YMCA that conducts both corporate and adult fitness programs, there may be two distinct departments with a director for each. These managers may work in equal line with a sports and recreation director. In a medium-size YMCA, one person may manage a combined health/fitness program and another a sports/recreation program. In a small YMCA that focuses primarily on family recreation, one person can manage both the health/fitness and the sports/recreation programs. The organizational relationships of different-sized YMCAs are illustrated in Figure 13.2.

■ **Figure 13.2** Sample YMCA organizational ■
structure for health/fitness programs.

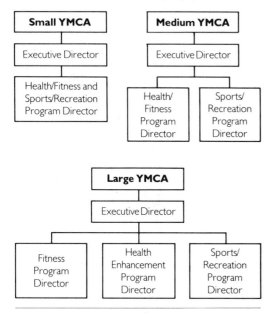

■ **Figure 13.3** Sample hospital organizational ■
structure for health/fitness programs.

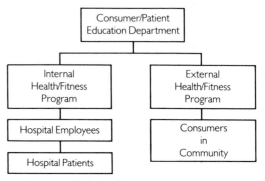

Hospitals can take several approaches to delivering health/fitness programs both to in-house hospital workers and to the outside community. In the past, health/fitness programs usually evolved from cardiac rehabilitation programs offered on an outpatient basis. The fitness components eventually were offered to hospital employees and to the community. In some hospitals, the health/fitness program now is under the administrative direction of the consumer/patient education department.[4] In others, it is placed under the personnel department's employee assistance program (EAP) or the recreation division. In some instances, it is directed by the physical therapy department.

An interesting trend facilitated by the American Hospital Association is to have health promotion services, including health/fitness programming, placed under the consumer/patient education department, with services delivered both internally to employees and patients of the hospital and externally to consumers in the community (Figure 13.3).

In a college or university that provides

health/fitness programs for individuals in the surrounding community, the health/fitness program may be offered through the continuing education department. In most cases, however, the program is organized within the department of health, physical education, recreation, and dance (Figure 13.4).

Commercial Setting

Comprehensive health/fitness programs are provided by private health care organizations, health spas, and health studios (Chapter 3). Usually, the medical, education, and activity directors all are responsible for delivering health/fitness programs to the community; they report directly to the chief executive officer (Figure 13.5).

In health spas and health studios, the promotion specialist, operations director, and activity director all share responsibility for the program (Figure 13.6). However, the burden of health/fitness delivery will probably be placed on the activity director, who is responsible for program development—that is, planning the types of activities to be offered. This individual usually has a background in health, physical education, or recreation.

The operations director is primarily responsible for the maintenance and safety of the facilities and equipment. The activity and operations directors should be familiar with each

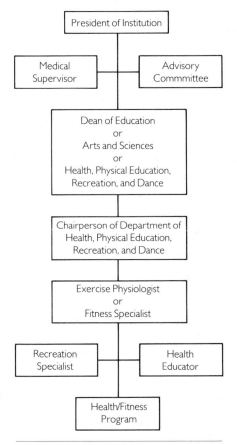

Figure 13.4 Sample organizational structure for health/fitness programs in the university setting.

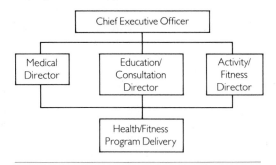

Figure 13.5 Sample private health-care facility organizational structure for health/fitness programs.

planning, implementation, and evaluation. Systematically following this process keeps the program organized and purposeful and ensures that the organization's mission is accomplished.

Needs Assessment

The first stage in the management process is needs assessment—defining where the organization is now and where it wants to be in the future.

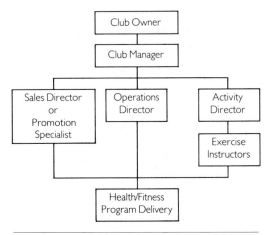

Figure 13.6 Sample health spa or club organizational structure for health/fitness programs.

other's responsibilities so they can cover for one another. The sales director or promotion specialist is in charge of selling memberships in the club by promoting its staff, programs, services, and facilities.

The Management Process

The major function of management is administrative planning and implementation of the organization's mission. The four-stage recyclable process includes needs assessment (input),

Figure 13.7 Sample needs assessment for low-back management.

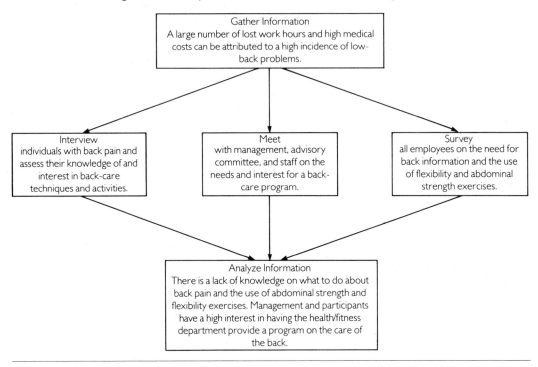

In the corporate setting, input data should be received from both target participants and management. You can obtain information by structured interviews, meetings, and surveys. Structured interviews involve talking to a representative sample of the target population to get opinions concerning the management and curricula of the health/fitness program. Hold meetings with management, the advisory committee, and the existing staff. Use surveys to solicit input from all employees. Appendix B is a sample survey form.

Analyze the data to define where the organization currently is concerning health/fitness and how the organization should implement the program. To illustrate how the input management process might operate, a low-back program needs assessment is shown in Figure 13.7.

In the community and commercial settings, needs assessment involves interviewing poten-

tial clients and conducting market surveys to assess the need for specific aspects of the health/fitness services. It also involves analyzing information from the organization's owner(s), manager(s), investor(s), or board of directors.

Planning

Planning involves taking the summary information from the needs assessment and defining program goals and objectives for both the organization and personnel. In the corporate setting, specific objectives should be placed in order of importance by answering several questions: Who is interested in the program? What goals are to be achieved? What are the community resources? What are the staffing needs? What are the inhouse capabilities? What are the program options? What are the anticipated

▮ Figure 13.8 Sample planning process for a ▮ low-back program in a corporate setting.

Define and Order the Objectives

1. Decrease lost work hours associated with low-back problems by 20% during next 12 months.
2. Decrease medical costs associated with low-back problems.

Define the Tasks

1. Test current flexibility and abdominal strength of employees.
2. Distribute educational material on low-back flexibility and abdominal strengthening exercises.
3. Conduct exercise classes emphasizing low-back flexibility and abdominal strength.
4. Test flexibility and abdominal strength after 6 and 12 months to detect changes.

obstacles? What is the estimated budget? What is the timing consideration? What are the long-term (3 years) goals? What will keep the participants involved in and excited about health/fitness?

Some general, easy-to-measure objectives might be: improvement in health/fitness levels of employees as measured by fitness tests; decreased heart disease risk as assessed by health hazard appraisals; decreased medical costs as determined by medical insurance claims; decreased absenteeism as documented by company sick leave records; and decreased turnover as represented by personnel records. Difficult-to-measure objectives are: improved morale; improved attitude; improved interpersonal relationships; improved ability to handle stress; and increased productivity.

After the objectives are put in order of priority, the tasks needed to carry out those objectives are defined. A *specific* example is presented in Figure 13.8.

The planning process in the community and commercial settings involves defining the target population for the health/fitness services, the specific types of programs to be delivered, and the cost for each health/fitness service. The timing of when certain aspects of the health/fitness services are to be provided and the personnel needed to deliver those services also are considered. The same tangible and intangible objectives defined in the corporate planning process are used by the community and commercial health/fitness services to explain the benefits companies can reap by purchasing their programs.

Implementation

Implementation of the health/fitness program in the corporate, community, and commercial settings involves five steps: (1) review the planned objectives for the program, (2) review the planned tasks for the staff, (3) delegate the tasks to the staff, (4) schedule the tasks for action, and (5) supervise the implementation of the programs to see that the tasks are accomplished. This model assumes that staff have already been hired in the organization and are available to implement the tasks assigned to them.

Implementation issues to address when delegating and scheduling tasks include: Who will develop and supervise the budget? Who will develop the time line for the implementation procedures? How and when will the participants be enrolled? How will the exercise and positive-living-habit programs be supervised? What facility resources will be used or developed? How and when will the participants be medically screened? How and when will other health/fitness assessments be administered? How and when will health, exercise, and other positive-living-habit information be presented? What educational strategies will be used in the program? What motivational techniques will be used? How will feedback be given to the participants? What special events will be conducted and when?

Figure 13.9 summarizes the implementation process for the low-back program.

■ **Figure 13.9** Sample implementation of the ■
low-back program in a corporate setting.

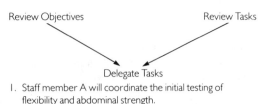

Review Objectives   Review Tasks

Delegate Tasks

1. Staff member A will coordinate the initial testing of
    flexibility and abdominal strength.
2. Staff member B will coordinate the distribution of
    educational materials.
3. Staff member C will conduct exercise classes emphasizing
    flexibility and abdominal strength.
4. Staff member A will coordinate testing of flexibility and
    abdominal strength after 6 and 12 months.

Schedule Tasks

1. Flexibility and abdominal strength testing will begin
    immediately.
2. Distribution of educational materials will begin immediately.
3. Exercise classes emphasizing flexibility and abdominal
    strength will begin immediately.
4. Flexibility and abdominal strength tests will be scheduled
    after 6 and 12 months.

Health/Fitness Manager Will Supervise
Implementation Of Program

Evaluation

Evaluation involves analyzing the implementation tasks that were assigned to the staff to see (1) if the tasks were accomplished and (2) if the objectives of the program were met. These two types of evaluation are called (1) *process evaluation* and (2) *outcome evaluation*; they can be used in all three settings.

Process evaluation assesses the techniques used during implementation of the program. Questions asked in process evaluation include: Was the operation of the program efficient? Were the assigned tasks reasonable? Was the time schedule reasonable? Were staff members prepared to carry out the tasks? Were staff members dependable and committed? Did staff

members have the proper resources to carry out the tasks? Did the staff members carry out the tasks? Was the budget adequate? Was the program fun? Was the program accessible? Was the program personalized?

Outcome evaluation assesses the effectiveness of the program. The questions asked in outcome evaluation include: How many participants received the program services? Did the program services meet the objectives set for the participants and organization alike? Was the program cost-effective (corporate setting)? Were the profits worth the effort (community and commercial settings)?

The process and outcome evaluations are then combined to see what effect the program had on the organization. If a health/fitness program has a positive effect on an organization, there should be positive changes in employees':

1. Behavior
    ■ activity levels increased
    ■ positive living habits adopted, such as blood pressure control, weight control, balanced nutrition, smoking abstinence, and substance-abuse elimination

2. Adherence
    ■ participation levels increased weekly
    ■ participation levels increased long-term

3. Health
    ■ individual health improved
    ■ coronary risks reduced
    ■ health care costs reduced

4. Fitness
    ■ fitness improved and maintained at good levels

5. Knowledge
    ■ health and fitness concepts understood

6. Attitudes
    ■ improved morale
    ■ improved self-confidence
    ■ positive attitude toward health/fitness

The procedure for the evaluation of the low-back corporate program is summarized in Figure 13.10.

■ **Figure 13.10** Sample evaluation process of the low-back program in a corporate ■ setting.

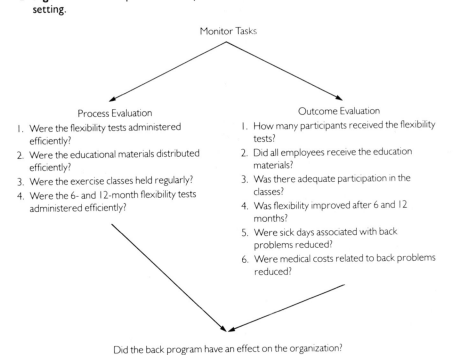

Monitor Tasks

Process Evaluation

1. Were the flexibility tests administered efficiently?
2. Were the educational materials distributed efficiently?
3. Were the exercise classes held regularly?
4. Were the 6- and 12-month flexibility tests administered efficiently?

Outcome Evaluation

1. How many participants received the flexibility tests?
2. Did all employees receive the education materials?
3. Was there adequate participation in the classes?
4. Was flexibility improved after 6 and 12 months?
5. Were sick days associated with back problems reduced?
6. Were medical costs related to back problems reduced?

Did the back program have an effect on the organization?

■ Summary

This chapter outlined generic models of the organizational structures and management processes of health/fitness programs within the corporate, community, and commercial settings. The major function of management is administrative planning and implementation of programs to meet the organization's objectives. The ultimate success of a health/fitness program depends on the selection of qualified, well-trained personnel to carry out the management process. Effective management involves a four-stage, recyclable process that includes needs assessment, planning, implementation, and evaluation.

References

1. American Heart Association (AHA). *Heart at work.* Dallas, TX: AHA, 1984.

2. American Heart Association (AHA), Texas Affiliate. *Employee fitness programs: Guidelines for implementation.* Austin, TX: AHA, 1983.

3. Recreation Canada (RC), Fitness and Amateur Sport Branch, National Health and Welfare. *Canadian home fitness test.* Ottawa, Ontario: RC, 1975.

4. American Hospital Association (AHoA). *Planning hospital health promotion services for business and industry: A decision-making and planning process for hospitals that are considering selling health promotion services.* Chicago: AHoA, 1982.

Corporate Needs Assessment Form

I. Participants

1. Total number of employees _____

2. Number of employees by job classification:
   Executive _____
   Middle-management _____
   Supervisory _____
   Labor _____
   Clerical _____

3. Number of employees by sex and age (in years) categories:

Women <30 _____	Men <30 _____
30–39 _____	30–39 _____
40–49 _____	40–49 _____
> 49 _____	> 49 _____

4. Three-year projection of employee turnover _____

II. Current activities in health/fitness program

1. Medical screening _____
   Number screened _____
   Cost _____

2. Fitness testing _____
   Number tested _____
   Cost _____

3. Activity programs _____
   Number active _____
   Cost _____

4. Health education _____
   Number contacted _____
   Cost _____

5. Special events _____
   Number involved _____
   Cost _____

6. Facilities _____
   Outside resources _____
   Cost _____

III. Identification of need

1. Total cost of medical claims _____

2. Medical costs by category:
   cardiovascular _____
   respiratory _____
   gastrointestinal _____
   back _____
   cancer _____
   accident _____
   other _____

3. Total sick days per year _____

4. Sick days by category:
   cardiovascular _____
   respiratory _____
   gastrointestinal _____
   back _____
   cancer _____
   accident _____
   other _____

A p p e n d i x ■ B

Participant Needs and Interest Survey

1. Rate your current level of general health.
   Poor _____   Good _____
   Fair _____   Excellent _____
   Average _____

2. Rate your current level of cardiovascular endurance.
   Poor _____   Good _____
   Fair _____   Excellent _____
   Average _____

3. Rate your current level of flexibility.
   Poor _____   Good _____
   Fair _____   Excellent _____
   Average _____

4. Rate your current level of strength.
   Poor _____   Good _____
   Fair _____   Excellent _____
   Average _____

5. How do you feel about your body weight and appearance?
   Poor _____   Good _____
   Fair _____   Excellent _____
   Average _____

6. What is your energy level after work?
   Poor _____   Good _____
   Fair _____   Excellent _____
   Average _____

7. Check the items you would like to improve.
   Your health _____
   Your fitness level _____
   Your weight/appearance _____
   Your energy level _____

8. Are you currently involved in any regular activity or program designed to improve or maintain your health?
   Yes _____   No _____
   If yes, describe _____
   _____
   _____
   Your goals? _____
   _____

9. Would you participate in a company-sponsored health/fitness program on a regular basis?
   Yes _____   No _____

10. If you answered *yes* to #9, check the activities that interest you the most and indicate the best time of day for you to participate.
    Walking _____
    Jogging _____
    Cycling _____
    Exercise classes _____
    Aerobic dance _____
    Weight training _____
    Racquetball _____
    Tennis _____
    Health-education seminars _____
    Other activities _____
    (please list)
    _____
    _____
    _____

(continued)

11. Would you participate in other aspects of the program such as: (if yes, indicate best time of day to offer)

Blood-pressure screening _____

Smoking cessation _____

Nutrition education _____

Weight-control classes _____

Stress management _____

Substance-abuse elimination _____

Back care _____

Cardiopulmonary resuscitation
classes _____

First aid _____

Other (please list)_____

_____

_____

_____

_____

12. Would you be willing to share the cost of health/fitness programs?
Yes _____ No _____
If yes, what would you be willing to pay?

13. To what extent should your family members be involved in the health/fitness programs? _____

14. Would you participate in medical screening tests if offered?
Yes _____ No _____

15. Would you be willing to share the cost of medical screening tests?
Yes _____ No _____
If yes, what would you be willing to pay? _____

16. What other suggestions do you have concerning a health/fitness program?_____

_____

_____

_____

MANAGEMENT ISSUES

This chapter will address the major issues confronting the manager of a health/fitness program. Some of these issues apply broadly to corporate, community, and commercial settings, but in most cases they apply specifically to an internal health/fitness program. Management issues in health/fitness programs may be classified into five categories:

1. General
   - Program philosophy
   - Management support
   - Participant support
   - Medical Support
2. Legal
   - Liability
   - Informed consent
   - Medical screening
   - Safety
3. Facility
   - Financing
   - Design
   - Equipment
   - Maintenance
4. Budget
   - Planning
   - Accounting
   - Evaluation

5. Office administration
   - Communications
   - Membership
   - Registration
   - Records

General Issues ■

The general management issues differ among the corporate, community, and commercial settings. In the corporate setting, the issues are internally solved with a blend of management and health/fitness goals. In the community and commercial settings, the delivery services must be flexible and molded to the goals of the contracting organization; the program must take on the management style of the organization.

In the corporate setting, the goals and philosophy of the company should be kept in mind at all times when planning the health/fitness program and when dealing with management issues and problems that arise. It is easier to get management's support for the health/fitness program when the company's goals are kept foremost. Health/fitness professionals should ensure that there is compatibility of philosophies between any organization with whom they contract and their companies.

Management's reason for starting a program may dictate the direction of the program. For example, if the major reason is health-care cost-containment, then the program impetus should be directed toward fast-return-on-investment programming such as hypertension screening. On the other hand, if employee productivity and satisfaction are major goals in the program's initiation, then programming that has long-term effects, such as exercise and nutrition, should be emphasized.

In the corporate setting, the health/fitness manager blends the program services into the company's mode of operation. For example, if a company has a strict 8-hour–workday policy with no extracurricular activities allowed, the manager must schedule the program before work, during lunch breaks, or after work. This makes it most convenient for the participants while following company policy. The staff uses other hours during the day for planning, record keeping, class preparation, facilities maintenance, and the many other duties required to keep the program running smoothly.

Health/fitness management issues are related to management issues in other departments within the company. For example, if communication with employees and staff morale are vital concerns with management in the operations department (and the company as a whole), then communications and morale also should be vital concerns in the health/fitness department. The health/fitness staff can make significant contributions to improving communication channels by bringing managers and employees together in the exercise setting. Some favorable business decisions are made in the locker rooms, where the participants communicate informally: bringing employees and management together in the exercise setting may help to improve morale by promoting informal communications. Thus, the health/fitness program may be used as a tool to address management issues in the entire company.

In the community and commercial settings, the management goals of the health/fitness delivery services are specifically molded to meet the goals of the organization buying the services. For example, if a company needs a smoking-cessation program because of numerous complaints from nonsmokers, then a health/fitness delivery service must plan to implement a program that will encourage the smokers to participate in the program without creating bad feelings among the employees, which might lower morale. The smoking-cessation program should be designed as a helpful resource rather than a vindictive tool to stamp out smoking in the company.

In some cases, the community and commercial agencies providing health/fitness services also must provide some management services to contracting organizations. For example, a company buying health-club memberships from a commercial enterprise expects the legal, facilities, budget, and office administration of the health/fitness program to be handled by the commercial club as part of the membership fee.

Well-organized, well-planned programs staffed by qualified health/fitness professionals will have few problems getting support from management, participants, and the medical community. Health/fitness staff can get good support from management by blending corporate goals with health/fitness goals, designing programs for the convenience of participants while observing company policies, and documenting results showing the cost–benefit ratio of the program.

Support from the employees will be enhanced by individualizing the program so that staff show personal and confidential concern for each participant. The program can be designed to involve the participant's family to reinforce the attitude of concern.

Support from the medical community can be obtained for the health/fitness program by consulting physicians, medical clinics, and hospital wellness programs. Communicating with the medical community demonstrates cooperation rather than competition. Health/fitness staff may need referral sources for participants with medical problems. Establishing good medical community relationships may speed up getting help for the participant, and this can create support for the program from both the participant and the medical community.

Health/fitness programs can exist harmoniously with traditional medical practice in the community by establishing a cross-referral system. A physician may refer a patient to a corporate, community, or commercial health/fitness program for a fitness evaluation, an exercise prescription, or implementation and monitoring of an exercise program. The fitness evaluation results and specifics of the exercise prescription and activity program can be relayed back to the personal physician for medical management. When participants with medical problems are identified in the health/fitness program and those people are referred to physicians for medical care, support for the health/fitness program from the medical community is enhanced.

Legal Issues

Each health/fitness program, whether in a corporate, community, or commercial setting, creates its own liabilities when the program is implemented. Those sponsoring health/fitness programs should neither ignore the possibility of legal problems nor be overly anxious about the potential injuries associated with exercise programs. Our society has a "sue syndrome," and injuries that occur in health/fitness programs are becoming part of the "injury industry."

The concern of legal liability includes not only the sponsoring organization of the health/fitness program but the professional staff as well. Legal liability can arise from acts of *omission*—failure to perform when performance could be reasonably expected—or *commission*—performance of an action in a negligent manner.[1] For example, if a staff member witnessed a participant collapse in an exercise area and then walked off, refusing to offer aid to the participant, this would be an act of omission negligence. Rendering first aid and administering emergency procedures are job responsibilities of health/fitness staff. If a staff member came upon a collapsed participant in the exercise area and grasped the arms of the victim to drag him or her from the area into another room without first ascertaining the cause of col-

lapse, this would be an act of commission negligence. Proper cardiopulmonary resuscitation, first aid, and emergency procedures should be followed. The victim may have head, neck, or spinal injuries, and dragging the person is not proper procedure in this case. Once a professional staff member accepts the responsibility for a health/fitness program participant, he or she also accepts the associated legal responsibility.

In general, negligence is defined as conduct that falls below the standard established by law for the protection of others against unreasonable risk of harm.[2] Negligence is failing to do something that a *prudent and reasonable person* would do or doing something that a prudent and reasonable person would not do. The mere existence of risk alone is not the basis of negligence liability. The law requires only that a person refrain from creating situations in which there is an *unreasonable* risk of injuring others. If a particular injury is unforeseeable or could not have been prevented by the exercise of reasonable care, it is an unavoidable accident, which is not considered actionable. There must be an unreasonable risk that has not been eliminated.[2] For example, a young man in an organized basketball league of the health/fitness program breaks an ankle bone during a game. Another participant landed on the foot of the victim, causing the latter to twist his ankle and break a bone. The health/fitness staff has made sure that the gym floor has been maintained free of dirt and dust, so the floor surface is safe—the accident has nothing to do with the floor. It was an unavoidable accident that someone happened to have landed on the player's foot.

The risk of having legal problems associated with the health/fitness program can be minimized by preparing carefully for the potential problems. Things you can do to reduce the chances of legal liability are shown in Figure 14.1.

The sponsoring organization should make sure that only qualified staff members are hired to deliver the health/fitness program. Ideally, the staff members should be certified by the American College of Sports Medicine[3] or any

■ **Figure 14.1** Tips for reducing legal problems. ■

1. Be aware of legal liabilities.
2. Select certified instructors to lead classes and supervise exercise on equipment.
3. Use good judgment in setting up programs and provide written guidelines for medical emergency procedures.
4. Inform participants about the risks and dangers of exercise and require written informed consent.
5. Require that participants obtain medical clearance before entering an exercise program.
6. Instruct staff not to "practice medicine" but instead to limit their advice to their own area of expertise.
7. Provide a safe environment by following building codes and a regular maintenance schedule for equipment.
8. Purchase adequate liability insurance for the staff.

other professionally associated body. Personnel should be mature, responsible individuals who are prudent in carrying out their duties and assignments. If you show lack of care by selecting unqualified personnel and if they then proximately cause participant injuries, two claims of negligence may be brought against the program—one for the direct negligence of the staff in causing the injuries and one for the negligence of the company in selecting an inadequately trained person.[1]

Written policies and guidelines, especially for emergency situations, should be established for the program. The procedures should be posted; they should be rehearsed and followed by all personnel. Examples of such program guidelines are available from the American College of Sports Medicine.[3]

Informed consent requires that you notify the participants of the risks and dangers of exercise as well as any medical or fitness tests given as part of the exercise program. You must ask if they have questions, answer any such questions, and make it clear they should ask any questions they have at any time during the program. Informed consent forms should be signed by the participants before they enter the program. Figure 14.2 is a sample consent form that you can adapt to your needs.

Consider requiring medical clearance and approval before you allow participation in the program. Medical clearance criteria based on age, disease, risk factors, and heredity factors help identify clients with high potential for health problems or injury in the program and minimize your liability by demonstrating that you exercised reasonable care.

The environment for the health/fitness program must be free from inherent dangers or defects, appropriate for the planned activity, and reasonably equipped for that activity. Environmental factors such as temperature and humidity should be monitored and controlled accurately in indoor facilities. In outdoor areas, warning flags or other devices should be used to inform participants of exact weather conditions.

Equipment must be in good working order, free from defects, and not inherently dangerous. Staff should test the equipment before it is used by the participants. Staff members can show that they are being responsible by inspecting and maintaining equipment and facilities on a regular basis and instructing participants in the proper use of the equipment. Accident report forms should be completed by staff as soon as possible after an accident/injury to document the circumstances and the first-aid/emergency procedures used. Figure 14.3 is a sample injury report form.

Misuse of the equipment by participants also can create legal problems. *Contributory negligence* refers to conduct by the injured party that falls below the standards necessary for his or her own protection. Contributory negligence may result from the injured party's having intentionally or unreasonably exposed him- or herself to the danger created by another person's negligence of which the injured party knew or had reason to know.[2] However, misuse of equipment also can be grounds for proving negligent liability if staff members have not provided adequate instruction.

The fact that injuries inevitably occur in an exercise program increases an organization's liability exposure; employees hurt in an inhouse

Figure 14.2 Sample informed consent for exercise form. (From American Heart Association (AHA). *Heart at work: Exercise program.* Austin, TX: AHA, 1984, p. 23. Used by permission.)

(This form should be submitted to legal counsel for review and modification to ensure that it conforms with the appropriate state and local laws governing consent.)

I desire to engage voluntarily in the _____ exercise program to attempt to improve my physical fitness.

I understand that these activities are designed to place a gradually increasing work load on my circulation and thereby attempt to improve its function. The reaction of the cardiovascular system to such activities cannot be predicted with complete accuracy. There is a risk of certain changes occurring during or following the exercise. These changes include abnormalities of blood pressure or heart rate, ineffective "heart function," and possibly, in some instances, a "heart attack" or "cardiac arrest."

I realize that it is necessary for me to report promptly to the exercise supervisor any signs or symptoms indicating any abnormality or distress. I consent to the administration of any immediate resuscitation measures deemed advisable by the exercise supervisor.

I have read the foregoing and I understand it. My questions have been answered to my satisfaction.

Participant signature _____

Date _____

Exercise Supervisor _____

program may be eligible for worker's compensation. Each state differs in the interpretation of its worker's compensation law; there are no general guidelines concerning how exercise injuries may be related to worker's compensation. If an organization has a strong commitment to health/fitness and encourages employees to exercise at an onsite facility, employees' exercise injuries may be subject to worker's compensation. However, if participation in a health/fitness program is considered an extracurricular event, the injury may fall outside of worker's compensation coverage.

Just how much and what type of insurance an organization should provide depends on the approach of the health/fitness program. Protection is much better in a supervised fitness program with well-qualified staff. Protection is less favorable in an unsupervised recreation program in which the injury risk is high, e.g., in sports activities such as softball and basketball. The determination of liability is related to whether management financed or supported the recreational activity, permitted the activity to take place on company property or during

work hours, derived any benefit from the activities, or made participation compulsory.[4] Some employers take steps to limit liability by imposing special rules on activities. For example, Corning Glass Works outlawed sliding, base-stealing, and spiked shoes in employee softball games and hired registered officials to control flag-football contests.[4]

We recommend that you become familiar with the legal issues associated with health/fitness programs; a list of selected references is presented in the Appendix.

Facility Issues

Facility considerations depend on whether the organization wishes to use outside resources to deliver a health/fitness program or develop its own facility. Information for judging the quality of outside resources and facilities was presented in Chapter 13. This section discusses facility considerations for inhouse programs, although some of the principles apply to judging the quality of outside resources. For example, both

■ Figure 14.3   Sample injury report form. ■

Name _____ Sex _____ Date _____

Time _____ Facility location _____

1. Suspected cause of injury
   _____ Blunt trauma   _____ Hyperextension
   _____ External object   _____ Hyperflexion
   _____ Fall   _____ Rotation (twist)
   _____ Heat stress   _____ Other (specify) _____

2. Site of injury
   _____ Abdomen   _____ Face   _____ Nose
   _____ Ankle(s)   _____ Finger(s)   _____ Pelvis
   _____ Arm(s)   _____ Foot   _____ Shoulder(s)
   _____ Back   _____ Forearm(s)   _____ Side(s)
   _____ Calf   _____ Hand(s)   _____ Thigh(s)
   _____ Chest   _____ Head   _____ Toe(s)
   _____ Ear(s)   _____ Knee(s)   _____ Wrist(s)
   _____ Elbow(s)   _____ Mouth   _____ Other (specify)
   _____ Eye(s)   _____ Neck   _____

3. Signs and symptoms
   _____ Abrasion   _____ Dislocation   _____ Pain
   _____ Bleeding   _____ Fracture   _____ Shock
   _____ Burn   _____ Hearing problem   _____ Sprain
   _____ Chest pain   _____ Heart involvement _____ Strain
   _____ Contusion   _____ Laceration   _____ Swelling
   _____ Convulsion   _____ Lung problem   _____ Visual problem
   _____ Crushed   _____ Nausea   _____ Vomiting
   _____ Discoloration   _____ Numbness
   _____ Other (specify) _____

4. Procedures used
   _____ Bandage   _____ Elevation
   _____ Bleeding control   _____ Ice
   _____ Compression   _____ Immobilization
   _____ CPR   _____ Oxygen
   _____ Dressing   _____ Other (specify) _____

5. Vital signs
   _____ Blood pressure   _____ Mental state
   _____ Heart rate   _____ Response to pain
   _____ Breathing rate   _____ Skin condition
   _____ Pulse strength   _____ Speech
   _____ Pupils   _____ Other (specify) _____

Signed _____

Date _____

inhouse and outside facilities should provide areas for the essentials of health/fitness programs, which are cardiorespiratory fitness, ideal body composition, flexibility, and strength testing.

Both outside and inside resources have their advantages and disadvantages. An organization should plan carefully the strategy of delivering the health/fitness program, utilizing the advantages and reducing or eliminating the disadvantages. One of the most important advantages an outside or inhouse resource might have is its convenience to the participants. Convenience of the program increases participation—it saves time for both the participant and the company.

A particular advantage of using an outside resource is to eliminate the costs of an onsite building and its maintenance. A program can be started at virtually no cost by simply recommending that participants consider using what already exists in the community.

If an organization decides to develop an inhouse health/fitness program and use an existing facility or construct a special area for exercise, the health/fitness director should meet with the architect to plan efficient use of the space. The provision of inhouse facilities demonstrates to participants that the organization is serious about and has a long-term commitment to the program. This increases participation. The health/fitness staff also may be more effective when implementing the program in facilities designed specifically for that purpose.

The first requirement for an inhouse facility is to provide separate shower and dressing areas for men and women. This involves minimal expenditure but goes a long way in making a program convenient. These facilities allow participants to dress for and clean up after exercise performed at the organization's facilities or at nearby community resources such as parks, jogging trails, tennis courts, and swimming pools.

Consider using a large room such as a cafeteria for group or individual exercise, such as calisthenic classes, aerobic dance programs, stationary cycling, and rope jumping. Or you can go a step further and construct and equip a specially designed room for the exercise program. This room could contain stationary bicycles, treadmills, rowing machines, and weight-training equipment; the organization should provide qualified staff to instruct the participants on the proper and safe use of the equipment.

You may wish to implement a more comprehensive program by providing an outdoor or indoor jogging track, a multipurpose gymnasium, courts for racquetball and tennis, and a swimming pool. Amenities for relaxation, such as steam baths, saunas, and whirlpools, may be added. Table 14.1 recommends which inhouse facilities and equipment you should consider on the basis of program size.

O'Donnell and Ainsworth provide excellent information on the configuration, size, and cost of inhouse facilities.[5] They emphasize that facilities should be configured to save participants time. Participants should travel the least amount of distance to get to the facility, change clothes in the locker rooms, warmup, exercise, cooldown, undress in the locker rooms, shower, dress, and leave.

The traffic flow in a facility should be organized to permit fast access to an exercise area without the participants stumbling over each other. Mesa Petroleum has an excellent traffic flow design. Figure 14.4 illustrates the facility plan, which allows easy access from the main hallway to the locker rooms, exercise room, racquetball courts, gymnasium, and juice bar area.

O'Donnell and Ainsworth also provide guidelines on the amount of space required for an exercise area based on the number of participants. For example, they estimate that each participant requires 60 square feet for circuit exercise. An exercise center with 600 members who attend an average of 3 days per week has 23 participants using the exercise circuits at any given time during peak hours: 1380 square feet are required for the exercise circuit area (60 square feet per participant × 23 participants = 1380 square feet). Space allocations for other areas of the health/fitness facility are presented in Table 14.2.

▌ T A B L E 1 4 . 1 ▌
Selection of Inhouse Facilities Based on Program Size

Facility	Program Size (based on number of participants)		
	Small (50 or less)	Medium (50–1000)	Large (1000 or more)
Community resources	+	+	+
Exercise area (e.g., cafeteria)	−	+	+
Shower and dressing areas	−	+	+
Exercise room with equipment	−	+	+
Outdoor track	−	+	+
Indoor track	−	−	+
Gymnasium	−	−	+
Courts	−	−	+
Swimming pool	−	−	+

Source: American Heart Association (AHA). Guidelines for exercise programs in the workplace. Austin, TX: AHA, 1984. Used by permission.
+ : recommended; −: not recommended.

Mechanical requirements of an inhouse facility include a plumbing system for the showers, sinks, lavatories, and laundry, and heating, ventilation, and air conditioning units. You may need special electrical systems for the gymnasium, testing room, exercise equipment, steam and sauna rooms, whirlpool areas, laundry room, and the heating, ventilation, and air conditioning units. Give special consideration to controlling heat and humidity in the locker rooms and exercise rooms. Showers, saunas, whirlpools, perspiration, heavy breathing, and traffic increase heat and humidity, especially if the rooms are small or confined. Heavy-duty, accurate ventilation equipment is required to keep the temperature and humidity at the recommended levels of 70°F and 40% for exercise facilities. Higher temperatures and humidities are uncomfortable and unsafe for vigorous exercise. In addition, use stainless steel and tile in wet areas to reduce maintenance problems, facilitate cleaning procedures, and ensure a safe, clean environment for the participants.

Ceilings in exercise areas should be more than 8 feet high if possible. This gives participants a feeling of open space and is psychologically more desirable. It also provides vertical space for special activities such as rope or mini-trampoline jumping. Sports courts, gymnasiums, and swimming pools require special high ceilings.

Heavy equipment such as weight-training machines should be located on the ground floor. If this is not possible, weight-bearing

▌ T A B L E 1 4 . 2 ▌
Space Allocations for an Inhouse Health/Fitness Center

Use	Percentage of Total Facility Space
Administrative	2–3
Circulation	3–9
Classrooms	3–5
Exercise circuits	35–45
Laundry	1–3
Lavatories	4–6
Locker rooms	20–25
Showers and drying	7–11
Storage	1–3
Warmup and cooldown	10–13

Source: O'Donnell, M. P., and Ainsworth, T. *Health promotion in the workplace.* New York: John Wiley & Sons, 1984, p. 599. Used by permission.

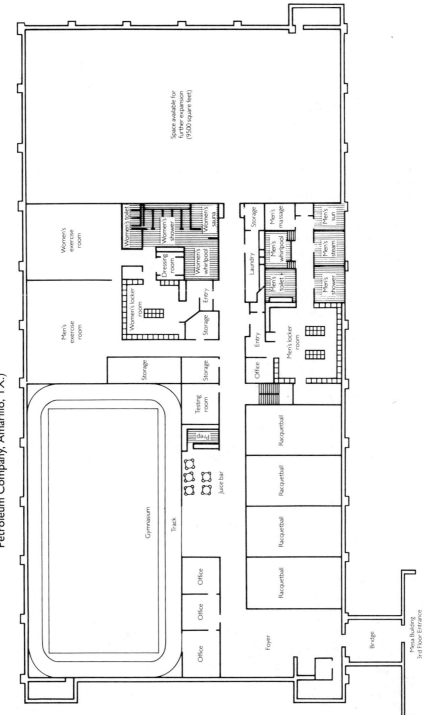

■ **Figure 14.4** Floor plan of T. B. Pickens, Jr. fitness center, Mesa Petroleum Company. *Scale:* 1 inch = 40 feet. (Reprinted with permission from the Mesa Petroleum Company, Amarillo, TX.)

Space available for further expansion (9500 square feet)

Women's exercise room

Women's toilet
Women's shower
Women's sauna
Women's whirlpool
Dressing room
Women's locker room

Men's exercise room

Storage
Men's massage
Men's whirlpool
Men's sun
Men's toilet
Men's steam
Men's shower

Laundry

Storage

Entry

Storage

Office
Entry
Men's locker room

Storage

Testing room

Prep

Racquetball

Racquetball

Racquetball

Racquetball

Juice bar

Gymnasium

Track

Office

Office

Office

Foyer

Bridge

Mesa Building
3rd Floor Entrance

tolerances greater than 100 pounds per square foot are required for exercise areas located on floors above ground level.

The cost of a facility depends on the options selected for the program. For example, a general-purpose room 50 feet by 50 feet can be cleaned, painted, lighted, and carpeted for approximately $5 to $10 per square foot: $12,500 to $25,000 for the 2500-square-foot area. Modification of existing space to provide showers, locker rooms, and special exercise areas may cost between $20 and $30 per square foot. If space allocated for these facilities totals 5000 square feet, then it will cost $100,000 to $150,000. Construction of a special building housing a health/fitness center may cost more than $50 per square foot. A fully developed facility with an exercise room, gymnasium, indoor track, swimming pool, nourishment center, members' lounge, two locker rooms, four racquetball courts, and four administrative offices may require 30,000 square feet and cost more than $1.5 million.

Equipment costs depend on the health/fitness program objectives and the facility selection. Cost ranges for typical equipment used in various areas of the health/fitness facility are listed in Table 14.3.

Good maintenance and custodial personnel can ensure a clean, safe environment for the program. As mentioned previously, regular maintenance schedules should be designed to keep all equipment operating correctly. Daily custodial services are mandatory to keep the health/fitness facility clean and attractive.

▌ Budget Issues

The health/fitness manager has responsibility for the budget. The financial management methods used in small business can be applied to budgeting the health/fitness program. In the corporate setting, the program director is primarily responsible for planning and allocating funds to the various program areas. In the community and commercial settings, the health/fitness manager is primarily responsible for the generation of revenues and cash management.

Budgeting for the health/fitness program involves the projection of how much money will be spent during a 1-year period and the allocation of the money among the various program components. Planning and controlling a budget are important for proving the cost-effectiveness of the program, demonstrating the importance of various program components, showing high-quality results, and evaluating the overall financial health of the organization.

The budget often is used as a decision-making guide throughout the year, determining which program components are emphasized. Some components may have financial allocations far above actual expenditures; other components may need more financial support to ensure their success. The budget should be flexible so that needed funds can be transferred.

Planning a budget involves estimating increases or decreases in the cost of operating existing programs and the initial cost of developing new programs. All costs should be included when planning the budget. The nonannual, noncash costs—sometimes the greatest expenditures in a program—are often overlooked; they include facility design, construction, and rental space. Design and construction costs can be amortized over 20 or 30 years.

In the corporate setting, the full costs of a health/fitness program should be clearly stated; they can be major expenditures within an organization. It may be difficult to justify the full costs of a health/fitness program because many of the benefits are intangible, such as morale, employer–employee relationships, self-confidence, or productivity. However, it is important to know the full costs of a program to understand its role and significance within the organization.

After the projected costs are reviewed by management, certain items probably will be negotiated. A program director should be well prepared to defend or compromise on each area of the budget with management. Corporate management often is reluctant to spend

▌ T A B L E 1 4 . 3 ▌
Approximate Costs for Equipment

Area	Cost Per Item (in dollars)	Area	Cost Per Item (in dollars)
Exercise room		Defibrillator	5000–7000
Weight machine		Spirometer	2000–10,000
Single station	500–3000	Pulsemeter	50–200
Multistation	3000–9000	Electrocardiograph	6000–20,000
Free-weight sets	300–900	Treadmill	3000–12,000
Stationary bicycle	250–3000	Bicycle ergometer	600–3000
Motorized treadmills	3000–12,000	Stepping bench	100–300
Minitrampolines	100–300	Laundry room	
Clock	50–200	Commercial washer	3500–5000
Gymnasium/indoor track		Commercial dryer	1000–2000
Pace clock	200–600	Folding table	100–500
Basketball backboard	200–1000	Juice bar	
Basketball	40–90	Refrigerator	700–1200
Volleyball net and holders	400–1000	Dishwasher	500–900
Volleyball	40–90	Trash compactor	400–800
Jumprope	1–5	Frozen-yogurt machine	1000–2000
Exercise mat (small)	20–100	Classroom	
Exercise mat (large)	300–600	Slide projector	300–500
Locker room		Movie projector	1000–2000
Locker (full size)	50–100	Screen	50–100
Locker (kit size)	20–40	Stand	100–200
Bench	100–200	Videotape system	2000–5000
Bath towel	3–6	Sound system	1000–2000
Hand towel	2–3	Chair	50–200
Washcloth	1–2	Table	100–400
Hair dryer	15–50	Podium	100–200
Testing room		Chalkboard	80–200
Stethoscope	10–50	Office	
Stopwatch	20–100	Desk	500–1000
Sphygmomanometer	200–1500	Chair	100–500
Skinfold calipers	200–500	File cabinet	150–800
Weight scale	200–400	Bookshelf	200–800
Metronome	30–80		

large amounts on staff salaries or upgrading of equipment because they generally are unfamiliar with the specific requirements of a health/fitness program. Most of the costs of a program involve the initial development, such as facility design, space rental, and program development. Staff salaries may represent a large percentage of the annual costs, but they probably will be a small percentage of the total budget when initial development of the program is considered: typically, staff salaries will be approximately 20% to 30% of the annual budget.

The program director has an important responsibility to act as a source of information to management, present the health/fitness program budget in a positive manner, and use the budget to analyze and improve the operation of the program. After negotiations are completed and the budget is approved, the planning stage is concluded.

■ T A B L E 1 4 . 4 ■
Sample Health/Fitness Program Line-Item Budget—1985

Item	1985 Projected Costs ($)	1984 Costs ($)	1983 Costs ($)
Staff salaries and fringe			
Director	50,000	45,450	41,318
Exercise specialists	30,000	27,273	24,794
Secretaries/clerical	27,000	24,545	22,314
Facilities			
Rent	200,000	200,000	200,000
Amortization construction	23,333	23,333	23,333
Utilities	30,000	27,900	25,947
Maintenance	30,000	28,500	27,075
Equipment			
New purchases	10,000	9,091	8,265
Amortization purchases	3,333	3,000	2,727
Maintenance	2,000	1,860	1,730
Supplies			
Testing	8,000	7,440	6,919
Educational	2,500	2,325	2,162
Exercise/sports	5,000	4,750	4,513
Office	2,500	2,325	2,162
Miscellaneous			
Special events	5,000	4,850	4,753
Publications and dues	2,000	1,960	1,901
Printing	4,500	4,320	4,234
Travel	3,000	2,940	2,852
Program promotion	1,000	950	931

The next stage involves monitoring the budget throughout the year. Actual expenditures are compared with the initial projections. Monthly or quarterly monitoring usually is adequate for health/fitness programs in the corporate setting, but programs in the community and commercial settings probably will want to monitor the budget daily or weekly because they are vitally concerned with cash flow and profit margins.

Deviations from projections signal potential problems; when they occur, the program director should reevaluate the budget and make appropriate changes. Close monitoring also can reveal positive aspects of the budget, such as savings being made in certain program areas.

Formats of budgets vary widely. The budget format in the corporate setting is designed more as a planning and monitoring budget of program areas, whereas that in the community and commercial settings is more a controlling budget over cash flow. Three types of format are outlined by O'Donnell and Ainsworth: line-item, functional-area, and impact-area.[5] Line-item budgets are the easiest to compile. Each item of expenditure is listed on one line of the budget and items are grouped into categories. An example of a line-item budget is presented in Table 14.4.

A functional-area budget organizes the items into functional areas of the program. For example, the line-item budget in Table 14.4 may be organized into a functional-area budget as illustrated in Table 14.5.

▌ T A B L E   1 4 . 5 ▐
Sample Health/Fitness Program Functional-Area Budget—1985

Item	1985 Projected Costs ($)	1984 Costs ($)	1983 Costs ($)
Program promotion			
Staff time	11,888	10,807	9,825
Materials	6,500	6,280	6,135
Advertising	5,000	4,850	4,753
Public relations	11,888	10,807	9,825
Other	1,000	950	931
Program management			
Staff supervision	11,888	10,807	9,825
Staff training	14,888	13,747	12,677
Financial management	11,888	10,807	9,825
Program planning	11,888	10,807	9,825
Facilities and equipment			
Rental	200,000	200,000	200,000
Amortization	26,666	26,333	26,060
Maintenance	32,000	30,360	28,805
Supplies	5,000	4,750	4,513
Services			
Testing	19,888	18,247	16,744
Classes	16,888	15,457	14,150
Counseling	11,888	10,807	9,825

An impact-area budget categorizes the expenditures into program components, as illustrated in Table 14.6. This type of budget can give an indication of the effectiveness of each component in the program in the use of its available resources.

All three formats can be combined into one system (Table 14.7). The funds allocated for the functional-area and impact-area budgets are estimated by the percentage of time/effort expended in each area.

In addition to budgeting for program delivery using the three formats, the health/fitness manager in the community and commercial settings must keep careful income records for proper analysis of the operation. The ultimate objective is to make a profit; only through careful budget analysis can this objective be met. It is not possible to conduct even the simplest of operations without proper record-keeping pro-

cedures. Record keeping is a mandatory operation for: (1) meeting legal requirements, such as filing income taxes, (2) safeguarding assets, such as assessing profits/losses, and (3) planning and controlling operations, such as marketing programs.[6]

A manager can use a simple accounting form, such as a checkbook, or a more complex balance sheet to record financial information. Regardless of the type of accounting method, the health/fitness manager is responsible for:[6]

▋ *Liquidity*: Forecast of the cash inflow and outflow is called a *cash budget*. The income must be kept higher than the expenses to make sure enough cash is on hand to pay the bills. Adequate records of disbursements must be kept to predict accurately the cash budget.

▋ *Profits:* Enough income must be generated to pay for the investment over a period of

T A B L E   1 4 . 6

Sample Health/Fitness Program Impact-Area Budget—1985

Item	1985 Projected Costs ($)	1984 Costs ($)	1983 Costs ($)
Evaluation			
Medical examinations	14,916	8,105	7,368
Fitness tests	4,972	2,702	2,457
Prescription			
Exercise	10,166	9,267	8,450
Nutrition	7,319	6,672	6,084
Weight control	7,319	6,672	6,084
Blood pressure	6,100	5,560	5,070
Smoking cessation	4,066	3,707	3,380
Stress management	3,660	3,336	3,042
Substance-abuse elimination	2,033	1,853	1,690
Followup Counseling	11,888	10,807	9,825
Education and Communication			
Newsletter	3,500	3,326	3,189
Materials	3,125	2,970	2,847
Audiovisual	2,750	2,613	2,505
Advertising	1,250	1,188	1,139
Public relations	1,250	1,188	1,139
Other	625	594	569
Motivation			
Special events	2,500	2,425	2,376
Awards	2,500	2,425	2,376
Documentation			
Computer	1,000	930	865

years. The objective is to maximize income and the return on the investment without endangering the liquidity of the organization. To accomplish these objectives, bookkeeping procedures are needed to prepare reports on: (1) daily cash income; (2) daily cash expenses; (3) weekly, monthly, and annual income and expense records; (4) profit/loss statements; (5) tax records; (6) mortgage and debt records; (7) payroll records; (8) balance sheet; (9) inventory records; and (10) financial statements.

The income and expenses of the profit-making health/fitness organization must be recorded daily. Normally, these items are posted in a general ledger journal. A profit/loss statement can then be prepared weekly, monthly, quarterly, and yearly to show the amount of

cash reserve. A sample profit/loss statement is provided in Table 14.8.

Record keeping is of little value unless the results are analyzed in light of the organization's objectives. Careful budgeting will enhance the success of the program. Keep accurate records. Assemble a line-item budget. Compare expenditures with projections. Look for trends in income/expenses. Relate budget to program objectives. Finally, know where you are going.

Office Administration Issues

Clerical details, maintenance, and custodial services of a health/fitness program often are overlooked by those involved in the planning

■ T A B L E   1 4 . 7 ■
Sample Health/Fitness Program Multiformat Budget

Line Items	Expenditures		
	Total Costs ($)	Functional Areas ($)	Impact Areas ($)
Staff salaries and fringe			
Director	50,000	25,000	25,000
Exercise specialist	30,000	15,000	15,000
Secretaries/clerical	27,000	20,250	6,750
Facilities			
Rent	200,000	200,000	0
Amortization construction	23,333	23,333	0
Utilities	30,000	30,000	0
Maintenance	30,000	30,000	0
Equipment			
New purchases	10,000	5,000	5,000
Amortization purchases	3,333	1,667	1,666
Maintenance	2,000	1,000	1,000
Supplies			
Testing	8,000	4,000	4,000
Educational	2,500	1,250	1,250
Exercise/sports	5,000	2,500	2,500
Office	2,500	2,500	0
Miscellaneous			
Special events	5,000	2,500	2,500
Publications and dues	2,000	1,000	1,000
Printing	4,500	2,250	2,250
Travel	3,000	3,000	0
Program promotion	1,000	500	500

process. It can be a costly oversight to assume that these office administration details will take care of themselves. Attention to efficient office-administration procedures cannot be overemphasized.

We have emphasized the importance of obtaining professionally qualified staff to lead the health/fitness program. It is also important to have excellent secretarial, clerical, maintenance, and custodial support to help make the program run smoothly.

Communications are vital to the operation of a well-run health/fitness program. The first line of communications between participants and the program staff often is handled by the secretary/receptionist in the department. This person should have excellent "people skills"; that is, he or she should be friendly, courteous, and adept at receiving people personally, receiving telephone calls, making appointments, and registering members and guests. The secretary/receptionist should have excellent typing and word-processing skills. Several software programs are available to help the secretary efficiently handle word processing, membership registration forms, membership lists, address files, accounts receivable/payable, and other business administrative procedures.

The secretary/receptionist should be able to keep accurate files. A well-organized filing system is needed to supplement any computer records kept on participants. Items that might

▮ T A B L E 1 4 . 8 ▮
Profit/Loss Statement—1985

Area	Dollar Amount
Income	
Club memberships	500,000
Wellness-program	
contracts	2,500
Consulting	1,000
Total income	503,500
Expenses	
Salaries and fringe	300,000
Utilities	50,000
Maintenance	9,000
Supplies	35,000
Advertising	10,000
Depreciation and	
amortization	3,500
Total expenses	407,500
Gross profit	96,000
Income taxes	20,000
Net profit	76,000

be kept in the files include registration or membership contracts, signed informed consent forms, medical clearance forms, fitness test results, medical examination results, exercise records, and correspondence.

The computer/filing system also can be used to maintain a current registration/membership list for the entire program. Financial records also can be maintained. Keep good records of the various program components with regard to dates and times scheduled, number of participants registered in each component, evaluation reports, and so on.

Summary ▮

This chapter described the major issues facing the manager of a health/fitness program. We suggested how to address the management issues of: program philosophy; management, participant, and medical support; legal liability; facility planning; budget planning, accounting, and evaluation; and office administration. The points we covered pertain to the inhouse corporate health/fitness program, but many of the suggestions could be used in the community and commercial settings.

References ▮

1. Herbert, D. L., and Herbert, W. G. *Legal aspects of preventive and rehabilitative exercise programs*. Canton, Ohio: Professional and Executive Reports and Publications, 1984.

2. Lowell, C. H. Legal responsibilities and sports medicine. *Physician and Sportsmedicine*, 60, 1977.

3. American College of Sports Medicine. *Guidelines for graded exercise testing and exercise prescription*, 2d ed. Philadelphia: Lea & Febiger, 1980.

4. Bureau of National Affairs. Charting worker's compensation shoals. *Bulletin to Management* 1665:1, 1982.

5. O'Donnell, M. P., and Ainsworth, T. *Health promotion in the workplace*. New York: John Wiley & Sons, 1984.

6. Epperson, A. F. *Private and commercial recreation: A text and reference*. New York: John Wiley & Sons, 1977.

A p p e n d i x

Selected References: Legal Aspects
of Exercise Testing and Prescription

- American College of Sports Medicine. *Guidelines for graded exercise testing and exercise prescription*, 2d ed. Philadelphia: Lea & Febiger, 1980.

- American Heart Association (AHA), Committee on Exercise. *Exercise testing and training of apparently healthy individuals: A handbook for physicians*. Dallas, TX: AHA, 1972.

- American Heart Association (AHA), Committee on Exercise. *Exercise testing and training of individuals with heart disease or at risk for its development: A handbook for physicians*. Dallas, TX: AHA, 1975.

- American Heart Association (AHA). *The exercise standards book*. Dallas, TX: AHA, 1980.

- Bacorn, R. W. Legal aspects of exercise stress testing and exercise prescription. In *Progress in cardiac rehabilitation: Medical aspects of exercise testing and training*, Zohman, L., and Phillips, R. E. (eds). New York: Intercontinental Book, 1973.

- Bureau of National Affairs. Charting worker's compensation shoals. *Bulletin to Management* 1665:1, 1982.

- Cooper, D. H., and Willig, S. H. Nonphysicians for coronary care delivery: Are they legal? *American Journal of Cardiology* 28:363, 1971.

- Dobrzensky, S. H. Legal aspects of exercise programs. In *Exercise and the heart: Guidelines for exercise programs*, Morse, R. L., et al. (eds). Springfield, IL: Charles C. Thomas, 1972.

- Epperson, A. F. *Private and commercial recreation: A text and reference*. New York: John Wiley & Sons, 1977.

- Haskell, W. L., et al. Law and cardiac rehabilitation. In *Exercise testing and exercise training in coronary heart disease*. Naughton, J., and Hellerstein, H. K. (eds). New York: Academic Press, 1973.

- Herbert, D. L. Legal considerations in cardiac rehabilitation and fitness programs. In *Exercise specialist workshop*. Blacksburg, VA: American College of Sports Medicine, August, 1982.

- Herbert, W., and Herbert, D. Exercise testing in adults: Legal and procedural considerations for the physical educator and exercise specialist. *Journal of Health, Physical Education, Recreation and Dance* 46:17–18, 1973.

- Herbert, D. L., and Herbert, W. G. *Legal aspects of preventive and rehabilitative exercise programs*. Canton, Ohio: Professional and Executive Reports and Publications, 1984.

- Ladimer, I. Professional liability in exercise testing for cardiac performance. *American Journal of Cardiology* 30:753, 1972.

- Lowell, C. H. Legal responsibilities and sports medicine. *Physician and Sportsmedicine* July, 1977.

- McNiece, H. F. The legal basis for awards in cardiac cases. *N.Y. State Journal of Medicine* 61:906, 1961.

- McNiece, H. F. Legal aspects of exercise testing. *N.Y. State Journal of Medicine* 72:1822, 1972.

■ O'Donnell, M. P., and Ainsworth, T. *Health promotion in the workplace.* New York: John Wiley & Sons, 1984.

■ Parr, R., and Kerr, J. *Liability and insurance in adult fitness and cardiac rehabilitation.* Baltimore: University Park Press, 1975.

■ Rochmis, P., and Blackburn, H. Exercise tests: A survey of procedures, safety and litigation experience in approximately 170,000 tests. *Journal of the American Medical Association* 217:1061, 1971.

■ Sagall, E. L. Legal implications of cardiac rehabilitation programs. In *Heart disease and rehabilitation.* Boston: Houghton-Mifflin, 1979.

■ Sagall, E. L., and Gumatay, R. R. Exercise testing, exercise training, and the law. In *Exercise and the heart,* Wenger, N. K. (ed). Philadelphia: F. A. Davis, 1978.

■ Van der Smissen, B. Legal aspects of adult fitness programs. *Journal of Health, Physical Education, Recreation and Dance* 45:55, 1974.

■ Wilson, P. K., et al. *Policies and procedures of a cardiac rehabilitation program: Immediate to long-term care.* Philadelphia: Lea & Febiger, 1978.

■ Wilson, P. K., et al. *Cardiac rehabilitation, adult fitness and exercise testing.* Philadelphia: Lea & Febiger, 1981.

Source: Herbert, D. L. Legal considerations in cardiac rehabilitation and fitness programs. In *Exercise Specialist Workshop.* Blacksburg, VA: American College of Sports Medicine, August 1982. Used by permission.

STAFFING CONSIDERATIONS

The three primary roles of the health/fitness professional are to motivate individuals, facilitate lifestyle changes, and manage and plan programs.

Effective management processes were discussed in Chapter 13. This chapter delineates more specifically the leadership skills needed for effective motivation and counseling of health/fitness participants. First, we will describe position qualifications and descriptions, as well as the selection, training, supervision, and evaluation procedures used for health/fitness staff. We then supply resource information on where health/fitness professional leadership can be found. The information on leadership skills in this chapter pertains to all three settings—corporate, community, and commercial.

Leadership is the key to a successful program. Jacobs observes that, despite agreement on the importance of leadership, the lack of a qualified leader frequently is the cause of an unsuccessful program.[1] Too often, organizations consider first which facilities and equipment they will purchase and then which staff they will hire to oversee the program. This can be a costly mistake; many organizations, wondering why employees are not using the expensive facilities and equipment provided for them, have learned this the hard way.

Staffing Needs

Most health/fitness programs in the corporate setting have a small number (one to five) of professional staff.[2] Nonetheless, program directors must coordinate many people involved with the program, such as student interns, consultants, subcontractors, participant volunteers, and members of the program advisory committee. Management of staff, consultants, and volunteers is different from management of program participants.

The number of health/fitness staff in community and commercial settings varies with the purpose of the service. For example, a large hospital wellness program may have more than ten staff members; a small commercial health club may have fewer than five.

In all settings, the staff may be either health-promotion or fitness/activity specialists, or a combination of both. Health-promotion specialists demonstrate competencies in needs assessment, planning, implementation, and evaluation of participants in areas such as medical evaluation, diet, nutrition, substance-abuse control, smoking cessation, safety, and stress management. They may be physicians, psychologists, health educators, nutritionists, or nurses. These are well-defined, familiar positions; the fitness/activity specialists are less well known. Some of the following descriptions of fitness/activity positions have been adapted from the American College of Sports Medicine.[3]

Program director: one who can demonstrate the competencies of the exercise specialist and exercise-test technologist plus demonstrate the knowledge and skills associated with administering preventive and rehabilitative exercise programs, educating the program staff and community, and designing and conducting research. Management skills should include supervision of health, physical fitness, and recreation programs within the business and industry settings. See also Figure 15.1.

Exercise specialist: one who can apply the knowledge and skills associated with exercise prescription and can lead exercise for individuals without medical limitations.

Exercise-test technologist: one who can demonstrate competencies in graded exercise testing, including knowledge of functional anatomy, exercise physiology, pathophysiology, electrocardiography, and psychology in order to perform such tasks as preparing the exercise-test station, screening participants, administering tests, recording data, interpreting data, and communicating test results to appropriate professionals.

Recreation specialist: one who can demonstrate competencies in recreation leadership skills associated with planning, supervising, and administering a fitness program.

The Conference Placement Center of the Association for Fitness in Business indicates that program directors typically possess a master's degree in exercise science or related fields and have a minimum of 3 years experience in the field. Corporate home offices tend to hire health/fitness professionals as program directors, whereas production-oriented workplaces tend to hire recreation specialists.

The health/fitness director in a highly organized program has competencies in management and skills in administering the following program components: health education, exercise, nutrition, weight control, blood-pressure control, smoking cessation, stress management, and substance-abuse elimination. Supporting staff should have abilities to implement these program components under the guidance of the director. The health/fitness staff collectively should know how to document procedures for evaluating the program.

The program director may be a health educator assisted by exercise specialists who can administer fitness tests and exercise programs; or the program director may be an exercise specialist assisted by health educators and health-promotion specialists such as nutritionists and psychologists.

❚ Figure 15.1 Characteristics of health/fitness program directors. (From **❚** Breuleux, C. E. *A profile of corporate fitness directors.* Ph.D. dissertation. Columbus, OH: Ohio State University, 1982. Used by permission.)

Age:	33 years average
	23–60 range
Sex:	62% male
	38% female
Education:	97% bachelor's degree
	53% master's degree
	16% doctorate
Specialization:	37% physical education
	18% exercise physiology
	10% health & physical education
	35% other (recreation, business administration, marketing, education, psychology, athletic training, public health, nursing, physical therapy, and sociology)

Some organizations employ as program directors recreation specialists who organize game activities such as bowling, softball, and golf for the participants. Although these activities may have some benefits, they do not always meet health/fitness needs. The field of recreation usually differs from that of the behavioral-change–based health/fitness field.

All health/fitness personnel should be trained and certified in cardiopulmonary resuscitation (CPR) and first aid. This is a vital safety feature in all programs, necessary to ensure the health and safety of participants.

▌ Selection Procedures

As the field of health/fitness continues to grow, the need for qualified personnel increases. The selection procedures used to find qualified health/fitness professionals include: (1) defining the needs of the program, (2) identifying the staff qualifications required to meet those needs, (3) reviewing personnel credentials for those qualifications, and (4) interviewing the most-qualified applicants.

Upper-level health/fitness personnel, such as program directors, usually are found by external, formal procedures, that is, by contact with placement services, national associations, and health/fitness professional consultants. Entry level staff, such as exercise instructors, are found using internal, local, informal procedures such as contacting local schools, universities, and YMCAs.

Hire professional staff with qualifications to deliver the components your program offers. The course areas in Figure 15.2 were recommended for relevant preparation by more than 50% of the corporate fitness directors in one survey. Only a few individuals currently in the health/fitness field have completed all the courses; those who have are extremely well qualified.

Many individuals who have had the traditional preparation programs in health, physical education, and recreation are not well prepared

▌ **Figure 15.2**   Course areas recommended for health/fitness staff. (From Breuleux, C. E. ▌ *A profile of corporate fitness directors.* Ph.D. dissertation. Columbus, OH: Ohio State University, 1982. Used by permission.)

Accounting
Adult fitness
Athletic facilities and management
Athletic training
Behavior modification
Cardiac rehabilitation
Cardiopulmonary resuscitation
Current health concepts
Exercise leadership
Exercise physiology
Financial management
First aid emergency care
Guidance and counseling
Health behavior
Health counseling
Health tests and measurements
High-level wellness
Holistic health
Human anatomy
Human motivation

Human movement theory
Human relations
Industrial and commercial recreation
Internship in fitness
Kinesiology
Leadership in recreation
Lifetime sports skills
Marketing management
Organization and administration of physical education
Organizational behavior
Personal health
Personnel management
Physical education
Psychological and social aspects of physical education
Psychology of the adult
Public relations
Research methods
Sport psychology
Stress testing

for the current health/fitness field. Breuleux suggests that curricula designed along the lines of the coursework listed in Figure 15.2 are needed to prepare health/fitness professionals adequately.[4] He also points out that there are competent individuals working in the health/fitness field despite the lack of quality education programs. Those who excel in corporate fitness positions seem to have inherent skills in communication, human relations, and organizational politics.

Employers reviewing personnel credentials and preparing to interview candidates for a health/fitness position should look for these characteristics:[5]

■ Positive image of good health and fitness—is a nonsmoker with less-than-average body fat, moderate eating habits, and high physical activity

■ Physically fit—scores better than average on fitness tests

■ Creative, enthusiastic, and adaptable in delivering programs—has a positive attitude with the ability to motivate people and be flexible in changing programs, if needed, for success

■ Dependable and trustworthy—is able to maintain confidentiality and follow through on commitments

■ Desires professional growth—is active in professional organizations, publication, and research

Health/fitness leaders should be both inspired and inspiring. They should be healthy and fit, and concerned about matters vital to human health. They should be well-rounded and have a good sense of humor.[1] They should understand and have the skills to undertake all the management processes and issues described in Chapters 13 and 14.

The selection of health/fitness professionals requires examination of the person's experience in the field—how long he or she has been implementing leadership skills. Contacting personal references helps to prevent later staff training problems.

The American College of Sports Medicine (ACSM) has established progressive certification levels for professionals in presentation and rehabilitation programs. The four certification classifications are fitness instructor, exercise-test technologist, exercise specialist, and exercise program director. To receive certification, individuals must demonstrate skills in techniques of health appraisal and risk-factor identification, administration and interpretation of graded exercise tests, exercise prescription and leadership, motivation, program administration, staff and community education, and research. Most graduate degree programs are designed to prepare students to meet the certification criteria.

The YMCA certifies its own health/fitness professionals. The categories fitness specialist and advanced fitness specialist have criteria similar to those of the ACSM.

A directory of universities providing graduate degree programs in industrial fitness, adult fitness, disease prevention, and cardiac rehabilitation can be obtained by contacting the National Office of the American College of Sports Medicine, P.O. Box 1440, Indianapolis, Indiana 46206.

Training Procedures ■

Regardless of how good the selection process is, some training of staff is needed to impleme the program according to the organization philosophy. Training includes orientation and continuing development in job skills, attitude, personal growth, and supervisory skills.

Orientation introduces new staff to the work environment, other staff members, facilities, programs, and participants; new employees also need to learn policies and procedures, job responsibilities, and staff reporting relationships. Orientation often is considered to be a probationary period.

Unlike orientation training, continuing development training need not have a formal structure. The latter can include: attendance at training courses, professional conferences, and continuing education classes; involvement in professional associations and committees; and assignments as understudies to experienced professionals. Continuing development involves communication. There are five attributes of effective communication.[6] Communication systems should be *informal*; encourage regular, casual meetings where staff members may share ideas. Communication intensity should be extraordinary; encourage decision making by peers—that is, create an open, confrontation-oriented management style that lets people go after issues bluntly, straightforwardly. Give communication physical supports; provide chalkboards, tables, rooms, and other facilities and equipment for the convenience of staff communication. Use forcing devices; encourage staff to experiment with new ideas—do not be afraid to be innovative. Finally, this intense, informal communication system should be tightly controlled; have people check informally to see how things are going.

Treat *people* as the primary source of the program's success. Extraordinary results can be achieved through ordinary people. Peters and Waterman emphasize this: "We are not talking about mollycoddling. We are talking about tough-minded respect for the individual and the willingness to train him, to set reasonable and clear expectations for him, and to grant him practical autonomy to step out and contribute directly to his job."[6]

their work, completing work on time, meeting deadlines for reports, and following safety procedures.

Motivation requires constant communication with staff so that they know what to do. Staff should have: (1) an understanding of tasks to be completed, (2) a match of abilities with responsibilities, (3) guidance from their supervisor, (4) professional growth opportunities, (5) personal rewards from working with participants, (6) incentives tied to performance, (7) feedback regarding performance, (8) participation in determining operating plans, and (9) competition with self and co-workers.[7] Most staff members are motivated by intrinsic rewards—that is, the self-satisfaction that comes from being recognized for a job well done. Reinforce good performance immediately with quick praise. Blanchard and Johnson suggest three techniques for successful supervision: (1) *1-minute goal setting*—have regular staff meetings and write down simple and short goals, review these goals often, and review and analyze accomplishments, problems, and strategies to solve problems; (2) *1-minute praising*—praise staff immediately for doing things right, be consistent; (3) *1-minute reprimand*—first confirm the facts, state the reprimand firmly, attack the mistake, not the person.[8]

∎ Supervision Procedures

A supervisor is responsible for hiring staff, developing their potential, delegating tasks, monitoring tasks to make sure they are completed, directing and coordinating staff responsibilities, motivating staff to perform and improve, and evaluating staff performance and making recommendations. Communication with other staff members is extremely important. Student interns, part-time staff, and volunteers need more supervision than do full-time professionals.

Good supervision involves constant evaluation of the program's activities. A supervisor should observe the staff to make sure they are doing their work, being responsible in

Evaluation Techniques ∎

The purpose of evaluating staff is to improve their performance and thus improve the program. After reviewing staff performance, the supervisor decides to (1) make no change, (2) change job design, (3) change variables affecting job performance, or (4) change the person's position (promote, demote, transfer, discharge). The process of evaluation should be positive and objective. Speak with staff, listen to their concerns, write them memoranda and notes and read theirs. Hold conferences to train staff in communication skills and practice face-to-face communicating.

Hold personal, confidential interviews with staff members for performance evaluations.

▌ **Figure 15.3** Areas that should be covered in ▐
staff performance evaluations.

Job knowledge, training, and experience
Willingness to accept responsibility
Planning and organization of work
Quality and quantity of work
Cost consciousness and control
Relationships with others
Leadership qualities
Initiative and resourcefulness
Originality and creativeness
Soundness of judgment
Dependability
Personal appearance, speech, habits
Attendance and punctuality
Support for organization goals and policies
Career objectives

Discuss areas of strength and weakness and suggest strategies for correcting problems and improving performance. Items discussed in the performance evaluation are listed in Figure 15.3.

Staff members should be rewarded for success. Various forms of reward are: salary increase, benefits, privileges, free time, ownership/membership, responsibility, recognition, title change, and learning opportunities.

▌ Using Resources

There are several staff resources available to a health/fitness program at low cost. They include student interns, part-time consultants, subcontractors, and participant volunteers. Most students in the health/fitness field are required to perform an internship during their bachelor's or master's degree program. Student interns usually are available at low-to-moderate compensation for part-time or full-time work.

Consultants and subcontractors may be available to provide certain aspects of the health/fitness program, such as health-hazard appraisal, medical testing, fitness testing, exercise-class leadership, or seminars and workshops. The use of outside consultants and subcontractors may reduce the need for a permanent, large, and diverse health/fitness staff. Use

of consultants and subcontractors also can reduce inhouse staff load and free more time for staff to plan and prepare for other aspects of the program, or to devote more time to individual counseling of participants. Participant counseling is one of the most important aspects of a health/fitness program; it is also one of the most time consuming and costly. Because it usually is private and confidential, it is not a visible part of the program.

Participant volunteers may be used to help plan, market, and budget the program; to recruit, encourage, and motivate other participants; to assist with special events, such as tournaments, leagues, fun runs, and seminars; and to help document and analyze program results by providing statistical or computer expertise. Participant volunteers represent a wealth of talent from which the program director can draw. Volunteers may be located by word of mouth or inhouse newsletters and bulletins.

Sources for locating paid staff, student interns, consultants, and subcontractors include: colleges and universities, professional associations, professional conferences, professional publications, word-of-mouth referral, newspapers, and telephone books. An extensive list of program consultants is available from the journal of *Corporate Fitness and Recreation*.[9] The following professional organizations also can help you locate health/fitness staff: the Association for Fitness in Business, 1312 Washington Boulevard, Stamford, CT 06902, (203) 359-2188; the American College of Sports Medicine, 1 Virginia Avenue, P.O. Box 1440, Indianapolis, IN 46206, (317) 637-9200; and the American Alliance for Health, Physical Education, Recreation and Dance, 1900 Association Drive, Reston, VA 22091, (703) 476-3400.

Summary   ▌

This chapter described the staffing considerations in a health/fitness program and the leadership skills needed for effective motivation of program participants. Leadership is the most important factor in a program's success.

Health-promotion specialists such as physicians, psychologists, health educators, nutritionists, and nurses provide competencies mainly in the program components of medical evaluation, diet, nutrition, substance-abuse control, smoking cessation, safety, and stress management. Fitness/activity specialists, such as fitness program directors, exercise specialists, exercise-test technologists, and recreation specialists, provide fitness testing, exercise and other positive living habit prescription, exercise leadership, counseling, education and motivation of participants, and documentation of program results. The qualifications for health/fitness positions were presented with information on selecting, training, supervising, and evaluating staff members.

To find qualified health/fitness professionals, (1) define the needs of the program, (2) identify the staff qualifications required to meet those needs, (3) review personnel credentials for those qualifications, and (4) interview the most-qualified applicants. Orientation and continuing development training are used to introduce new staff members to the health/fitness program and further their professional development. Emphasize treating people with respect and providing opportunities for staff to grow professionally.

Supervision procedures include hiring staff, developing their potential, delegating tasks, monitoring tasks to make sure they are completed, directing and coordinating staff responsibilities, motivating staff to perform and improve, and evaluating staff performance and making recommendations. Supervisors should have personal and confidential interviews with staff members to discuss performance evaluations. Discuss areas of strength and weakness and suggest strategies for correcting problems and improving performance.

The chapter concluded with information on inside and outside staff resources available to help conduct health/fitness programs. Inside resources may be found in participant volunteers and members of the program's advisory committee. Outside resources include student interns, consultants, and subcontractors.

References

1. Jacobs, D. T. *Getting your executives fit.* Mountain View, CA: Anderson World, 1981.

2. *Survey of corporate fitness and recreation programs.* Mt. Kisco, NY: Fitness Systems, 1983.

3. American College of Sports Medicine. *Guidelines for graded exercise testing and exercise prescription.* Philadelphia: Lea & Febiger, 1980.

4. Breuleux, C. E. A profile of corporate fitness directors. Ph.D. dissertation. Columbus, OH: Ohio State University, 1982.

5. Institute for Aerobics Research. *Workshops and certificate of proficiency in the management of exercise and fitness programs.* Dallas, TX: Division of Continuing Education, The Aerobics Center, 1981.

6. Peters, T. J., and Waterman, R. H., Jr. *In search of excellence.* New York: Warner Books, 1982.

7. O'Donnell, M. P., and Ainsworth, T. *Health promotion in the workplace.* New York: John Wiley & Sons, 1984.

8. Blanchard, K., and Johnson, S. *The one minute manager.* New York: Berkley Books, 1982.

9. Spector, H., and Waldman, M. H. (eds). 1984 buyer's guide. *Corporate Fitness and Recreation* 3:31, 1984.

FACILITY DESIGN

The topics of facility design and equipment selection were introduced in Chapter 14. This appendix provides a detailed presentation of typical facility designs in the corporate, commercial, community, and clinical settings. Each setting has special design features necessitated by the clientele and program objectives.

The corporate setting, which focuses on programming for adults only, generally has excellent facility and equipment provisions. These conditions are equally true of commercial settings such as exclusive health clubs. Although the clientele is similar, program objectives, particularly profit motivation, require differences in facility design.

Urban community facilities share some features of the corporate and commercial settings. However, suburban community programs such as Ys and community recreation facilities are larger in scope to accommodate families.

Clinical programs include either a wellness program, which mimics the corporate-type design, or a special-population program, such as cardiac or drug rehabilitation.

In determining the typical design for each setting, the following guidelines were considered.

Traffic

- Traffic flow proceeds from one entrance to the control area to the lockers to the exercise area.
- The control area faces the entrance and provides for user screening, personal contact with all entrants, secondary supervision of programming, documentation of adherence via members logging in and out, and towel and/or uniform services.
- Certain exits are for use in an emergency only; normal exits are through a single entrance area.

Administration

- Central offices are close to the control areas and have visual access to most areas.
- The testing area is adjacent to the administrator's office.
- Laundry facilities are close to the locker rooms and exits.
- The warm-up and cool-down areas are good spaces for stretching and should be centralized in the exercise area (coed); they also serve to separate the strength and cardiovascular areas well.

Resistive exercise area

- Beginners and children's areas do not have free weights.
- A variety of strength-development equipment (e.g., rack-mounted weights and hydraulic and cam-loaded machines) are available.
- The free weights are separated from the other strength areas.
- Built-in circuits are established through proper placement of resistive and cardiovascular exercise equipment.
- Mirrored walls are standard features.

Miscellaneous

- The indoor track is as large as the facility perimeter allows, has a banked turn and composition surface, and attempts to provide good scenery.

- The aerobics or gym area is a multipurpose area with a wood floor surface on suspension, if possible, that allows 60 square feet per class member. A good sound system with acoustical separation from other areas is a must.

- The aquatics area has separate ventilation systems and is separated from other areas for sound and humidity control.

- The storage area is decentralized and adjacent to areas that require equipment storage.

- For high-density space utilization allow 5 square feet per active participant; for moderate-density space utilization allow 10 square feet per active participant; and for optimal-density space utilization allow 15 square feet per participant.

Features of the Corporate Setting

- The facility is designed exclusively for health/fitness and does not include areas for court games or recreational activities.

- An educational area includes a kitchen/staff lounge that can be used for nutrition, stress management, weight-control, and other behavioral classes.

- The locker rooms are equally divided into men's and women's areas. The men's and women's showers are individualized. Separate wet areas (steam, sauna, whirlpool) are provided for privacy. A separate mini-fitness center for private workouts is recommended, particularly for special population groups such as pregnant women and the obese.

- Areas inside the track area are designated for aerobics activity and strength equipment.

■ Corporate facility. ■

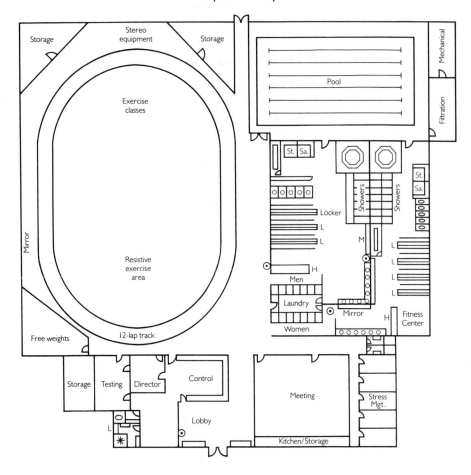

0 10 20 30 40 50 feet

Features of the Community Setting

▌ The facility is designed for a variety of ages, interests, and programs, primarily family oriented.

▌ Profit-making areas such as a snack bar, nursery, or recreation room are designed for expanded services.

▌ Multipurpose gym areas are designated for recreation and fitness activities. Court games are located close to the control area for supervision. Multiple gyms accommo-date the various populations (e.g., adults and children). Weight areas are kept separate to avoid injury and intimidation. The elevated track affords an overview of the exercise area.

▌ Locker rooms are separated by age and sex: boys, men, girls, and women each have separate locker areas. Women's showers are individualized; men's are ganged. Separate mini-fitness centers are provided for special-interest groups. Whirlpools are provided in each area.

Community facility.

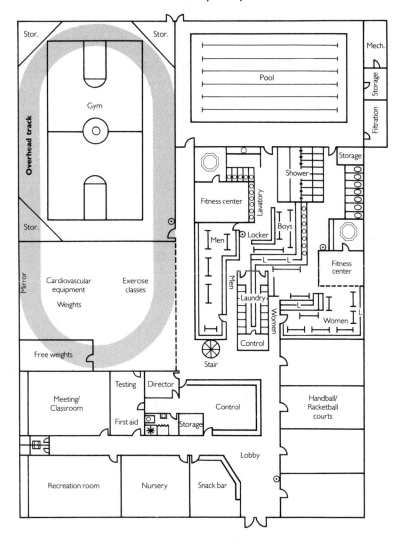

| 0 | 10 | 20 | 30 | 40 | 50 feet |

Features of the Commercial Setting

▪ The commercial facility is designed primarily for profit.

▪ Profit-making areas such as a nursery and snack bar and areas for meetings, testing, and court games are available for expanded services.

▪ The gym includes a separate strength area for team activities.

▪ Areas for court games are essential as a draw for membership.

▪ A large rooftop track accommodates many individuals and permits expanded membership numbers.

▪ Locker areas have complete wet areas (e.g., Jacuzzi, steam, sauna).

▪ A variety of equipment and services are essential to provide broad market appeal.

▌ Commercial facility. ▌

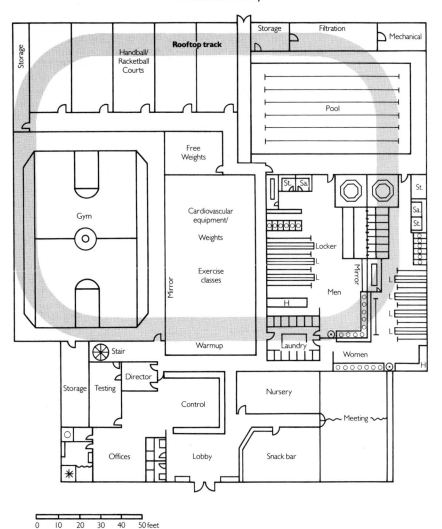

Storage

Handball/
Racketball
Courts

Rooftop track

Storage Filtration Mechanical

Pool

Free
Weights

Gym

Cardiovascular
equipment/

Weights

Exercise
classes

St. Sa.

St.

Sa.

St.

Locker

L

L

Mirror

L

Mirror

Men

L

L

H

L

L

Warmup

Laundry

Women

H

Stair

Director

Testing

Storage

Nursery

Control

Meeting

Offices

Lobby

Snack bar

0 10 20 30 40 50 feet

Features of the Clinical Setting (Cardiac Rehabilitation)

▌ The facility is designed for both inpatients and outpatients (Phases I–III, with emphasis on a Phase III outpatient program).

▌ Multipurpose rooms such as a kitchen/staff lounge, which works as a nutrition education setting and a meeting/classroom area for patient education programs, are available.

▌ Locker rooms are needed for outpatient participants. The men's area is larger because of the greater number of male participants. Wet areas are not included because of the potential dangers.

▌ The administration area is central. It is accessible to the control area, in view of the exercise area, and adjacent to the testing area.

▌ The exercise area includes cardiovascular and stretching areas only. The indoor track is in full view of the supervisor. The exercise areas can be small due to space use: inpatients during the workday and outpatients before and after the workday.

■ Clinical facility. ■

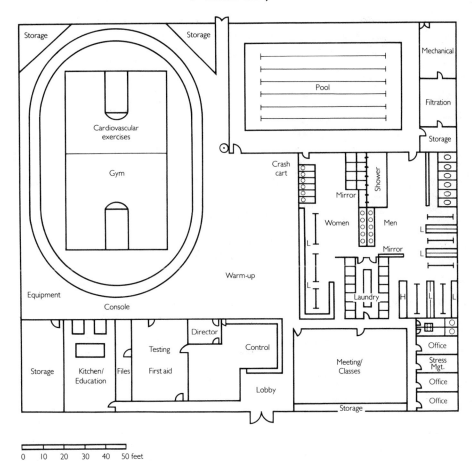

Space Allocations in Health/Fitness Settings (square feet/% of total)*

Area	Corporate	Community	Commercial	Cardiac/Pulmonary; Clinical
Administration (testing, control, offices)	2109–5%	1659/4%	3095/8%	1758/5%
Exercise circuits	18,050/49%	16,806/43%	16,419/42%	18,688/49%
Warm up/Cool down	4050/11%	3450/9%	3895/10%	4895/13%
Multipurpose rooms	2461/7%	2475/6%	1375/4%	3403/9%
Locker rooms	6466/18%	7087/18%	6450/17%	4950/13%
Storage	963/3%	858/2%	1027/3%	1631/4%
Laundry	422/1%	450/1%	422/1%	675/2%
Nursery	—	900/2%	774/2%	—
Snack bar	—	675/2%	844/2%	—
Circulation	2350/6%	4061/13%	4458/11%	1800/5%
Total sq. ft.	36,871	38,421	38,729	37,800

*Similar total square footages were adopted for ease of comparison of space use.

Program Components and Activities in Health/Fitness Settings

Activities	Corporate	Community	Commercial	Cardiac/Pulmonary; Clinical
Jogging	■	■	■	■
Swimming	■	■	■	■
CV equipment	■	■	■	■
Exercise classes	■	■	■	■
Testing	■	■	■	■
Weight training	■	■	■	*
Wellness classes	■	■		■
Wet area	■	■	■	
Team sports	■	■	■	■ (III)
Stress management	■			■
Nursery	■	■	■	
Snack bar		■	■	
RB/HB/Squash courts		■	■	
Recreation activities		■		

*Some cardiac rehabilitation programs are now beginning low-resistance weight-training classes.

Membership Options in Health/Fitness Facilities

Type of Membership	Corporate*	Community	Commercial	Cardiac/Pulmonary; Clinical †
Individual	■	■	■	■
Separate fees for men and women		■	■	
Family		■		■ (III)
Individual and spouse	(■)	■	■	■ (III)
Junior < 26 years	(■)	■	■	
Children's		■		
Student		■	■	
Corporate		■	■	
RB/HB only		■	■	
Lower summer rates	(■)	■	■	
Pool only		■	■	
Fitness (testing, CV, weights)		■	■	
Allows visitors	(■)	■	■	■ (III)

*Corporate membership options depend on the philosophy of the management and whether or not the program is free to the employee.

† Spouse, family, and visitor memberships apply only to those cardiac-rehabilitation participants in Phase III of rehabilitation.

Hours of Operation at Health/Fitness Facilities

	Corporate	Community	Commercial	Cardiac/Pulmonary; Clinical
Mon.–Fri.	6a–7p (65)	6a–10p (80)	6a–10p (80)	6a–7p (65)
Sat.	—	8a–10p (14)	8a–10p (14)	9a–5p (8)
Sun.	—	9a–6p (9)	9a–6p (9)	—
Total hours per week	65	103	103	73

Peak Hours*

	Corporate	Community	Commercial	Cardiac/Pulmonary; Clinical
Mon.–Fri.	6–8a, 11–1p, 5–7p	6–8a, 5–7p	6–8a, 5–7p	6–8a, 10–12n, 5–7p
Sat.	—	10a–6p	10a–6p	1–5p
Sun.	—	12n–6p	12n–6p	—

*Peak hours determination: Commercial/community program peak hours in a typical suburb, residential, noncorporate location will be before and after work and on weekend afternoons. Corporate program peak hours will be before work, during lunch, and after work if it is an on-site program; it is closed on weekends. Clinical–cardiac/pulmonary program peak hours depend on the stages involved. Stages I and II peak hours are 10 a.m. to 12 noon because the participants have not returned to work yet. Stage III peak hours are before and after work hours, comparable to other adult programs.

BUYER'S GUIDES

Buyer's guides, which are very useful to health/fitness profession-als, provide information on commercially available equipment and materials. Two of the more popular guides are presented here.

▌ Athletic Business
1842 Hoffman Street
Suite 201
Madison, WI 53704
(608) 249-0186

Annual Buyer's Guide, 1985 edition, 199 pp.
Topics: Athletic Equipment

Conditioning, Training, and Testing equipment

Transportation and Travel Accommodations

Building and Facility Components

Manufacturers and Suppliers Directory

Trainer's Supplies

Fund-Raising

Directory of Professionals (facility architects, builders, and consultants

Directory of Advertisers

Directory of Associations

Article Index, Athletic Business

▌ Corporate Fitness and Recreation
Brentwood Publishing Corporation
825 Barrington Avenue
Los Angeles, CA 90049
(213) 826-8388

Annual Buyer's Guide, 1985 edition, 86 pp.
Topics: Facility Planning

Fitness/Strength/Conditioning

Health and Wellness Programs/Consultants

Product Index

DIRECTORY OF ASSOCIATIONS

Amateur Athletic Union AAU House
3400 W. 86th Street
Indianapolis, IN 46268

Amateur Basketball Association of the U.S.
1750 E. Boulder Street
Colorado Springs, CO 80909

Amateur Hockey Association of the U.S.
2997 Broadmoor Valley Road
Colorado Springs, CO 80906

Amateur Softball Association
2801 Northeast 50th Street
Oklahoma City, OK 73111

**American Academy of Podiatric
Sports Medicine**
P.O. Box 31331
San Francisco, CA 94131

American Academy of Sports Physicians
28222 W. Agoura Road, #105
Agoura, CA 91301

**American Alliance of Health,
Phys. Ed., Rec. & Dance**
1900 Association Drive
Reston, VA 22091

American Amateur Baseball Congress
215 East Green, Box 467
Marshall, MI 49068

American Amateur Racquetball Association
815 N. Weber, Suite 203
Colorado Springs, CO 80903

**American Association for
Leisure & Recreation**
1900 Association Drive
Reston, VA 22091

American Athletic Association of the Deaf
3916 Lantern Drive
Silver Spring, MD 20902

**American Athletic Trainers Assn.
& Certification Board**
660 W. Duarte Road
Arcadia, CA 91006

American Baseball Coaches Association
605 Hamilton Drive
Champaign, IL 61820

American Bowling Congress
5301 South 76th Street
Greendale, WI 53129

American Cancer Society
777 Third Avenue
New York, NY 10017

American College Health Association
15879 Crabbs Branch Way
Rockville, MD 20855

American College of Sports Medicine
P.O. Box 1440
Indianapolis, IN 46206

American Dietetic Association
430 N. Michigan Avenue
Chicago, IL 60611

American Health Foundation
320 East 43rd Street
New York, NY 10017

American Heart Association
7320 Greenville Avenue
Dallas, TX 75231

Source: Adapted from *Athletic Business*, February, 1985, pp. 161–166. Used by permission.

American Hockey League
P.O. Box 100
218 Memorial Avenue
West Springfield, MA 01089

American Hospital Association
840 N. Lake Shore Drive
Chicago, IL 60611

American Medical Association
535 North Dearborn Street
Chicago, IL 60610

**American Orthopaedic Society
for Sports Medicine**
70 West Hubbard Street
Chicago, IL 60610

**American Osteopathic Academy
of Sports Medicine**
1551 NW 54th, Suite 200
Seattle, WA 98107

American Physical Therapy Assn.
2036 Cowley Hall
La Crosse, WI 54601

American Platform Tennis Assn.
P.O. Box 901
248 Lorraine Avenue
Upper Montclair, NJ 07043

**American Professional Racquetball
Organization**
8303 E. Thomas Road
Scottsdale, AZ 85251

American Public Health Association
1015 Fifteenth Street, NW
Washington, D.C. 20005

American Running and Fitness Association
2420 K Street NW
Washington, DC 20037

American Society of Landscape Architects
1733 Connecticut Avenue, NW
Washington, DC 20009

American Swimming Coaches Association
One Hall of Fame Drive
Fort Lauderdale, FL 33316

American Tennis Association
475 Riverside Drive
Suite 439
New York, NY 10115

American Water Ski Association
P.O. Box 191
Winter Haven, FL 33882

American Youth Soccer Association
5403 W. 138th Street
Hawthorne, CA 90250

Army Sports (Phys. Act. Div.)
HQDA, DAAG-MSP
Alexandria, VA 22331

Association for Fitness in Business
1312 Washington Boulevard
Stamford, CT 06902

Association of Physical Fitness Centers
5272 River Road, Suite 500
Bethesda, MD 20816

**Assoc. of Phys. Plant Admin.
of Univer. and Colleges**
1 Dupont Circle, Suite 250
Washington, DC 20036

Association of School Business Officials
720 Garden Street
Park Ridge, IL 60068

Association of Tennis Professionals
319 Country Club Road
Garland, TX 75040

Athletic Institute
200 N. Castlewood Drive
North Palm Beach, FL 33408

Athletics Congress of the USA
200 South Capitol Avenue
Suite 140
Indianapolis, IN 46225

Babe Ruth League, Inc.
P.O. Box 5000
1770 Brunswick Avenue
Trenton, NJ 08638

Baseball Canada
333 River Road
Vanier, Ontario, CN K1L 8H9

**Boy Scouts of America National
Exploring Div.**
P.O. Box 61030
Dallas, TX 75261

Boys Clubs of America
771 First Avenue
New York, NY 10017

Canadian Amateur Rowing Assn.
333 River Road
Tower C, 10th Floor
Ottawa, Ontario, CN K1L 8H9

Canadian Amateur Wrestling
333 River Road
Ottawa, Ontario, CN K1L 8H9

Canadian Assoc. for Health;
Phys. Ed./Recreation
333 River Road
Ottawa, Ontario, CN K1L 8H9

Canadian Association of Sports Sciences
333 River Road
Ottawa, Ontario, CN K1L 8H9

Canadian Colleges Athletic Association
333 River Road
Ottawa, Ontario, CN K1L 8H9

Canadian Figure Skating Assn.
333 River Road
Tower A, 3rd Floor
Ottawa, Ontario, CN K1L 8H9

Canadian Football League
11 King Street, W.
Suite 1800
Toronto, Ontario, CN M5H 1A3

Canadian Intramural Recreation Association
333 River Road
Vanier, Ontario, Canada
K1L 8H9

Canadian School Sport Federation
Colonel Gray High School
Charlottetown, Prince Edward
Island, CN C1A 4S6

Canadian Sporting Goods Assn.
1315 deMasionneuve
Boulevard W
Suite 702
Montreal, Quebec, CN
H3G 1M4

Canadian Track & Field Assoc.
333 River Road
Tower B, 11th Floor
Ottawa, Ontario, CN K1L 8H9

Center for Health Promotion
American Hospital Association
840 N. Lake Shore Drive
Chicago, IL 60611

Coaching Assn. of Canada
333 River Road
Ottawa, Ontario, CN K1L 8H9

College Athletic Business
Managers Association
Athl Dept.-U. of OK
Norman, OK 73019

College Athletic Conference
University of the South
Sewanee, TN 37375

College Sports Information
Directors of America
Box 114, Texas A & I Univ.
Kingsville, TX 78363

College Swimming Coaches
Association of America
1000 W. Laurel
Ft. Collins, CO 80521

Commonwealth Games Assoc. of Canada Inc.
P.O. Box 3763, Station C
Hamilton, Ontario, CN L8H 7N1

Executive Fitness Newsletter
33 E. Minor Street
Emmaus, PA 18049

Field Hockey Association of America, Inc.
1750 East Boulder Street
Colorado Springs, CO 80906

Fitness and Amateur Sport
365 Lauier Avenue West
General Tower South
Ottawa, Ontario, Cn K1A 0X6

Girl Scouts of the U.S.A.
830 3rd Avenue at 51st Street
New York, NY 10022

Golden Gloves Association of America
9000 Menaul, N.E.
Albuquerque, NM 87112

Ice Skating Institute of America
1000 Skokie Boulevard
Wilmete, IL 60091

Intercollegiate Association of
Amateur Athletes of Amer.
P.O. Box 3
Centerville, MA 02632

Intercollegiate Soccer Association of
America
Marist College
Poughkeepsie, NY 12601

Intercollegiate Tennis Coaches Association
P.O. Box 71
Princeton, NJ 08544

International Amateur Boxing Association
135 Westervelt Place
Cresskill, NJ 07626

International Amateur Swimming Federation
2000 Financial Center
Des Moines, IA 50309

International Association of Auditorium Managers
500 N. Michigan Avenue
Chicago, IL 60611

International Badminton Fed.
24 Winchcombe House
Winchcombe Street,
Cheltenham
Gloucestershire, EN GL52 2NA

International Collegiate Sports Foundation, Inc.
P.O. Box 866
Plano, TX 75074

International Dance-Exercise Association
4501 Mission Bay Drive
Suite 2F
San Diego, CA 92109

International Golf Association
60 East 42nd Street
Room 746
New York, NY 10165

International Racquet Sports Association
112 Cypress Street
Brookline, MA 02146

International Softball Congress, Inc.
6007 E. Hillcrest Circle
Anaheim Hills, CA 92807

International Sports Exchange
5982 Mia Court
Plainfield, IN 46168

Jewish Welfare Board
15 E. 26th Street
New York, NY 10010

Lacrosse Foundation, The Inc.
Newton H. White
Athletic Center
Baltimore, MD 21218

Ladies Professional Golf Association
1250 Shoreline Drive
Sugar Land, TX 77478

Lawn Tennis Association, The
Palliser Road, Barons Court
W. Kensington
London, EN W14 9EG

Little League Baseball, Inc.
P.O. Box 3485
Williamsport, PA 17701

National Amateur Baseball Federation
2201 North Townline Road
Rose City, MI 48654

National Archery Association
1750 E. Boulder Street
Colorado Springs, CO 80909

National Association of Employers on Health Care Alternatives
1134 Chamber of Commerce Boulevard
15 S. 15th Street
Minneapolis, MN 55402

National Association for Girls and Women in Sports
1900 Association Drive
Reston, VA 22091

National Association for Sport and Physical Education
1900 Association Drive
Reston, VA 22091

National Assoc. of Basketball Coaches of the U.S.
P.O. Box 307
Branford, CT 06405

National Assoc. of Collegiate Directors of Athletics
1229 Smith Court, Box 16428
Cleveland, OH 44116

National Association of Concessionaires
35 E. Wacker Drive, #1849
Chicago, IL 60601

National Association of Educational Buyers
180 Froehlich Farm Boulevard
Woodbury, NY 11797

National Association of Intercollegiate Athletics
1221 Baltimore Street
Kansas City, MO 64105

National Association of Sports Officials
1700 N. Main Street, 2nd Floor
Racine, WI 53402

National Athletic Equipment Reconditioners Assoc.
West Hills Road #2
Stroudsburg, PA 18360

National Athletic Health Institute, Inc.
575 East Hardy Street
Inglewood, CA 90301

National Athletic Trainers Association, Inc.
1001 East 4th Street
Greenville, NC 27834

National Baseball Congress, Inc.
P.O. Box 1420
Wichita, KS 67201

National Basketball Association
645 Fifth Avenue
New York, NY 10022

National Basketball Players Association
15 Columbus Circle
New York, NY 10023

National Board YWCA
726 Broadway
New York, NY 10003

National Bowling Association
377 Park Avenue S.
7th Floor
New York, NY 10016

National Bowling Council
1919 Pennsylvania Avenue, NW
Suite 504
Washington, DC 20006

National Christian College Athletic Association
1815 Union Avenue
Chattanooga, TN 37404

National Collegiate Athletic Association
P.O. Box 1906
Mission, KS 66201

National Council on Alcoholism
2 Park Avenue
New York, NY 18016

National Employee Services and Recreation Association
2400 S. Downing Avenue
Westchester, IL 60155

National Fed. for Catholic Youth Ministry
3025 4th Street, N.W.
Washington, DC 20017

National Federation of State High School Associations
P.O. Box 20626
11724 Plaza Circle
Kansas City, MO 64195

National Fitness Association
P.O. Box 1754
Huntington Beach, CA 92647

National Football League
410 Park Avenue
New York, NY 10022

National Football League Players Association
1300 Connecticut Avenue NW, #407
Washington, DC 20036

National Golf Foundation
200 Castlewood Drive
North Palm Beach, FL 33408

National Health Information Clearing House
1555 Wilson Boulevard
Rosslyn, VA 22209

National High School Athletic Coaches Association
3423 E. Silver Springs #9
Ocala, FL 32670

National Hockey League
500 Fifth Avenue
34th Floor
New York, NY 10110

National Hockey League Players Association
65 Queen Street, W-Suite 210
Toronto, Ontario, CN M5H 2M5

National Institute on Parks & Ground Management
P.O. Box 1936
Appleton, WI 54913

National Institution on Alcohol Abuse and Alcoholism
5600 Fishers Lane
Rockville, MD 20852

National Intercollegiate Soccer Officials Assoc.
131 Moffitt Boulevard
Islip, NY 11751

National Intercollegiate Women's Fencing Assoc.
235 McCosh Road
Upper Montclair, NJ 07043

National Interscholastic Athl. Administrators Assn.
P.O. Box 20626
11724 Plaza Circle
Kansas City, MO 64195

Nat. Intra.-Rec. Spts. Assoc.
Dixon Recreation Center
Oregon State University
Corvallis, OR 97331

National Junior College Athletic Association
12 E. 2nd Street
Hutchinson, KS 67504

National Junior Tennis League
P.O. Box 1586
25 W. 39th Street
Suite 1105
New York, NY 10018

National League of Prof. Baseball Clubs, The
350 Park Avenue, 18th Floor
New York, NY 10022

National Little College Athletic Association
RD #1
Princeton, IN 47670

National Outdoor Volleyball Assn.
936 Hermosa Avenue, Ste 109
Hermosa Beach, CA 90254

National Recreation & Park Association
3101 Park Ctr Drive, 12th Floor
Alexandria, VA 22302

National Rowing Foundation
P.O. Box 6030
Arlington, VA 22206

National School Board Assn.
1680 Duke Street
Alexandria, VA 22314

National School Supply and Equipment Association
1500 Wilson Boulevard, Ste 609
Arlington, VA 22209

National Senior Sports Association
317 Cameron Street
Alexandria, VA 22314

National Ski Areas Assoc.
20 Maple Street, P.O. Box 2883
Springfield, MA 01101

National Ski Patrol System, Inc.
2901 Sheridan Boulevard
Denver, CO 80214

National Soccer Coaches Association of America
RD #5, P.O. Box 5074
Stroudsburg, PA 18360

National Spa and Pool Institute
2111 Eisenhower Avenue
Alexandria, VA 22314

National Sporting Goods and Dealers Association
714 Pierce Street
Sioux City, IA 51101

National Sporting Goods Association
1699 Wall Street
Mt. Prospect, IL 60056

National Strength & Conditioning Association
P.O. Box 81410
Lincoln, NE 68501

Nat'l. Wheelchair Athl. Assn.
2107 Templeton Gap Road
Suite C
Colorado Springs, Co 80907

National Wheelchair Basketball Association
110 Seaton Bldg.-U. of KY
Lexington, KY 40506

Nat'l. Wrestling Coaches Assn.
P.O. Box 8002
Foothill Station
Salt Lake City, UT 84108

National Youth Sports Coaches Association
2611 Old Okeechobee Road
West Palm Beach, FL 33409

North American Boxing Federation
708 Colorado, Suite 804
Austin, TX 78701

North American Soccer League
1133 6th Avenue, Suite 3400
New York, NY 10036

Participaction
80 Richmond Street West
Suite 805
Toronto, Ontario, CN M5H 2A4

PGA Tour
Sawgrass
Ponte Verda, FL 32082

Pony Baseball, Inc.
P.O. Box 225
Washington, PA 15301

Pop Warner Football
1315 Walnut Street Bldg.
Suite 606
Philadelphia, PA 19107

**President's Council on Physical
Fitness & Spts.**
450 5th Street NW #7103
Washington, DC 20001

Professional Bowlers Association of America
1720 Merriman Road
Akron, OH 44313

Professional Golfers' Association of America
100 Avenue of the Champions
Palm Beach Gardens, FL 33410

Recreation Vehicle Industry Association
P.O. Box 204
Chantilly, VA 22021

Road Runners Club of America
1224 Orchard Village
Manchester, MO 63011

Roller Skating Rink Operators Association
P.O. Box 81846
7700 "A" Street
Lincoln, NE 68501

Scholastic Rowing Association of America
Saint Andrew's School
Middletown, DE 19709

Ski Industries of America
8377-B Greensboro Drive
McLean, VA 22102

Softball Canada
333 River Road
Vanier, Ontario, CN K1L 8H9

Special Olympics Inc.
1305 New York Avenue
Suite 500, N.W.
Washington, DC 20005

Sporting Goods Agents Association
P.O. Box 998
Morton Grove, IL 60053

Sporting Goods Manufacturers Association
200 Castlewood Drive
North Palm Beach, FL 33408

Sports Ambassadors
25 Corning Avenue
Milpitas, CA 95035

Sports and the Courts
P.O. Box 2836
Winston-Salem, NC 27102

Sports Medicine Council of Canada
333 River Road
Ottawa, Ontario, CN K1L 8H9

Tennis Foundation of North America
200 Castlewood Drive
North Palm Beach, FL 33408

Texas Intercoll. Athl. Assn.
Tarleton State University
Box T-309
Stephenville, TX 76402

U.S. Association for Blind Athletes
55 W. California Avenue
Beach Haven Park, NJ 08008

U.S. Badminton Association
P.O. Box 456
Waterford, MI 48095

U.S. Baseball Federation
4 Gregory Drive
Hamilton Square, NJ 08690

U.S. Collegiate Sports Council
Univ. of South Carolina
Blatt PE Center
Columbia, SC 29208

U.S. Cycling Federation
1750 E. Boulder Street
Colorado Springs, CO 80909

U.S. Diving Inc.
901 W. New York Street
Indianapolis, IN 46202

United States Fencing Association, Inc.
1750 East Boulder Street
Colorado Springs, CO 80909

U.S. Field Hockey Assn. (Women)
1750 E. Boulder Street
Colorado Springs, CO 80909

U.S. Gymnastics Federation
200 S. Capitol Avenue
Suite 110
Indianapolis, IN 46225

U.S. Intercollegiate Lacrosse Association
Washington College
Chestertown, MD 21620

U.S. Luge Association
P.O. Box 651
Lake Placid, NY 12946

United States Olympic Committee
1750 E. Boulder Street
Colorado Springs, CO 80909

U.S. Paddle Tennis Association
189 Seeley Street
Brooklyn, NY 11218

U.S. Professional Tennis Assn.
P.O. Box 7077
3113 Mill Pond Road
Wesley Chapel, FL 34249

U.S. Rowing Association
Four Boathouse Row
Philadelphia, PA 19130

U.S. Rugby Football Union Ltd.
27 East State Street
Sherburne, NY 13460

U.S. Ski Association
U.S. Olympic Complex
1750 E. Boulder Street
Colorado Springs, CO 80909

U.S. Ski Coaches Association
P.O. Box 1747
Park City, UT 84060

U.S. Ski Education Foundation
P.O. Box 100
255 Main Street
Park City, UT 84060

U.S. Soccer Federation
350-5th Avenue 4010
New York, NY 10118

U.S. Sports Academy
P.O. Box 8650
Mobile, AL 36689

U.S. Squash Racquets Association
211 Ford Road
Bala-Cynwyd, PA 19004

United States Swimming Inc.
1750 E. Boulder Street
Colorado Springs, CO 80909

United States Table Tennis Association
1750 E. Boulder Street
Colorado Springs, CO 80909

U.S. Team Handball Federation
1750 E. Boulder Street
Colorado Springs, CO 80909

U.S. Tennis Association
51 E. 42nd Street
New York, NY 10017

U.S. Tennis Court and Track Builders Association
223 W. Main Street
Charlottesville, VA 22901

United States Volleyball Association
1750 E. Boulder Street
Colorado Springs, CO 80909

U.S. Weightlifting Federation
1750 E. Boulder Street
Colorado Springs, CO 80909

U.S. Women's Curling Association
2792 Fairmount Boulevard
Cleveland Heights, OH 44118

U.S. Women's Lacrosse Association
339 Plain Street
Mills, MA 02054

U.S. Wrestling Federation
405 W. Hall of Fame Avenue
Stillwater, OK 74074

Washington Business Group on Health
1555 Wilson Boulevard
Rosslyn, VA 22209

Women's International Bowling Congress, Inc.
5301 South 76th Street
Greendale, WI 53129

Women's Sports Foundation
195 Moulton Street
San Francisco, CA 94123

Women's Tennis Association
1604 Union Street
San Francisco, CA 94123

World Amateur Golf Council
Golf House
Far Hills, NJ 07931

World Championship Tennis
2340 Thanksgiving Tower
Dallas, TX 75201

World Professional Squash Association
12 Sheppard St.-Suite 500
Toronto, Ontario, CN M5H 3A1

YMCA of the USA
101 N. Wacker Drive
Chicago, IL 60606

INDEX